T0220666

Changing the Global Approach to Medicine

Volume I

New Perspectives on Treating AIDS, Diabetes, Obesity, Aging, Heart Attacks, Stroke and Cancer

Lane B. Scheiber II, MD

Lane B. Scheiber, ScD

iUniverse, Inc.
New York Bloomington

Changing the Global Approach to Medicine, Volume 1
New Perspectives on Treating AIDS, Diabetes, Obesity, Aging, Heart Attacks, Stroke and Cancer

The information, ideas, and suggestions in this book are not intended as a substitute for
professional medical advice. Before following any suggestions contained in this book,
you should consult your personal physician. Neither the author nor the publisher shall
be liable or responsible for any loss or damage allegedly arising as a consequence of
your use or application of any information or suggestions in this book. At the time of
publication the authors believed that certain concepts set forth in this text to be unique
and different from any other previous work present in the general published literature.

iUniverse books may be ordered through booksellers or by contacting:
iUniverse
1663 Liberty Drive
Bloomington, IN 47403
www.iuniverse.com
1-800-Authors (1-800-288-4677)

Because of the dynamic nature of the Internet, any Web addresses or links contained in
this book may have changed since publication and may no longer be valid. The views
expressed in this work are solely those of the author and do not necessarily reflect the
views of the publisher, and the publisher hereby disclaims any responsibility for them.

ISBN: 978-1-4401-1212-6 (sc)
ISBN: 978-1-4401-1213-3 (ebook)

Printed in the United States of America
iUniverse rev. date: 1/23/09

Additional Reading:

IMMORTALITY: QUATERNARY MEDICINE CODE

by Anthony Scheiber

THE HUMAN COMPUTER

by Anthony Scheiber

EARTH PRO

by Anthony Scheiber

Dedication

Thanks to our wives, Karin and Mary Jane
for all of their love and support.

Forward

After decades of research and development, and countless billions of dollars, the medical community still finds itself without cures for many illnesses that plague the world's population such as AIDS, diabetes, obesity, and most cancers. A new approach is called for. This book introduces one such approach; the development and use of medically therapeutic viruses. While currently viruses are generally considered and treated as threats, they, like many other substances, have potential beneficial uses. It is the beneficial uses that need to be developed and exploited. Medically therapeutic viruses have, as described in this book, not only the potential to provide physicians around the world with the ability to cure even the most difficult diseases, but in some cases may be utilized to eradicate the causes of the diseases themselves. In our research we have looked upon viruses as treatment tools. In this book we explain how we envision these tools as being used to treat such illnesses as AIDS and diabetes as well as to treat obesity, chronic fatigue, forestall aging, improve management of heart attacks and strokes, and advance the treatment of cancer. Understanding how to develop and use these tools will bring about a vigorous change to the global approach to medicine.

Viruses do not represent life; they carryout no biologic function on their own. A virus is simply a shell equipped with a genetic code that facilitates the virus in forcefully commandeering the faculties of animal[1] or plant cells for the sole purpose of replicating itself. Viruses can be thought of much like building blocks. The basic components of a virus include an outer shell, search probes mounted on the outer shell, genetic material carried inside the shell, and enzymes that assist the genetic material in commandeering a host. Rearranging the properties of these building blocks leads to the wide variety of

---

1 In medical terms, the word animal includes humans.

viruses that infect humans as well as other animal and plant life. Deciphering the pathophysiology of viruses teaches us that they are simply a vehicle aimed at engaging a specific type of target cell, taking command of the target cell and enslaving the target cell to act as a host for purposes of manufacturing copies of the virus.

Thus, understanding that changing the exterior probes of a virus potentially alters the cell type the virus will target and by changing the payload the virus carries, this age-old nemesis can be transformed into one of the most powerful therapeutic tools ever developed for the medical profession. Gene therapy has to date been an effort to use common viruses to insert a specific DNA gene into the cells the common virus targets as its host. Medically therapeutic viruses could be fashioned by altering a virus's exterior probes to target a specific cell type and to carry instruction code such as powerful protein building RNA genetic code or drugs or energy molecules to these specific target cells to conduct a predetermined form of medical therapy. Viruses could be fashioned to deliver a means to terminate unwanted cells whether they are cancer cells or infectious pathogens invading the body. Medically therapeutic viruses could aide doctors in treating patients in times of crisis such as a heart attack or stroke by bypassing the blood stream and delivering oxygen or energy molecules directly to essential tissues at risk of dying by alternative means.

Recognizing the intricacies of how viruses are constructed and how they function leads to viable medical means to defend the population from lethal viruses by filtering blood, combating viruses on their own level, devising effective vaccines against aggressive viruses, or by slightly altering the genetics of precursor cells in a person to make individuals at high risk impervious to specific infections. The prodigy of the next fatal virus is at this moment mutating somewhere on the planet in a host, be it birds, rodents or swine, incessantly evolving until it becomes an infectious threat to humans. HIV rarely leaves natural survivors except for those carrying a homologous genetic flaw in the CCR5 cell-surface receptor gene and the only thing preventing HIV from challenging all of humanity is its lack of ability to exist outside the safe harbor of body fluids. If it morphs into a form that can be transmitted through the air - like the influenza virus - or in water, it will quickly become the most devastating plague the world has ever seen. The opportunity exists now to develop the means to protect the population from future, disastrous worldwide panepidemics. In evolutionary terms, if we fail to procure an effective means of combating deadly viral infections, a goal which we have not yet accomplished, these smallest of pathogens could eliminate the human race from the face of the globe in what might be considered 'an instant' with regards to the time-line of the planet's 4.5 billion year existence.

Table of Contents

Forward ix

INTRODUCTION 1

I: Strategy to Eradicate AIDS 5

❖ BASIC CONSTRUCT OF HIV.................................... 6
❖ TRADITIONAL APPROACH TO TREATING INFECTIONS........11
❖ REASONS WHY HIV IS SO DIFFICULT TO ERADICATE 19
❖ PROGRESSION OF HIV INFECTION TO AIDS...................... 22
❖ CURRENT APPROACH TO COMBATING HIV...................... 22
❖ SEVEN ENTIRELY NEW MEDICAL TREATMENT
  STRATEGIES TO ERADICATE AIDS: 29
  ➢ STRATEGY NUMBER ONE: FILTER PATIENT'S BLOOD ... 30
  ➢ STRATEGY NUMBER TWO: TREAT WITH SMART
    VIRUS TECHNOLOGY 34
  ➢ STRATEGY NUMBER THREE: ELIMINATION OF
    INFECTED T-HELPER CELLS 38
  ➢ STRATEGY NUMBER FOUR: NEW APPROACH FOR
    A VACCINE FOR HIV... 40
    ▫ TESTING TO DEMONSTRATE A VACCINE'S
      EFFECTIVENESS 57
  ➢ STRATEGY NUMBER FIVE: FUSION AND CHIMERIC
    ANTIBODIES AGAINST HIV 65
  ➢ STRATEGY NUMBER SIX: UTILIZING VIRUSES TO
    DELIVER DRUG THERAPY..71
  ➢ STRATEGY NUMBER SEVEN: A CURE FOR AIDS 71
❖ CONCLUSION 75

II: Curing Diabetes, Eliminating Obesity and Fatigue,
and Halting the Aging Process 78

III: Innovative Means for Intervention in Heart Attacks,
Stroke, Diabetic Crisis, and Cancer 88

IV: Vision for the Future of Medicine 95

Addendum: Drafting an Entirely New Approach to
    Medicine & Technology 101

Epilogue.. 115

APPENDIX A: Patent Applications to Eradicate AIDS 116

A1: ANTI-HUMAN IMMUNODEFICIENCY VIRUS SURROGATE
    TARGET AGENT TECHNOLOGY FILTER INTENDED TO
    NEUTRALIZE OR REMOVE HUMAN IMMUNODEFICIENCY VIRUS
    VIRIONS FROM BLOOD 116

A2: ANTI-HUMAN IMMUNODEFICIENCY VIRUS SURROGATE
    TARGET AGENT TECHNOLOGY FILTER INTENDED TO
    TERMINATE T-HELPER CELLS INFECTED WITH THE HUMAN
    IMMUNODEFICIENCY VIRUS CIRCULATING IN BLOOD......... 138

A3: SCIENTIFICALLY MODULATED AND REPROGRAMMED
    TREATMENT (SMART) VIRUS TECHNOLOGY INTENDED TO
    NEUTRALIZE THE HUMAN IMMUNODEFICIENCY VIRUS 166

A4: UNIVERSAL BARRIER TO PREVENT INFECTIONS FROM
    HUMAN IMMUNODEFICIENCY VIRUS............................... 179

A5: FEMALE BARRIER TO PREVENT INFECTIONS FROM HUMAN
    IMMUNODEFICIENCY VIRUS...................................... 198

A6: SCIENTIFICALLY MODULATED AND REPROGRAMMED
    TREATMENT (SMART) FAS/FASL VIRUS TECHNOLOGY
    INTENDED TO NEUTRALIZE T-HELPER CELLS INFECTED
    WITH THE HUMAN IMMUNODEFICIENCY VIRUS 221

A7: A VACCINE COMPRISED SPECIFICALLY OF PROTEIN
    SUBUNITS OF HUMAN IMMUNODEFICIENCY VIRUS'S
    GLYCOPROTEIN 120 PROBE TO PREVENT AND TREAT AN
    INFECTION CAUSED BY THE HUMAN IMMUNODEFICIENCY
    VIRUS... 234

A8: MEDICAL TREATMENT DEVICE FOR TREATING AIDS BY
    UTILIZING MODIFIED HUMAN IMMUNODEFICIENCY
    VIRUS VIRIONS TO INSERT ANTI-VIRAL MEDICATIONS
    INTO T-HELPER CELLS 255

A9: METHOD FOR CURING AND PREVENTING ACQUIRED IMMUNE DEFICIENCY SYNDROME BY ALTERING CELL-SURFACE RECEPTORS IN PRECURSOR T-HELPER CELLS AND MATURE T-HELPER CELLS TO PREVENT HUMAN IMMUNODEFICIENCY VIRUS VIRIONS ACCESS TO MATURE T-HELPER CELLS 270

APPENDIX B: Patent Applications to Cure Diabetes, Eliminate Obesity and Fatigue, and Halt Aging 299

B1: ADAPTABLE MESSENGER RIBONUCLEIC ACID MEDICAL TREATMENT DEVICE TO MANAGE DIABETES MELLITUS 299

B2: METHOD FOR TREATING DIABETES MELLITUS, OBESITY, CHRONIC FATIGUE, AGING, AND OTHER MEDICAL CONDITIONS BY UTILIZING MODIFIED VIRUS VIRIONS TO INSERT MESSENGER RIBONUCLEIC ACID MOLECULES INTO CELLS 319

B3: A MEDICAL DEVICE FOR TREATING DIABETES MELLITUS, OBESITY, CHRONIC FATIGUE, AGING, AND OTHER MEDICAL CONDITIONS BY UTILIZING MODIFIED VIRUS VIRIONS TO INSERT MESSENGER RIBONUCLEIC ACID MOLECULES INTO CELLS 357

APPENDIX C: Patent Applications for Innovative Means for Intervention in Heart Attacks, Stroke, Diabetic Crisis, and Cancer... 396

C1: METHOD FOR TREATING HEART ATTACKS, STROKES AND DIABETIC CRISIS BY UTILIZING MODIFIED VIRUS VIRIONS TO INSERT NECESSARY PROTEIN MOLECULES AND VITAL NUTRIENTS INTO TARGETED CELLS 396

C2: METHOD FOR TREATING CANCER, RHEUMATOID ARTHRITIS AND OTHER MEDICAL DISEASES BY UTILIZING MODIFIED VIRUS VIRIONS TO INSERT MEDICATIONS INTO TARGETED CELLS 426

INTRODUCTION

This document represents a series of dramatic new perspectives aimed at advancing the practice of medicine for the good of all. Forging together principles of science and engineering, the approach described in this book is aimed at eradicating the worldwide threat of Acquired Immunodeficiency Syndrome (AIDS), curing diabetes, eliminating obesity, re-energizing those that suffer from chronic fatigue, halting the aging process, intervening in times of crisis such as heart attack and stroke to improve the survival of essential tissues, and improving the treatment of cancer. All of these subjects are intimately tied together and are extremely challenging problems that can be solved. The Human Immunodeficiency Virus (HIV), an RNA virus, the root cause of AIDS, provides a critically important teaching tool, from which one can unlock many of nature's secrets which facilitates the pursuit of practical solutions to the above-mentioned problems.

Viruses have always posed a threat to the health and survival of mankind. These obligate parasites are simply a shell carrying one or more strands of genetic material with the sole purpose of replication. By itself, a virus is incapable of carrying out any of life's processes. A virus requires a host to complete its replication cycle. Viruses pilfer the resources and production capacity of living cells in order to propagate themselves. Once a virus replicates, the copies of the virus scour the environment in search of additional suitable hosts. Viruses appear to play no valuable role in the food chain other than a narcissistic role of self-propagation. Viruses are playing an important role in teaching us about the intricate biologic building blocks of life and how to best utilize them. They also show us that it is of the utmost importance for us to understand these concepts.

1

On a microscopic scale, humans face a constant threat of disease. Over eons, viruses have evolved and continue to evolve. Some viral strains have been equipped with means to defeat the immune system protecting the average human. Various strains of influenza virus have swept the globe at different times, infecting and killing hundreds of thousands of people. Small pox and polio represent devastating viruses that killed or maimed a significant portion of the population until vaccines were developed to protect people from these pathogens. Hepatitis viruses A, B, C, D and others remain a persistent threat, always poised to emerge at times of disaster and infect mass quantities of the population. The Human Immunodeficiency Virus (HIV), responsible for Acquired Immunodeficiency Syndrome (AIDS), remains one of deadliest and persistent viruses challenging mankind; HIV presently infecting an estimated 41 million people worldwide. HIV represents a deadly infectious agent that the body's immune system is apparently incapable of ridding itself of and thus leaves no survivors other than a few individuals that possess a genetic defect that provides an innate immunity to the virus.

Though various strains of viruses are responsible for illness that range from the common cold to an incapacitating 24-hour stomach flu to lethal forms such as the influenza virus, the human immunodeficiency virus, SARS, and Ebola, these submicroscopic pathogens could shed the dark aura that currently cloaks their image and be transformed into modern medicine's elite workhorses. Viruses soon could be thought of in a more positive manner as they offer the possibility of a very effective means of treating some of mankind's most challenging illnesses.

The overall concept of a virus is rather simple, being that it is merely a shell that carries genetic material to a specific cell with the intent of replicating itself. Most viruses target a specific cell type as its 'host' cell which the virus will use to replicate itself. A virus utilizes probes mounted on the surface of its outer shell as its means to identify and engage the host cell that offers the virus the appropriate biologic machinery to successfully replicate copies of itself.

Given the fact that a virus is a vehicle that carries a payload of genetic material, naturally occurring viruses can be reconfigured to carry nearly any medically therapeutic payload to any type of cell in the body. Powerful RNA molecules could be transported by viruses to target cells throughout the body to act as genetic templates to produce all types of cellular proteins. In order to accomplish this objective, a host cell would be programmed to manufacture copies of a virus with specific cell seeking probes attached to the modified virus's surface. The host cell would be further programmed to place into the virus vehicle any of a variety of molecular payloads. A medically therapeutic virus could carry drug molecules to a specific type of cell, or carry ribonucleic acid molecules to up-regulate a cell's capacity to produce proteins. A modified virus could deliver to specific cells nutrients or energy molecules in times of a crisis.

Utilizing Medically Therapeutic Viruses (MTV), modified in a manner to produce a medically beneficial effect, diabetes and obesity could be treated by up-regulating the utilization of blood sugar by inserting RNA to produce metabolically active enzymes in specific target cells of the body. Using modified viruses, aging and chronic fatigue could be treated by stoking the metabolic processes inside the cytoplasm and the mitochondria, the powerhouses of the cell, to produce additional energy molecules for cells to utilize to enhance function, maintenance and growth.

The use of antibiotics, medicine's traditional approach to combat infections, has not been an effective or practical means to eradicate viruses which are parasitic pathogens that hide inside cells in order to evade detection and to replicate. To successfully combat aggressive viral infections the virus needs to be managed in a manner that capitalizes on exploiting the

3

needs of the virus. Trapping a deadly virus, neutralizing a virus, or creating an effective barrier to prevent infection by a virus requires developing management techniques designed to engage one of a virus's weak spots, its exterior probes. For example, utilizing surrogate targets designed to engage HIV's exterior probes, in a manner similar to how HIV engages a T-Helper cell, provides a means to prevent the spread of the virus. A means for curing patients of a virus like HIV would be to make the vulnerable T-helper cells in the body impervious to being engaged by the virus's exterior probes.

The following sections describe many new and innovative concepts. The fourteen medical patent applications which follow represent a diverse array of new ideas that will change the manner by which the medical profession approaches tough problems beginning with the eradication of AIDS, by eliminating the threat of HIV. Others medical treatment objectives include an innovative management of diabetes, obesity and chronic fatigue as well as pro-actively forestalling the aging process, interceding in heart attacks and strokes to increase survivability, and a new approach to treating cancer. Although the work has been ongoing at Viresoft for a number of years, all patent applications presented in this document were submitted during the period from late December 2007 through May of 2008. At the time this book was published, the authors believed the key concepts presented in this work to be applicable, unique and quite different from existing prior art.

I: Strategy to Eradicate AIDS

'HIV provides a critically important teaching tool from which to learn many of nature's most valuable secrets.'

HIV poses a significant threat to the health and well-being of the world's population. HIV is but one lethal viral infection that exists in the world. A number of fatal viruses have appeared throughout history, some such as the global influenza outbreaks have repeatedly resulted in dramatic mortality rates.

The current medical approach to treating infectious agents is not sufficient in its means for either eliminating HIV infections or controlling the spread of HIV. The primary medical management tools presently available act only to slow HIV's replication process, they do not eliminate HIV's presence in the body. Vaccines are meant to expose the body to the presence of a pathogen to generate an immune response capable of repelling such an intruder if the pathogen is encountered at a later time. To date, a vaccine to protect the population from HIV has yet to be successfully developed.

HIV possesses a predator-like capacity to transform its host cell, an infected T–Helper cell, into an instrument that has the capability of killing noninfected T-Helper cells. The elimination of T-Helper cells leads to a decline in the body's capability to defend itself from other environmental pathogens. When the number of T-Helper cells declines to the point the body is unable to effectively ward off common infectious agents the clinical picture of Acquired Immunodeficiency Syndrome (AIDS) ensues.

In the United States it is estimated that 900,000 people are infected with HIV; this estimate is possibly lower than the actual number of people infected since medical records are kept confidential and mass screening of the population for the presence of HIV is not currently being done. Further, it has been estimated that HIV infects over forty-one million lives around the globe.

After over twenty-five years of research and investigation, combating the ever-growing global humanitarian crisis posed by the HIV remains an elusive goal for the medical community. New strategies intended to treat the effects of viral infections and protect the population from the spread of infection by lethal viruses are most certainly needed. Incorporating blood filtering techniques, developing scientifically modified medically therapeutic viruses to combat viral infections on their own terms, and redefining the construct of vaccines, provides a new and innovative arsenal of treatment options with which to fight deadly viral infections.

BASIC CONSTRUCT OF HIV

HIV is a very ingeniously designed, deadly virus. Viruses, in general, have been difficult to contain and eradicate due to the fact they are obligate parasites and tend not to carry out biologic functions outside the cell the virus has targeted as its host. A virus, when it exists as a single entity outside the boundaries of a cell, is generally referred to as a 'virion' (Figure 1).

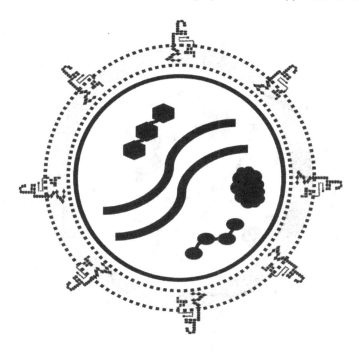

Figure 1: Human Immunodeficiency Virus virion[2]

An HIV virion is comprised of an exterior envelope, an inner shell and a payload carried inside the inner shell. The payload of the HIV virus consists of the genome and proteins that facilitate the genome in infecting the host cell. HIV is an RNA virus. Its genome consists of two strands of ribonucleic acid (RNA) molecules. The purpose of the RNA genome is to take command of the T-Helper host cell and redirect the host cell to produce copies of the virus. The proteins include reverse transcriptase, protease and integrase (Figure 2).

---

2 The figures in this document are intended to be cartoon approximations representing actual complex three dimensional biologic structures; the figures are not intended to be detailed enough to represent said biologic structures in their exact form, but rather are meant to provide a visual image of the concepts put forth in this document.

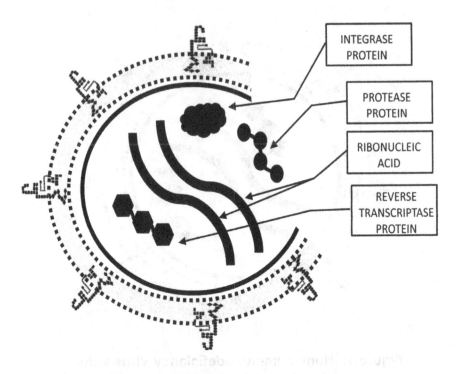

INTEGRASE PROTEIN

PROTEASE PROTEIN

RIBONUCLEIC ACID

REVERSE TRANSCRIPTASE PROTEIN

Figure 2: HIV virion inner structures

The outer structure of the HIV virion is comprised of an external envelope, probes mounted on this external envelope and an inner shell (Figure 3). The external envelope consists of a bilayer lipid membrane, which the virus acquires from its host, the T-Helper cell. As the fledgling copy of the HIV virus buds out and leaves an infected T-Helper cell, the virus wraps itself in a portion of the exterior membrane of the T-Helper cell. Mounted on the exterior envelope are the probes glycoprotein 120 (gp120) and glycoprotein 41 (gp41). The HIV virion utilizes these probes to seek out and attach to a T-Helper cell that it may infect. The inner shell of the virion is comprised of repeating copies of protein molecules termed capsid proteins. The inner shell is constructed of p24 core proteins and p17 matrix proteins.

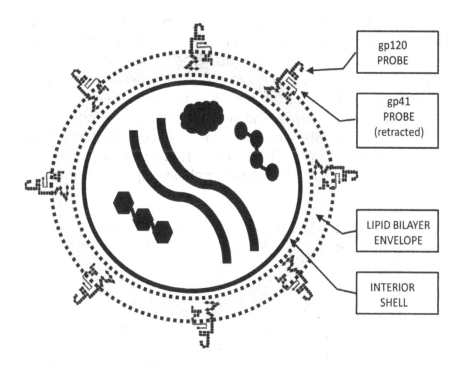

gp120
PROBE

gp41
PROBE
(retracted)

LIPID BILAYER
ENVELOPE

INTERIOR
SHELL

Figure 3: HIV virion outer structures

HIV utilizes its gp120 probe to attach to a T-Helper cell's CD4 cell-surface receptor to make initial contact with a potential host cell. Once HIV's gp120 probe has successfully attached to a CD4 cell-surface receptor, HIV's gp41 probe makes contact with the T-Helper cell's CCR5 or CXCR4 cell-surface receptor. Once both probes have successfully engaged their respective cell-surface receptors, HIV inserts its RNA genome and support proteins into its host cell. Inside the T-Helper cell the proteins assist in preparing the virus's genetic material to take command of the T-Helper cell's function. The reverse transcriptase protein changes the RNA genome into deoxyribonucleic acid (DNA). The protease protein assists in changing the viral DNA into its final form. The integrase protein escorts the viral DNA into the nucleus of the T-Helper cell and then inserts the viral DNA into the T-Helper cell's chromosomes. HIV's viral DNA may lay dormant for a considerable period of time residing in the T-Helper cell's chromosomes. When activated, HIV's viral DNA is read by the cell's nuclear polymerase molecules. HIV's viral DNA re-directs the T-Helper cell's internal machinery to make copies of the pieces of the virus. The copies of the pieces of the virus aggregate at a site near the outer membrane of the T-Helper cell. After the pieces of the virus have clustered near the outer membrane, the viral copies are assembled. As the copies of the HIV virion exit the T-Helper cell, the copies acquire a portion of the T-Helper cell's outer membrane and utilize this as the HIV virion's external envelope (Figure 4).

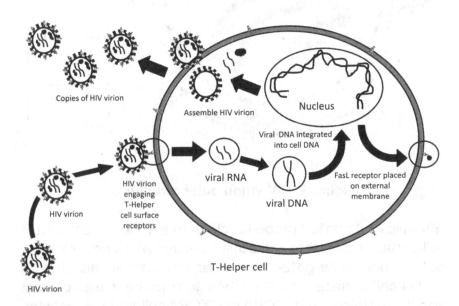

Figure 4: HIV virion infects T-Helper cell with viral RNA, which redirects T-Helper cell to generate copies of HIV and places FasL receptor on outer wall

When the HIV viral DNA is read by a polymerase molecule, the T-Helper cell is directed to place FasL receptors on its own exterior membrane. The purpose of the FasL receptor is to kill any noninfected T-Helper cells that the infected T-Helper cell might encounter while circulating about the body.

HIV virions posses several attributes that make this form of virus very elusive and especially difficult to destroy.

TRADITIONAL APPROACH TO TREATING INFECTIONS

A bacterium is approximately 100 times larger than a virus virion, though various types of both entities vary considerably in size. Bacterial infections have posed a much easier target for the medical community to kill than viral infections. Not only are bacterial agents much larger than viral virions, but generally bacteria live and reproduce outside animal cells. Viruses use host cells to conduct replication. A bacterium divides to reproduce. Bacteria, like animal cells, depend upon respiration to produce energy and engage in biologic functions. Outside of a host cell, viruses do not produce energy, nor do they conduct biologic processes.

A large multi-celled organism such as the human body combats a bacterial infection with a combined force of: mobile circulating white cells, collections of white cells resident in lymph nodes and the spleen, antibodies, complement and the lymphatic system. White cells, which are also referred to as leukocytes, white blood cells and white corpuscles, are divided into three differing groups. Leukocytes may be grouped as lymphocytes, granulocytes and monocytes. Lymphocytes tend to engage in a defense against viruses and cancer cells. Granulocytes may be further subdivided into cell types including neutrophils, eosinophils and basophils. Neutrophils circulate tending to seek out bacteria, eosinophils combat parasitic infections and basophils tend to participate in noninfectious allergic reactions. Monocytes tend to transform into macrophages which act as scavenger cells that circulate the body intending to ingest infectious agents, red blood cells and/or large particles.

Lymphocytes tend to be divided into two groups recognized as T-lymphocytes and B-lymphocytes. T-lymphocytes derive their name from being dependent upon maturation in the thymus. B-lymphocytes were first named in relation to having been found in a bursa in birds. T-lymphocytes are generally classified as either CD4 T-helper cells that act to either coordinate immune responses against pathogens or CD8 cytotoxic cells that kill viruses, infected cells or cancer cells. B-lymphocytes generate immunoglobulins, immune proteins that act as antibodies to combat infectious agents.

The origin of T-lymphocytes begins as offspring of stem cells in the bone marrow. Precursor lymphocytes migrate to the thymus. In the precursor form, lymphocytes express neither the CD4 nor CD8 cell-surface receptor. In the thymus lymphocytes undergo significant maturation presumably to learn the proper signals of what constitutes innate body tissues in order to insure the T-lymphocytes are able to properly distinguish the body's own cells from foreign invaders. Most maturing T-lymphocytes die in the thymus. Lymphocytes that are allowed to mature develop into either T-Helper cells which carry a CD4 cell-receptor or cytotoxic T-cells which carry a CD8 cell-surface receptor. Once the CD4 T-Helper cell leaves the thymus its job is to coordinate the immune response to defend the body against invasion by various microorganisms. Cytotoxic T-cells are intended to engage and kill viruses, cells infected by a virus and some cancer cells.

Certain cells, such as macrophages, scour the body in search of foreign substances called antigens. Macrophages are one form of a functional class of cells termed antigen presenting cells (APC). Antigens may be associated with a virus, a bacteria, a parasite, a protein structure not normally present in the body, or any object that is foreign to the tissues of the body. When a macrophage detects a foreign antigen, the macrophage ingests the antigen, decodes the antigen and expresses part of the antigen (decoded antigen) on its surface. The macrophage uses Major Histocompatibility Complex (MHC) receptors located on its surface to present the decoded antigen to a T-Helper cell.

Major Histocompatibility Complex is divided into two classes. MHC Class I molecules are expressed on the surface of most cells in a body. The MHC Class I molecules are used as a code by the majority of the cells in an organism to identify each cell that is resident in the body as a cell innate to that body. By having MHC Class I molecules present on the surfaces of the majority of cells in the body the immune system is able to determine which cells are suppose to reside in the body and which cells may represent an invader, and thus a danger to the body. Every individual possesses their own unique MHC class I code which is expressed on the surface of the cells in their body. In the event an individual requires an organ transplant, the medical team attempts to match the organ donor's MHC Class I code as close as possible to the recipient's MHC Class I code in order to reduce the occurrence of rejection of the donated organ by the recipient's immune system. Major Histocompatibility Complex Class II molecules are utilized by certain cells comprising the immune system as a means of communication.

T-Helper cells query macrophages and other cells that are classified as antigen presenting cells. The T-Helper cell searches for both a decoded antigen being expressed on the surface of the APC and Major Histocompatibility Complex Class II molecules. When a T-Helper cell finds both a decoded antigen and MHC Class II molecule being expressed together on the surface of an APC, the T-Helper cell connects its surface receptors to the decoded antigen and the MHC Class II molecules present on the APC.

When a T-Helper cell's receptors engage and read the decoded antigen expressed on the surface of the macrophage the T-Helper searches for a secondary signal. Such a secondary signal can be either a chemical signal termed a 'cytokine' or the macrophage connects its B7-1(CD80), B7-2 (CD86) cell-surface receptor to the T-Helper cell's CD28 cell-surface receptor. If the T-helper cell detects a secondary signal while reading the decoded antigen then the T-Helper cell will become activated. Once activated, the T-Helper cell changes into a

T-Helper 1 (TH1) cell or T-Helper 2 (TH2) cell. TH1 cells secrete various chemicals termed cytokines, which stimulate cytotoxic T-cells and macrophages to engage the antigen the scavenger macrophage has found and decoded. TH1 cells secrete cytokines such as gamma interferon, tumor necrosis factor beta (TNFβ) and Interleukin 2 (IL-2) as stimulatory chemical signals. TH2 T-Helper cells stimulate B-cells to divide and generate antibodies to seek out and engage the decoded antigen the scavenger macrophage has found. TH2 cells secrete the cytokines IL-4, IL-5, IL-6, IL-9, IL-10, and IL-13 as stimulatory chemical signals.

Once stimulated by a TH2 cell, B-cells divide creating a new subset of B-cell that will generate antibodies specific to the antigen the scavenger macrophage has detected. Antibodies traverse the blood and body tissues in search of the specific antigen or bacterium they were created to engage. Antibodies, also called immunoglobulins, generally are classified as IgM, IgG, IgA, IgD and IgE. Immunoglobulins are comprised of molecular chains. The chains contain both variable regions and constant regions. Antibodies tend to bind to the antigen they are created to interact with by means of the variable regions located on a pair of heavy and light chains. The immunoglobulins are generally classified on the basis of the construction of the constant domain (structure) of the antibody's heavy chain. A heavy chain is a long protein molecule. There are generally at least two heavy chains comprising an immunoglobulin.

IgM antibodies are large pentamer molecules with ten antigen binding sites. IgM antibodies are usually generated by B-cells as the initial response to an infection. The large IgM molecules bind to the exterior of microorganisms and cause them to clump together inhibiting the migration of the microorganisms and making it easier for immune cells to engage the microorganisms.

IgG antibodies are the most common immunoglobulins. IgG antibodies are comprised of four chains consisting of two heavy chains and two light chains (Figure 5). Both the light chains and the heavy chains contain variable and constant regions. The head of an IgG antibody is made of both variable and constant regions of the heavy and light chains and has two antigen binding sites. The binding sites represent the functional end of the IgG antibody and are where the antibody is intended to latch onto an antigen. The tail of the antibody is comprised of the constant region of the two heavy chains.

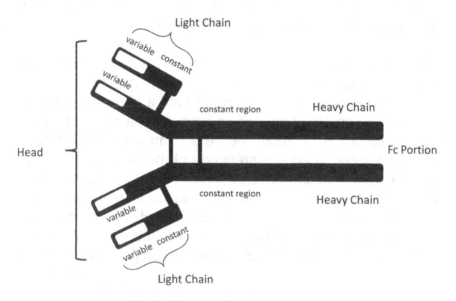

Figure 5: General schematic of IgG antibody

IgA antibodies are usually present in body secretions such as saliva, tears, respiratory secretions, intestinal secretions and breast milk. IgA immunoglobulins tend to be generated only by B-cells located in the mucous membranes of the body. Very little IgA circulates in the blood stream.

IgD is present on the surface of most B-cells. IgD antibodies are not released into circulation. The function of IgD antibodies may include regulating the activation process B-cells exhibit toward antigens.

IgE antibodies circulate in low concentrations in the blood. The IgE antibodies assist in defending the body from parasitic infections. IgE antibodies are also capable of attaching to basophils and acting to stimulate allergic reactions.

The IgG antibodies are generated following the initial response to an infection and tend to confer a long-lasting immunity against the antigen or microorganism that the IgG antibody was generated to respond to by the B-cells.

When an antibody encounters a bacterium it was created to repel, the antibody attaches to the bacterium's outer wall by way of a pair of variable regions at the head of the antibody (Figure 6). The effect antibodies have on coating the surface of a bacterium is to assist the cells comprising the immune system in recognizing the presence of the bacterium so that appropriate action can be taken against the bacterium. Some antibodies, in addition to coating the bacterium outer wall, work in concert with complement molecules, which act to punch holes through the bacterium's outer wall. If the integrity of the bacterium's cell wall is breached, this action generally leads to the death of the bacterium. Complements are primitive protein structures that circulate the blood stream in search of anything that appears consistent with a bacteria cell wall. Complements are indiscriminant. Once the complement proteins detect any form of bacterium cell wall, the complement proteins organize, and act in concert to punch a hole though the bacterium's cell wall to compromise the viability of the bacterium. The lymphatic system, which includes lymph nodes and the spleen in a human, screen the blood in search of bacteria. When a bacterial pathogen is identified, such as by antibodies coating the surface of the pathogen, it is removed from circulation and terminated.

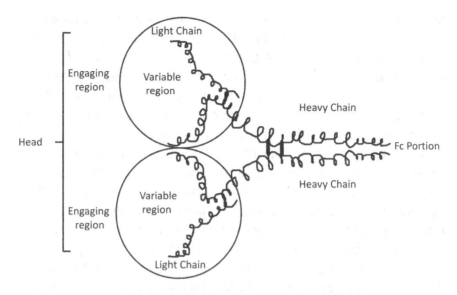

Figure 6: Variable region of the IgG antibody is used to engage an antigen

As noted above, viruses pose a much different challenge to the body's defense system than bacteria. Since viruses do not carry out biologic processes outside their host cell, the survival of a virus is not dependent upon the individual virions converting glucose and oxygen into energy. A virus can be physically destroyed, but since no active life process is conducted inside the virus's virion, viruses are resistant to being killed in the conventional sense of the term. A virus is simply comprised of an external shell with probes to locate a host, possibly an internal shell, a portion of genetic material and enzymes to assist the genetic material in commandeering a host cell.

The virus's genetic information is carried in the core of the virion. Antibodies can coat the exterior of a virus to make it easier for the white cells in the body to identify the pathogen, but the action of punching holes in the virus's external shell by antibodies or complement proteins may not kill the virus. Many viruses only briefly circulate in the blood and tissues of the body, thus they exist for only a limited time as an exposed and vulnerable entity. Using its exterior probes, a virus virion hunts down a cell type in the body that will act as an appropriate host so that the virus can replicate. Once the virus has found a proper host cell, the virus virion inserts its genome into the host cell. The virus's genetic material takes command of cellular functions and the virus's genetic material causes the host cell to manufacture replicas of the virus. Once a virus's genome has gained access to the interior of the host cell, the virus's genetic material is shielded from the body's immune system by the host cell. A virus which has infected a host cell is generally only represented as 'genetic information' that often becomes intimately incorporated into the host cell's own DNA. Often, following the action of a virus's virion infecting a cell in the body, the presence of the virus can only be eradicated if the host cell is destroyed. Antibodies and complements are generally designed not to attack the tissues innate to the body; though some infected host cells do signal that they have been compromised. Circulating white cells and other cells comprising the immune system may or may not recognize that a cell, which has become a host for a virus, is infected with a virus. A host cell in selected circumstances may mount a marker on its surface membrane in attempt to signal the immune system that its outer wall has been breached by a microorganism. If the immune system is capable of detecting such a marker on the surface of an infected cell then cytotoxic T-cells or natural killer cells may respond and destroy the infected cell.

If the immune system fails to identify a cell that has become infected with a virus, the virus's genetic material can proceed unimpeded and force the infected cell to make copies of the virus. Since a virus is in essence simply a segment of genetic material, time is of no consequence to the life-cycle of the virus and in some cases a virus's genome may exist for years or even decades without a need to activate, and only becomes active when the pathogen's genetic programming senses the time is right to initiate the virus's replication process. The only opportunity then for the immune system to destroy a latent virus is when copies of the virus virions leave the host cell and circulate in the blood or tissues in search of other perspective host cells to continue the virus's life-cycle.

The traditional medical approach to combating infectious agents such as bacteria and cellular parasites, therefore, has limited value in managing or eradicating aggressive viral infections. Synthetic antibiotics, generally used to augment the body's capacity to produce naturally occurring antibodies against 'bacterial' infections, have had little success in combating stealthy viral infections. Stimulating the body's immune system recognition by administering a vaccine also has limited value in combating elusive viral infections. Vaccines generally are intended to introduce to the body's immune system an attenuated, noninfectious intact form of a bacteria or virus or pieces of a bacteria or virus so that the immune system is able to recognize and process the infectious agent and generate antibodies directed to assist in killing the pathogen. Once the immune system has been primed to recognize an intruder, antibodies are generally produced by the immune system in great quantities in an effort to repel an invader. Since antibodies have limited value in combating some of the more elusive viruses, the current approach to deriving a vaccine to prevent or treat an infection by HIV has met with limited success in controlling such a latent virus.

REASONS WHY HIV IS SO DIFFICULT TO ERADICATE

The Human Immunodeficiency Virus demonstrates at least four factors that make this pathogen particularly elusive and a difficult infectious agent to eradicate from the body.

First: the host for HIV is the T-Helper cell. The T-Helper cell is a key element in the immune system's response since it acts as a pivotal member of the immune system to coordinate the body's defensive actions against various pathogens seeking to invade the body's tissues. In cases of a bacterial infection versus a viral infection, T-Helper cells actively direct which immune cells will rev-up in response to the infectious agent and engage the particular pathogen. Since HIV infects and disrupts T-Helper cells, coordination of the immune system's defensive response against the virus is compromised. By HIV targeting the T-Helper cell as its host, the body's capacity to mount an effective response to the presence of the virus and successfully eradicate the virus is crippled. When an antigen presenting cell, such as a scavenger macrophage, detects the presence of an HIV antigen and signals for T-Helper cells to migrate to the area in which the the macrophage is residing, this action may actually aid HIV in locating T-Helper cells to infect. The initial T-Helper cell response to the presence of the virus may work to the HIV virion's advantage. By clustering T-Helper cells and providing HIV virions the option to quickly infect these first responder T-helper cells and become cloaked inside the T-Helper cells, HIV is afforded the opportunity to evade the defense mechanisms comprising the immune system.

Second: latent viruses such as HIV have a strategic advantage. When the immune system first recognizes a pathogen has breached the body's perimeter and begins to generate antibodies against a particular pathogen, the response is generally robust. Once time has passed and the immune system fails to detect an active threat, the production of antibodies against the particular pathogen diminishes. When HIV infects a T-Helper cell, the viral genome may lay dormant, sometimes for years before taking command of the T-Helper cell's biologic functions. Therefore, HIV may indeed generate a vigorous initial immune response to its presence, but if the virus sits dormant inside a T-Helper cell for months or years, the antibody response to the virus will diminish over time. There may not be an adequate quantity of circulating antibodies to actively engage the copies of the HIV virion as they migrate from the T-Helper cell that generated the copies to uninfected T-Helper cells that will serve as new hosts to support further replication. If the immune system's response is insufficient during the period while the virus is exposed and vulnerable, it becomes extremely difficult for the body to successfully eradicate the virus.

Third, when replicas of the Human Immunodeficiency Virus are released from their host cell, during the budding process that releases the HIV virion into circulation, the HIV virion coats itself with an exterior envelope comprised of a portion of the plasma membrane from the T-Helper cell that acted as the host for the virus. A T-Helper cell's plasma membrane is comprised of a lipid bilayer; a double layer of lipid molecules oriented with their polar ends at the outside of the membrane and the nonpolar ends in the membrane interior. The virus thus, in part, takes on an external appearance of a naturally occurring cell in the body. The portion of the cell membrane taken from the T-Helper cell may carry the MHC Class I molecules which might serve to fool immune cells, such as cytotoxic T-Cells, into thinking the virus is an innate part of the body and should not be attacked. Cloaked in an exterior envelope that has characteristics of a T-Helper cell, the HIV virion possesses a tremendous stealth advantage in eluding the body's natural defense mechanisms as it migrates through the body in search of a T-Helper cell to infect.

Fourth, the Human Immunodeficiency Virus exhibits a very elusive mode of action which the virus readily utilizes to actively defeat the body's immune system. HIV carries in its genome a segment of genetic material that directs an infected T-Helper cell to create and mount on the surface of the plasma membrane a FasL cell-surface receptor. Healthy T-Helper cells carry on the surface of the T-Helper cell's plasma membrane Fas cell-surface receptors. The Fas cell-surface receptor when engaged by a FasL cell-surface receptor on another cell, initiates apoptosis in the cell carrying the Fas cell-surface receptor. Apoptosis is a biologic process that causes a cell to terminate itself. A T-Helper cell infected with the HIV virus carrying FasL cell-surface receptors is therefore capable of killing noninfected T-Helper cells that the infected T-Helper cell encounters as it circulates the body. The occurrence of AIDS is therefore propagated not only by the number of T-Helper cells that become incapacitated due to direct infection by HIV, but also by the number of noninfected T-Helper cells that are eliminated by coming in direct contact with infected T-Helper cells.

PROGRESSION OF HIV INFECTION TO AIDS

Acquired Immune Deficiency Syndrome (AIDS) occurs as a result of the number of circulating T-Helper cells declining to a point where the immune system's capacity to mount a successful response against opportunistic infectious agents is significantly compromised. The number of viable T-Helper cells declines either because they become infected with the HIV virus or because they have been killed by encountering a T-Helper cell infected with HIV. When there is an insufficient population of non-HIV infected T-Helper cells to properly combat opportunistic infectious agents such as Pneumocystis carinii or cytomegalovirus or other pathogens, the body becomes overwhelmed with the opportunistic infection and the patient becomes ill. In cases where the combination of the patient's compromised immune system and medical assistance in terms of synthetic antibiotics intended to combat the opportunistic pathogens, fluids, intravenous nutrition and other treatments are not sufficient to sustain life, the body succumbs to the opportunistic infection and death ensues.

CURRENT APPROACH TO COMBATING HIV

The human immunodeficiency virus (HIV) locates its host, the T-Helper cell, by utilizing probes located on its exterior envelope. The HIV virus has at least two different glycoprotein probes attached to the outer surface of its exterior envelope. HIV utilizes a glycoprotein probe 120 (gp120) to locate a CD4 cell-surface receptor on a T-Helper cell. After connecting its gp120 probe to the T-Helper cell's CD4 receptor, the HIV virion utilizes its glycoprotein 41 (gp41) probe to engage a CCR5 cell-surface receptor or a CXCR4 cell-surface receptor located on the outer membrane of a T-Helper cell.

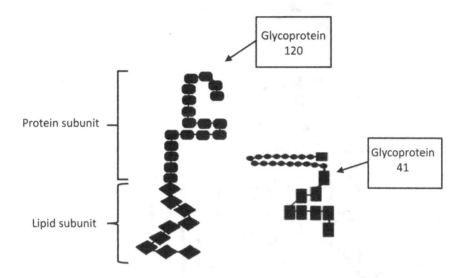

Figure 7: HIV glycoprotein 120 and 41 probes

The gp120 probe is comprised of a protein subunit and a lipid subunit (Figure 7). The protein subunit is used to attach to the T-Helper cell's CD4 cell-surface receptor. The lipid subunit anchors the probe into the HIV virion's exterior envelope (Figure 8). While the lipid subunit remains embedded in the wall of the exterior envelope, the protein subunit projects itself away from the surface of the virion and seeks to engage a CD4 cell-surface receptor.

The HIV gp41 probe is located near the gp120 probe. The gp41 probe is also anchored in the exterior envelope of HIV's surface envelope. The gp41 probe exists in a retracted mode until the gp120 probe makes successful contact with a CD4 cell-surface receptor. Once the gp120 probe does properly engage a CD4 cell-surface receptor a conformational change occurs in the probes and the gp41 probe is allowed to expose itself in order to make proper contact with a CCR5 or CXCR4 cell-surface receptor.

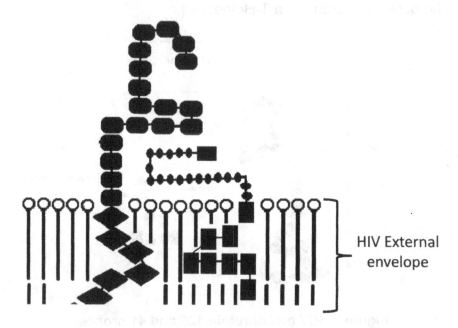

Figure 8: Glycoprotein 120 and 41 probes showing the lipid portion of the probes embedded in exterior envelope of HIV virion

When a HIV virion locates a T-Helper cell that it might infect, the first step to a successful breach of the T-Helper cells requires the HIV gp120 probe to make contact with the CD4 cell-surface receptor located on the T-Helper cell (Figure 9). The CD4 cell-surface receptor has a protein subunit extending away from the T-Helper cell's external membrane, while the lipid portion anchors the CD4 cell-surface receptor to the external membrane.

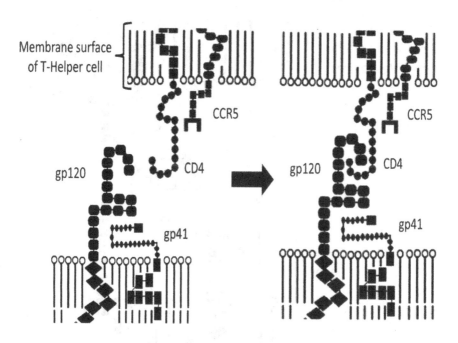

**Figure 9: HIV gp120 probe making contact with
T-Helper cell CD4 receptor**

Following the occurrence of an HIV gp120 probe having successfully engaged a CD4 cell-surface receptor on a T-Helper cell, a conformational change occurs in the probe and a
gp41 probe is exposed on HIV's exterior envelope. The gp 41
probe's intent is to engage a CCR5 cell-surface receptor or a
CXCR4 cell-surface receptor mounted on the exterior membrane on the same T-Helper cell (Figure 10).

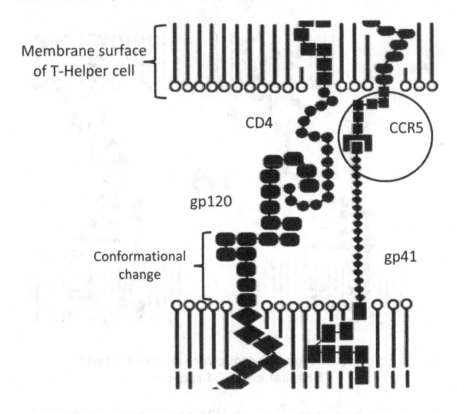

Membrane surface
of T-Helper cell

CD4

CCR5

gp120

Conformational
change

gp41

**Figure 10: HIV gp41 probe making contact with
T-Helper cell's CCR5 receptor**

Once the connection between the HIV gp120 probe and the T-Helper cell's CD4 cell-surface receptor are secure and HIV's gp41 probe makes contact with a CCR5 cell-surface receptor or CXCR4 cell-surface receptor on a T-Helper cell, HIV burrows an access port through the T-Helper cell's outer membrane (Figure 11). The access port through the T-Helper cell's outer membrane provides a tunnel through which the HIV virion is able to insert into the T-Helper cell the RNA genome and support proteins the virion is carrying.

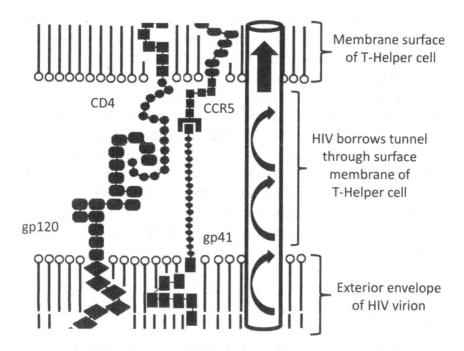

CD4

CCR5

gp120

gp41

Membrane surface of T-Helper cell

HIV borrows tunnel through surface membrane of T-Helper cell

Exterior envelope of HIV virion

Figure 11: Following HIV gp41 probe making successful contact with T-Helper cell's CCR5 receptor, HIV virion burrows tunnel into T-Helper cell to facilitate delivering its RNA payload[3]

When the HIV virion has successfully penetrated the T-Helper cell's outer membrane and opened an access portal into the T-Helper cell, the HIV virion inserts two positive strand RNA molecules, approximately 9500 nucleotides in length, into the T-Helper cell. Inserted along with the RNA strands are the support proteins: reverse transcriptase, protease and integrase. Upon reaching the cytoplasm on the interior of the T-Helper cell, the pair of RNA molecules is transformed into deoxyribonucleic acid (DNA) by the reverse transcriptase protein. The viral DNA is further modified by the protease protein. Following completion of the transforming process that converts viral RNA

---

3 Tunnel shown in figure is for illustrative purposes. When contact is made by both gp120 and gp41 probes with T-Helper cell's cell surface receptors an access port is created such that the virus's RNA and support proteins can be inserted into the T-Helper cell.

into viral DNA the virus's genetic information migrates to the host cell's nucleus. In the nucleus, with the assistance of the integrase protein, the virus's DNA is inserted into the T-Helper cell's native DNA. The viral DNA may sit dormant residing in the T-Helper cell's chromosomes for a variable amount of time. When the timing is appropriate, the integrated viral DNA is read by a host cell's polymerase molecule. The polymerase molecule activates the virus's genetic information as if it represented a segment of native human DNA genes. The result is that the virus's genetic instructions take command of the cell's functions, distracting them from their normal duties and redirecting them to carry out the replication processes necessary to construct copies of the HIV virion.

Present anti-viral therapy has been designed to target the proteins that assist the HIV genome with the replication process. Anti-viral therapy has been devised to interfere with the action of these replication proteins. Part of the challenge of eradicating HIV is that once the virus inserts its genome into a T-Helper cell host, the viral genome may lay dormant until appropriate circumstances evolve. The virus's genome may sit idle inside a T-Helper cell for years before becoming activated, causing drugs that interfere with HIV's life cycle to have limited effect on eliminating the virus from the body. Further, arresting the replication process does not thwart the T-Helper cells infected with HIV that are expressing an FasL receptor on their outer membrane from circulating the body and continuing to actively kill noninfected T-Helper cells. Thus, despite treatment with such an anti-viral agent or combination of anti-viral agents, the individual's healthy T-Helper cell population may progressively decline and the patient may continue to progress to a clinically apparent state of Acquired Immunodeficiency Syndrome and eventually succumb to an opportunistic infection resulting in a fatal outcome.

The outer layer of the HIV virion is comprised of a portion of the T-Helper cell's outer cell membrane. In the final stage of the replication process, as a copy of the HIV capsid, carrying the HIV genome, buds through the host cell's outer membrane, the capsid acquires as its outermost shell a wrapping of lipid bilayer from the host cell's plasma membrane. Traditional vaccines are often comprised of copies of the entire virus or bacterium weakened to the point the pathogen is incapable of causing an infection. Some traditional vaccines are comprised of pieces of a virus or bacteria. The copies of a nonvirulent pathogen or pieces of a pathogen comprising the vaccine serve generally to prime the immune system such that a traditional vaccine causes B-cells in the vaccinated body to produce antibodies that are programmed to seek out the surface characteristics of the pathogen. In the case of HIV, since the surface of the pathogen is an envelope comprised of lipid bilayer taken from the host T-Helper cells, a vaccine might not only cause the vaccinated individual's immune system to target HIV virions, but might also have deleterious effects on the T-Helper cell population. Antibodies produced to combat HIV infections may not be able to differentiate between the surface of an infectious HIV virion and a noninfected T-Helper cell, and such antibodies may act to coat and assist in the elimination of both targets. In such a scenario, since the vaccine might result in a decline in the number of available T-Helper cells, it is conceivable that such a vaccine might paradoxically induce clinically apparent AIDS in a patient that received the vaccine.

SEVEN ENTIRELY NEW MEDICAL TREATMENT STRATEGIES TO ERADICATE AIDS:

It is clear that the approach of utilizing antibiotics or providing traditional forms of a vaccine to stimulate the immune system to produce endogenous antibodies are, by themselves, an ineffective strategy to manage a virus as elusive and deadly as HIV. Drugs that interfere with the replication process of HIV generally slow progression of the infection by the virus, but do not eliminate the virus from the body. Since infected T-Helper cells may continue to circulate the body unimpeded, they may continue to kill healthy T-Helper cells and thus the patient may continue to progress to a state of clinically apparent AIDS despite treatment. A new set of strategies is desperately needed in order to successfully combat HIV and prevent the occurrence of AIDS.

STRATEGY NUMBER ONE: FILTER PATIENT'S BLOOD

Dialysis is generally regarded as a means of removing waste products in patients whose kidneys are no longer capable of effectively filtering the blood and eliminating water-soluble waste from the body. One option immediately available to reduce a portion of the load of HIV circulating in the blood is to physically remove HIV from the blood. Dialysis utilizes the fact that waste products in the blood are smaller in size than blood cells and large protein molecules; therefore by passing blood across a porous filter, blood cells and large protein molecules can be retained, while waste products pass through the holes in the filter and are effectively removed from the blood.

A strategy to combat the Human Immunodeficiency Virus could incorporate a means to trap HIV virions and removed them from a patient's blood stream. HIV virions seek out their host cell by utilizing the gp120 and gp41 probes mounted on the surface of the virus. By bating HIV virions with a surrogate target that engages the surface probes located on the surface of HIV virions, the virus can be removed from the blood (Patent Application A1).

HIV is much smaller in size than the red cells and white cells that circulate in the blood. When blood cells are separated from the blood, the remaining fluid portion is referred to as plasma. The fluid portion of the blood could be filtered and HIV separated from the plasma by trapping the HIV virions in a filter. The gp120 and gp41 probes located on the surface of HIV are seeking to engage the CD4 and a CCR5 cell-surface receptor or a CXCR4 cell-surface receptor located on the surface of T-Helper cells.

A filter mechanism could be fashioned to be comprised of a chamber of circulating exogenous T-Helper cells made of a collection of T-Helpers previously removed from the patient, a collection of T-Helper cells pooled from blood bank donors, or a quantity obtained by other means. Plasma taken from a patient infected with HIV would be introduced into the filter chamber as simultaneously fluid would be removed from the filter chamber. As blood plasma passed through the filter chamber, HIV would come in contact with the collection of T-Helper cells resident in the filter chamber. As HIV's glycoprotein probes engage the cell-surface receptors mounted on the exogenous T-Helper cells, the HIV virions would adhere to the exogenous T-Helper cells and either become stuck to the T-Helper cells and thus are retained in the filter chamber as the plasma exited, or by the action of the HIV probes engaging the T-Helper cell's cell-surface receptors, the HIV virion would eject its genome thus making it incapable of infecting an endogenous T-Helper cell in the patient (Figure 12). The patient's plasma, now cleared of infectious HIV virions, would be infused back into the patient.

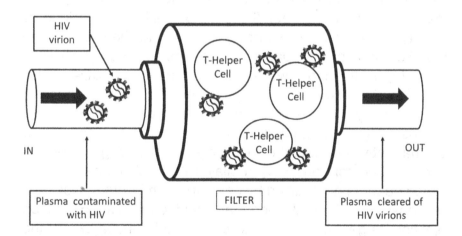

Figure 12: Inside filter chamber T-Helper cells engage HIV virions and HIV virions are cleared from the blood plasma

The technology to construct such a filtering mechanism is readably available and could be quickly implemented for worldwide use to treat HIV.

A quantity of T-Helper cells has a limited life span and requires specially handling to insure the T-Helper cells do not become metabolically inactive and then deteriorate to a point where they are ineffective as a filtering medium. A method to accomplish the same task, without having to incorporate a special storage or handling of healthy T-Helper cells, would be to construct a filter mechanism that houses a material that emulates the surface of naturally occurring T-Helper cells, since it is the cell-surface receptors that the HIV virion's probes are seeking. Sheets of lipid bilayer constructed with a large quantity of CD4, CCR5, and CXCR4 cell-surface receptors could be utilized as a filter medium in place of T-Helper cells.

A filter could be constructed in a manner where one or more sheets of lipid bilayer constructed with a large quantity of CD4, CCR5 and CXCR4 cell-surface receptors would be placed inside a filtering chamber (Patent Application A1). Blood or blood plasma would pass through the filtering chamber. As the blood or blood plasma passes across the surface of a sheet of lipid bilayer, HIV virions would come in contact with CD4, CCR5 and CXCR4 cell-surface receptors present on the surface of the lipid bilayer and engage the cell-surface receptors. HIV virions making contact with the lipid bilayer would either permanently adhere to the lipid bilayer or by engaging the cell-surface receptors on the lipid bilayer the HIV virion's genome would become neutralized by cell-surface receptors evoking a response from the HIV virion that would result in the HIV virion ejecting its genome. The blood or blood plasma exiting the filter chamber would be cleared of intact HIV virions capable of infecting a T-Helper cell (Figure 13). The blood or blood plasma would then be reintroduced back into the patient's body.

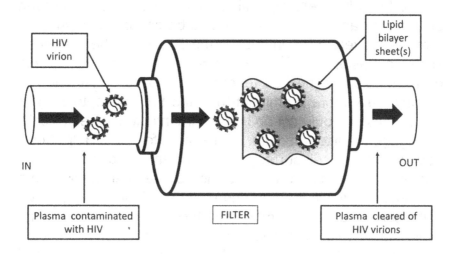

Figure 13: Within the filter chamber material with CD4, CCR5 and CXCR4 cell-surface receptors capture HIV virions and clear them from the blood plasma

The filter technique could be utilized as a dynamic process whereby a patient's blood is removed, filtered and returned to the patient in real-time. The filter technique could be utilized as a static process, where specimens in a blood-bank are filtered to remove HIV virions as they wait to be donated to patients. Filtering blood bank specimens would help to eliminate the threat of HIV to trauma and surgical patients.

It may be considered one day to place a filter inside a patient with known HIV; any artery or vein could potentially be used. If HIV were triggered to eject its genome upon successful engagement of CD4 cell-surface receptor and a CCR5 or CXCR4 cell-surface receptor, then a tiny filter placed in the blood stream, that triggered HIV to eject its genome upon contact with the filter medium would in fact reduce the load of HIV virions circulating in the blood stream. HIV might remain in some tissues, but would not be able to circulate freely in the blood.

Infected T-Helper cells circulating in the blood could be removed by a similar approach. A filter could be constructed whereby a medium fixed to the interior of the filter could be fashioned such that Fas and FasL receptors were present on the surface of the medium. The Fas receptors could be constructed to be physically more prominent than the FasL receptors. The Fas receptors would act as bait to lure infected T-Helper cells to engage the filter medium. When an infected T-Helper cell, bearing a FasL cell-surface receptor came in contact with a Fas receptor located on the surface of the filter medium, the T-Helper cell would then be engaged by a FasL receptor fixed to the surface of the filter medium. Once a FasL receptor on the filter medium makes contact with a Fas receptor on an infected T-Helper cell, the Fas cell-surface receptor on the infected T-Helper cell would trigger the biologic signal for the T-Helper cell to destroy itself. The T-Helper cell would pass through the filter, but later the infected T-Helper cell would be terminated by the process of apoptosis (Patent Application A2).

STRATEGY NUMBER TWO: TREAT WITH SMART VIRUS TECHNOLOGY

White blood cells or leukocytes are generally approximately the size of red blood cells or larger than red blood cells. Bacteria are generally much smaller than red blood cells. An HIV virion is physically much smaller in size than a bacterium. Due to the small size of the HIV virion, HIV can potentially maneuver into places in the body's tissues where mobile leukocytes are unable to easily make their way into; thus the virus's small size tends to protect the virus from being killed by circulating leukocytes.

An approach to managing HIV would be to create a product designed to intercept and neutralize HIV that is relatively the same size as the HIV virion so that the product could penetrate into every location that an HIV virion might migrate to inside the body or outside on the skin surface or mucosal surfaces.

HIV's probes are perpetually seeking the CD4 and CCR5 or CXCR4 cell-surface receptors of a T-Helper cell, thus a mobile product to challenge HIV could be equipped with the same cell-surface receptors as would be found on a naturally occurring healthy T-Helper cell.

HIV is generated by a T-Helper cell being forced to make copies of the virus's genome and internal core capsid. Once the package of the HIV genome and replication enzymes are loaded into a capsid, the capsid buds through the cell membrane of the T-Helper cell and as the capsid emerges it confiscates a portion of the T-Helper cell's outer cell membrane and utilizes this as an envelope to act as an outer covering. The gp120 and gp41 probes are mounted on the surface of the virion's outer envelope.

Utilizing genetic machinery and a colony of modified, hybrid T-Helper cells, a product approximately the size of a HIV virion could be manufactured in a similar manner as HIV is known to replicate, except the product would carry T-Helper cell cell-surface receptors rather than the glycoprotein probes found on a naturally occurring HIV virion. The product would be constructed either with no genetic information present inside the capsid or genetic material that is inert and incapable of carrying out any useful function (Patent Application A3).

Such scientifically modulated and reprogrammed treatment (SMART) viruses could be utilized in several different fashions to combat HIV (Figure 14). SMART viruses could be manufactured and pooled together into a liquid medium that could be utilized as a cleaning solution (Patent Application A4). As such a liquid is introduced onto a surface where HIV virions reside, the copies of the SMART virus would come in contact with the HIV virions. The clusters of CD4 and CCR5 cell-surface receptors and clusters of CD4 and CXCR4 cell-surface receptors located on the surface of the SMART viruses would engage the HIV virions' gp120 and gp41 probes. The SMART viruses would latch on to the HIV virions.

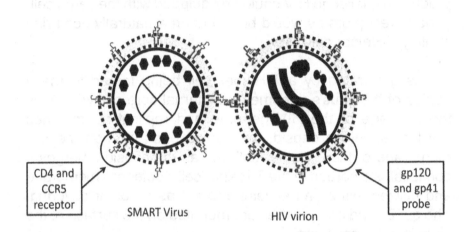

CD4 and CCR5 receptor

SMART Virus

HIV virion

gp120 and gp41 probe

Figure 14: A SMART virus engaging a HIV virion

The action of SMART viruses adhering to HIV virions would either make HIV incapable of properly engaging T-Helper cells, make HIV more visible to the immune system for body's defenses to detect and destroy, or cause the HIV virion to eject its genome harmlessly into the environment, making the HIV virions unable to infect a healthy T-Helper cell (Figure 15).

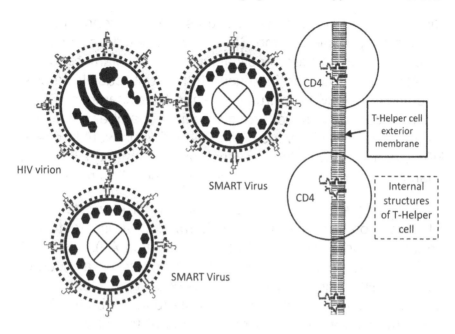

**Figure 15: SMART Viruses blocking HIV virion
from engaging T-Helper cell**

SMART viruses could be pooled together into a gel and utilized by women as a surface defense mechanism. Women commonly apply spermicidal gels into their vagina as a means to prevent pregnancy. Women could utilize a topical vaginal gel containing a quantity of copies of a SMART virus as a means of preventing infection by HIV during sexual intercourse. Semen deposited by a man would make contact with the vaginal gel. If a proper quantity of the gel was present in the vagina, the HIV virions introduced into the vagina would come in contact with SMART viruses present in the gel. HIV virions making contact with the gel would be neutralized by the SMART virus. The residual of the gel could be washed out of the vagina at a later time. The gel containing SMART virus would provide an effective barrier where HIV virions would be unable to breach the skin of the vagina or gain passage through the cervix and into the uterus in a form that could result in an HIV infection in the woman (Patent Application A5).

Similar to the approach described as the filter concept in the first strategy, copies of the SMART virus could be placed in a filter chamber (Patent Application A1). The diameter of the SMART virus could be increased to make it feasible to easily contain the SMART virus inside the filter chamber. Blood plasma could be passed through the filter chamber containing a quantity of SMART virus. The SMART virus would engage HIV virions as the blood plasma passed through the filter chamber and neutralize the virulence of the HIV virions.

A more aggressive use of the SMART virus would be to introduce copies of the medically therapeutic virus directly into an infected person's body (Patent Application A3). SMART viruses could be constructed in a similar size as a naturally occurring HIV virion. SMART viruses could circulate the body and travel anywhere HIV might migrate to in the body. Being the same size as an HIV virion, copies of the SMART virus could disseminate throughout the body and engage HIV virions anywhere they might be found in the blood stream or tissues of the body. In effect, in the treatment of an individual infected with HIV, such SMART viruses would act much like a sophisticated antibody by engaging and neutralizing its virus target. Being constructed in a similar manner as naturally occurring HIV virions, but with nearly identical physical characteristics of the outer membrane of a T-Helper cell, the SMART virus would have a low risk of generating a neutralizing antibody response by the patient's immune system.

STRATEGY NUMBER THREE: ELIMINATION OF INFECTED T-HELPER CELLS

Engaging HIV virions as they circulate the blood and tissues of the body does not attack or in any manner neutralize the reservoir of HIV, the infected T-Helper cells, as it exists in the body. Until both the HIV virions migrating through the body and the T-Helper cells infected with HIV are neutralized or destroyed AIDS remains a threat to the individual infected with HIV. It becomes imperative that, for a strategy intended to combat HIV to be successful, the population of infected T-Helper cells needs to be identified and effectively terminated and eliminated from the body.

As mentioned earlier, HIV carries in its genome a segment of genetic material that directs an infected T-Helper cell to create and mount on its surface a FasL receptor. T-Helper cells carry, on the surface of their cell membrane, Fas receptors. The Fas receptor, when triggered, initiates apoptosis in the cell. Apoptosis is a biologic process that causes a cell to terminate itself, thus ending the cell's life. A T-Helper cell infected with the HIV virus is therefore capable of killing noninfected T-Helper cells that the infected T-Helper cell encounters as it circulates the body. The occurrence of AIDS is therefore enhanced not only by the number of T-Helper cells that become incapacitated due to direct infection by the HIV virus, but also by the number of noninfected T-Helper cells that are eliminated by coming in contact with infected T-Helper cells.

A scientifically modified and reprogrammed treatment (SMART) virus could be created to possess, on its surface, both Fas and FasL receptors (Patent Application A6). This version of a SMART virus could be fashioned such that the Fas receptor could be physically more prominent than the FasL receptor. The Fas receptor on the surface of the SMART virus could be physically mounted further out from the FasL receptor, or in a manner likened as to how HIV is constructed with the gp120 and gp41 probes, the Fas receptor may hide the FasL receptor and a conformational change in the Fas receptor would be required before the FasL receptor is exposed. On the surface of a naturally occurring HIV virion, the gp120 probe hides the gp41 probe. When the gp120 probe engages a CD4 cell-surface receptor a conformational change occurs in the gp120 probe such that the gp41 probe becomes exposed so that the gp41 probe can engage either a CCR5 cell-surface receptor or a CXCR4 cell-surface receptor. On the surface of the SMART virus, the Fas receptor would be fashioned to be engaged first, and once engaged, the FasL receptor would become available to be readily engaged.

A SMART virus constructed with both Fas and FasL receptors would have the capacity to terminate HIV infected T-Helper cells. An infected T-Helper cell is armed with FasL cell surface receptors. The infected T-Helper cell's FasL cell-surface receptors are in search of Fas cell-surface receptors located on noninfected T-Helper cells. The SMART virus would act as a decoy, baiting infected T-Helper cells with its Fas surface receptors. The Fas receptor on a SMART virus would lure and engage the FasL receptor located on an infected T-Helper cell. Once the Fas receptor on the SMART virus has been engaged by an HIV infected T-Helper cell, the FasL receptor on the SMART virus would then engage a Fas cell-surface receptor on the infected T-Helper cell. With the SMART virus's FasL receptor engaging the Fas cell-surface receptor on an infected T-Helper cell this action would cause 'apoptosis' to be triggered in the infected T-Helper cell. Triggering apoptosis in such a cell will cause the cell to terminate itself. SMART viruses equipped with Fas and FasL receptors could be introduced into the body of a person infected with HIV in order to eliminate T-Helper cells infected with HIV and thus actually avert the patient from progressing to the clinical state of AIDS. With infected T-Helper cells eliminated from the body's tissues, the body's immune system could replenish the numbers of circulating noninfected T-Helper cells and allow the patient infected with HIV to return to a state of normality.

STRATEGY NUMBER FOUR: NEW APPROACH FOR A VACCINE FOR HIV

Once a patient's HIV infection has been treated and stabilized by filtering the blood to reduce the viral load, utilizing SMART viruses or other surrogate targets to eliminate circulating HIV virions and to neutralize the reservoir of HIV by terminating infected T-Helper cells, a strategy needs to be put into place to prevent further infection by HIV. At the point where the HIV infection is being actively managed, a vaccine might be introduced. Of course, conceptually, vaccines administered to healthy individuals are meant to prevent an infectious agent from ever gaining a foothold in a patient. Vaccines are intended to alert the immune system to the presence of a pathogen. Once the immune system has been sensitized to a pathogen, antibodies are generated with the mission to intercept and terminate the invading pathogen.

Most vaccines are comprised of whole units or pieces of a virus or bacterium with the intention that the vaccinated individual's immune system will recognize the pathogen resulting in the vaccinated individual's B-cell population producing an effective neutralizing antibody response to the pathogen. Newer versions of vaccines have attempted to introduce HIV's genetic material into T-Helper cells, with the intention of stimulating an immune response.

It has been reported that even the latest vaccines designed to prevent HIV infections have had limited success. There may be several reasons for the poor performance of a traditional vaccine. First: HIV, utilizing T–Helper cells as their host, cripples the immune system's response. Second: HIV's capacity to turn infected T-Helper cells into killing machines represents a direct means for the virus to combat the body's innate immune response. Third: The outer layer of the HIV virion is comprised of a portion of the T-Helper cell's outer cell membrane. A vaccine comprised of simply pieces of HIV's exterior envelope or a vaccine comprised of an intact but weakened HIV virus, might not only cause an antibody response to target HIV virions, but such antibodies might also attack the T-Helper cell population believing they represent HIV virions, thus paradoxically accelerating a patient's development of AIDS. Any means that results in a decline in the number of healthy T-Helper cells will result in the clinical development of AIDS.

HIV has also been regarded as a pathogen that possess the capacity to create a high rate of genetic mutation and thus copies of the virus can readily adapt to the effects of the antiviral drugs utilized to interfere with the viral replication process that are currently in use to combat the disease. It has been reported that given the length of time HIV infects an individual, new, more resistant strains of the virus will appear in the same patient as a result of the introduction of current anti-viral therapies, to the point that single drug therapy is well recognized as 'not' being an effective treatment strategy. Combination therapy is currently targeted to slow down HIV virion replication.

Genetic variability may assist HIV in resisting the effects of currently available anti-viral medications, but despite the possibility of genetic variation, an HIV virion's probes must remain compatible with the T-Helper cell's cell-surface receptors. This is clearly an inherent weakness of HIV. If the T-helper cell's cell-surface receptors changed due to genetic variation then genetic variation would benefit HIV. As long as the design of cell-surface receptors mounted on the surface of T-Helper cells remain relatively constant HIV is bound to keep its surface probes a standard design in order to retain the capacity to gain access to its host cell. Genetic variation in HIV's surface probes only hinders the virus's capacity to infect healthy T-Helper cells, rather than aiding the virus in resisting strategies to eradicate the virus by attacking the virus's exterior probes.

It is understood that the B-cells of the immune system, when activated, are capable of generating antibodies directed against viruses, bacteria, cellular parasites and foreign proteins. If a snake or insect venom, which generally consists of one or more proteins, is injected into a body, the body will, if sufficient time is allowed, generate antibodies against the venom. Injectable medications that consist of one or more proteins may stimulate the B-cells of the immune system to generate antibodies against the medication. Often protein-based medications such as insulin are therefore designed to appear to the immune system as identical as possible to the naturally occurring human protein, so as to avoid generating a neutralizing immune response against the medication. A robust and effective immune response to a drug like insulin negates the medically therapeutic effect of the insulin.

The physical structure of the molecule which initiates an immune response by a body is important to the construction of the physical structure of the antibody generated by the immune system in response to the stimulus molecule.

In the treatment of rheumatic diseases there are three biologic agents currently utilized to suppress inflammation by engaging the TNF alpha molecule. The TNF alpha molecules bind to specific receptors (p55 and p75) on cells to stimulate an inflammatory response. Once the TNF alpha molecule binds to a naturally occurring cell surface receptor located on the surface of a cell, the biologic signal to propagate the inflammatory response is transmitted to that cell. Of the two receptors, receptor p75 appears to be more biologically sensitive for treating rheumatic diseases. The three biologic agents that act as TNF alpha blocking agents by binding to the TNF alpha molecule and thus act as a surrogate p75 receptor are known as etanercept, inflixamab and adalimumab. Each biologic agent acts in a likened manner to engage and neutralize the TNF alpha molecule. The three biologic agents are constructed differently. Etanercept is a dimeric fusion protein consisting of the extracellular ligand binding portion of the human 75 kilodalton (p75) tumor necrosis factor receptor (TNFR) linked to the FC portion of human IgG1. Adalimumab is a recombinant human IgG1 monoclonal antibody specific for tumor necrosis factor alpha and blocks its interaction between TNF alpha molecule and the naturally occurring p55 and p75 TNF cell-surface receptors. Inflixamab is a chimeric protein comprised of part human and part mouse proteins that, as a unit, engage

TNF alpha, blocking the TNF alpha molecule from interacting with the naturally occurring TNF cell surface receptors.

The introduction of these three protein structures individually results in an immune response. It has been reported that etanercept causes 6% antibody response, inflixamab results in a 10% immune response and adalimumab causes approximately a 12% antibody response.

Neutralizing antibodies are defined as antibodies that interfere with the function of the structure the antibodies have been generated to respond to by the immune system. The 6% antibody response caused by etanercept tends not to be neutralizing antibodies and therefore do not interfere with the function of etanercept. Both inflixamab and adalimumab produce neutralizing antibodies as part of the immune response to the introduction of these biologic agents into the body and this results in either the biologic agent being ineffective in some patients or requires in some patients an increase in dose to produce the desired anti-inflammatory effect by the biologic agent.

The point is that though protein structures may act in a similar manner, their physical construction can lead to a varied response by the immune system when such proteins are introduced into the body. The immune system may generate antibodies that are effective against a stimulus protein created with one design, while the same immune system may produce a different antibody response to a protein that performs the same biologic action as the first but is constructed with differing physical characteristics.

Since the introduction of a protein alone into the body may generate an immune response and cause antibodies to be formed, using the glycoprotein probes alone, which are unique to HIV, might act as the basis for an effective vaccine. The two HIV probes gp120 and gp41 are constructed of a combination of protein and lipid structures. Injecting a quantity of intact or partially intact gp120 and gp41 probes into the body, like one would inject a traditional vaccine, in theory might produce an immune response by the B-cells directed solely against the presence of these probes. Since the gp120 and gp41 probes only occur on the surface of HIV virions, antibodies created by the B-cells of the immune system against such probes would target HIV virions and not T-Helper cells. The B-cell's action need not destroy the virion, just make HIV's exterior glycoprotein probes interoperable to the point where HIV virions are unable to properly engage T-Helper cells (Patent Application A7). If an HIV virion is unable to infect a healthy T-Helper cell, the HIV virion will fail to complete its life-cycle requirements, be made impotent and will eventually be detected and destroyed by the body; this is the desired outcome for an antibody response generated against HIV.

Attempts to develop a vaccine for HIV have included using the entire gp120 probe. The IgG antibody presented in Figure 16 is

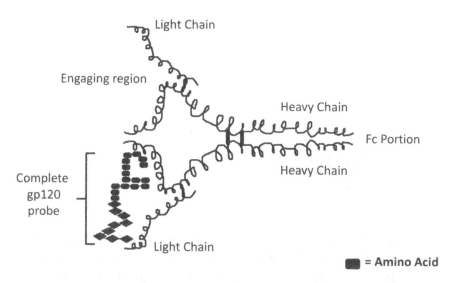

Figure 16: IgG antibody generated to latch onto the complete or nearly complete HIV gp120 probe utilizing a variable region located in the head of the IgG antibody

generated by the immune system and intended to latch onto the complete or nearly complete HIV gp120 probe as it exists.

The IgG antibody generated to engage the complete HIV gp120 probe is physically too large and therefore unable to properly latch on to the engagable portion of the protein subunit of the HIV gp120 probe when the HIV gp120 probe is embedded in the exterior envelope of the HIV virion (Figure 17). This form of antibody response, though generated as a result of the immune system being challenged with the complete HIV gp120 probe molecule, is ineffective in attaching to the HIV gp120 probe and therefore ineffective in preventing the HIV virion from engaging and latching onto a T-Helper cell; this is not the desired antibody response.

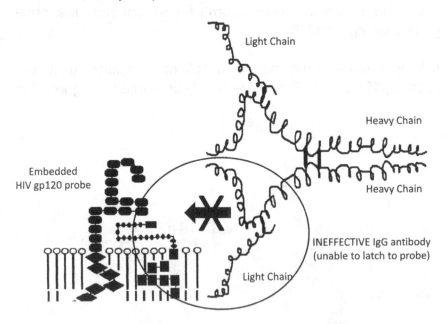

Light Chain

Heavy Chain

Embedded
HIV gp120 probe

Heavy Chain

INEFFECTIVE IgG antibody
(unable to latch to probe)

Light Chain

Figure 17: IgG antibody is <u>ineffective</u> against embedded HIV gp120 probe due to IgG antibody being too large to successfully latch to embedded HIV gp120 probe

Removal of the lipid subunit from the intact HIV gp120 probe leaves the complete protein subunit of the HIV gp120 probe. A vaccine comprised of the entire portion of the HIV gp120 probe will produce antibodies generated to engage the entire protein subunit of the HIV gp120 probe and such antibodies will be designed with a variable region that is intended to engage the entire protein subunit structure (Figure 18).

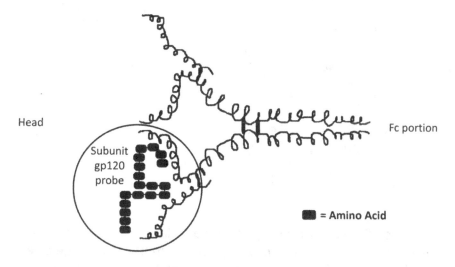

Head

Subunit gp120 probe

Fc portion

■■ = Amino Acid

Figure 18: IgG antibody generated to engage the entire protein subunit of HIV gp120 probe

As shown in Figure 19, the antibody generated to engage the complete protein subunit of the HIV gp120 probe is also physically too large and therefore unable to properly latch on to the engagable portion of the protein subunit of the HIV gp120 probe when the HIV gp120 probe exists in its natural state embedded in the exterior envelope of the HIV virion. Such an antibody will not properly attach to the HIV gp120 probe and therefore will not inhibit or prevent the HIV gp120 probe from engaging the CD4 cell-surface receptor on a vulnerable T-Helper cell; this again is not a desired antibody response.

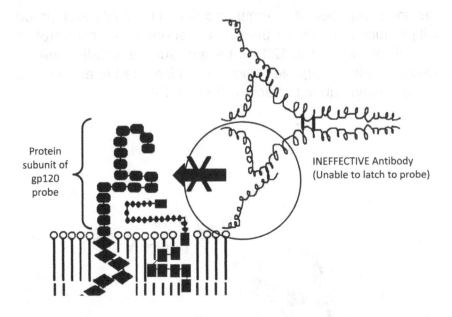

Protein
subunit of
gp120
probe

INEFFECTIVE Antibody
(Unable to latch to probe)

Figure 19: IgG antibody generated to latch onto the entire protein subunit of HIV gp120 probe is unable to engage due to IgG antibody being too large to properly latch onto the HIV gp120 probe

The ideal antigen to produce an effective antibody is to use the portion of the protein subunit of the HIV gp120 probe that is engagable when the gp120 probe exists in its natural state embedded in the exterior envelope of the HIV virion (Figure 20).

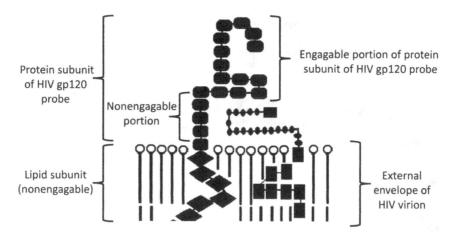

Figure 20: HIV gp120 probe protein subunit is comprised of an engagable portion and a nonengagable portion

To determine the construct of the antigen to be used to stimulate the most effective antibody response by the immune system to HIV that will latch on to the HIV virion and prevent the HIV virion from interacting with a T-Helper cell, a regimented removal of amino acids from the amino acid sequence comprising the gp120 probe protein subunit would be performed (Figure 21). Eventually an effective engagable portion of the gp120 probe protein subunit will be determined. This effective engagable portion of the gp120 probe protein subunit can then be utilized to create an effective vaccine.

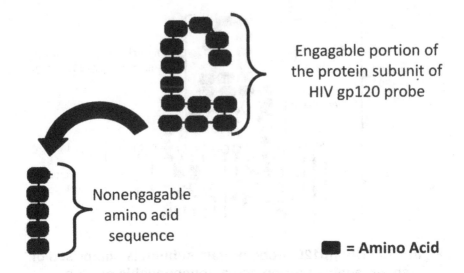

Engagable portion of the protein subunit of HIV gp120 probe

Nonengagable amino acid sequence

■ = Amino Acid

Figure 21: Removal of selected amino acid sequence from protein subunit of HIV gp120 probe produces an antigenic form of the HIV gp120 probe that will result in an antibody that is able to effectively engage the embedded HIV gp120 probe

The effective engagable portion of the gp120 probe protein subunit can then be utilized as an antigen to stimulate the body's immune system to create antibodies directed at and successfully engaging HIV virions (Figure 22).

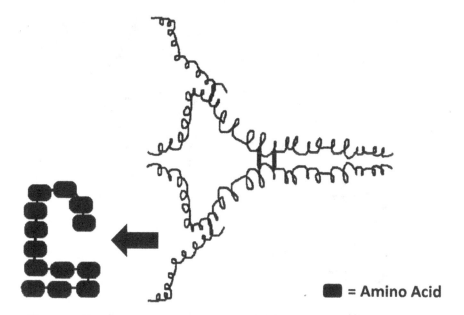

= Amino Acid

Figure 22: IgG antibody generated in response to the presence of the engagable portion of the protein subunit of HIV gp120 probe

Antibodies generated by the immune system that are capable of latching on to the engagable portion of the HIV gp120 probe protein subunit will prevent HIV virion gp120 probes from successfully engaging a T-Helper cell's CD4 cell-surface receptors (Figure 23).

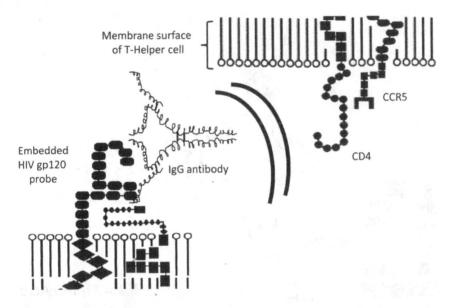

Figure 23: IgG antibody designed to latch onto the <u>engagable</u> portion of the HIV gp120 probe is <u>effective</u> in preventing HIV gp120 probe from connecting with CD4 receptor

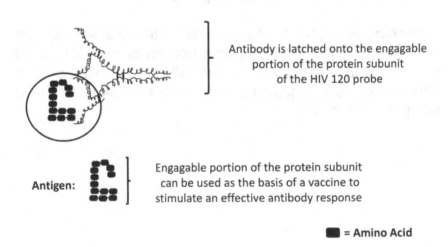

Figure 24: An EFFECTIVE vaccine is comprised of the engagable portion of the protein subunit of the HIV gp120 probe

An effective vaccine will be comprised of antigens that are constructed of only that portion of the HIV gp120 probe that is engagable by an antibody when the HIV gp120 probe is embedded in the exterior envelope of an HIV virion (Figure 24).

The vaccine to prevent and treat HIV infections will be comprised of antigens that are constructed of only that portion of the HIV gp120 probe that is engagable by an antibody when the HIV gp120 probe is embedded in the exterior envelope of an HIV virion and suspended in a hypoallergenic medium (Figure 25).

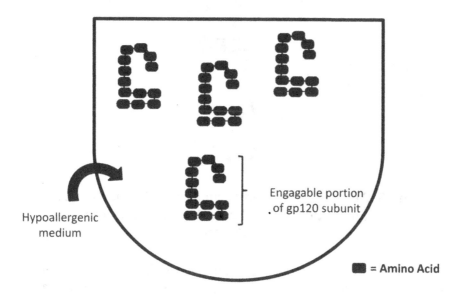

Hypoallergenic medium

Engagable portion of gp120 subunit

■ = Amino Acid

Figure 25: Vaccine comprised of engagable portion of the protein subunits of the HIV gp120 probe intended to stimulate an effective antibody response

Though represented as a two dimensional structure in the diagrams presented in this work, the probes, cell-surface receptors and antibodies are indeed three-dimensional structures. The gp120 probe mounted on the surface of the HIV virion may have more than one binding site where an antibody might latch onto and thus prevent the HIV gp120 probe from being able to successfully engage a T-Helper cell CD4 cell-surface receptor. Thus, the possibility of alternative binding sites suggests that differing antibodies might be useful. Further, an antibody successful in preventing HIV virions from infecting T-Helper cells may have its variable region designed to latch onto a segment of the HIV gp120 probe that is smaller than the entire engagable portion of the protein subunit of the HIV gp120 probe (Figure 26).

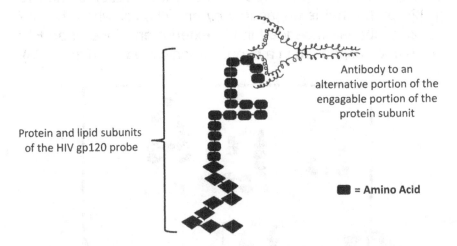

Antibody to an alternative portion of the engagable portion of the protein subunit

Protein and lipid subunits of the HIV gp120 probe

■ = Amino Acid

Figure 26: Antibody attached to an alternative portion of the engagable portion of the protein subunit of the HIV gp120 probe[4]

An antibody generated to latch onto a smaller segment of the entire engagable portion of the protein subunit of the HIV gp120 probe may be equally as effective or even more effective than an antibody generated to latch onto the entire engagable portion of the protein subunit of the HIV gp120 probe (Figure 27).

---

4 The size of the IgG antibody has been reduced in order to sufficiently demonstrate the concept of the alternative binding site on the HIV gp 120 probe.

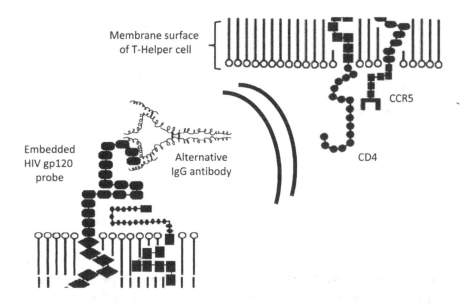

Membrane surface of T-Helper cell

CCR5

CD4

Embedded HIV gp120 probe

Alternative IgG antibody

Figure 27: Alternative IgG antibody designed to latch onto an alternative segment of the <u>engagable</u> portion of the HIV gp120 probe is <u>effective</u> in preventing HIV gp120 probe from making contact with the CD4 receptor

An effective alternative vaccine will be comprised of antigens that are constructed of a smaller alternative segment of the engagable portion of the protein subunit portion of the HIV gp120 probe when the HIV gp120 probe is embedded in the exterior envelope of an HIV virion (Figure 28). The vaccine would be comprised of such antigens suspended in a hypoallergenic medium for storage and transport purposes.

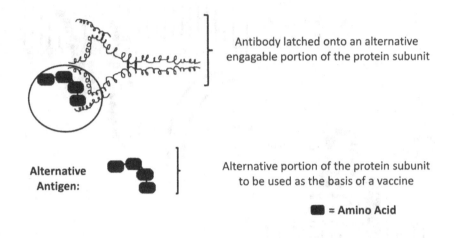

Antibody latched onto an alternative engagable portion of the protein subunit

Alternative Antigen:

Alternative portion of the protein subunit to be used as the basis of a vaccine

■ = Amino Acid

Figure 28: An EFFECTIVE vaccine may be comprised of an alternative segment of an engagable portion of the protein subunit of the HIV gp120 probe

The antibody generated in response to the antigen representing an alternative binding site to the HIV gp120 probe will attach only to the portion of the HIV gp120 probe that it has been

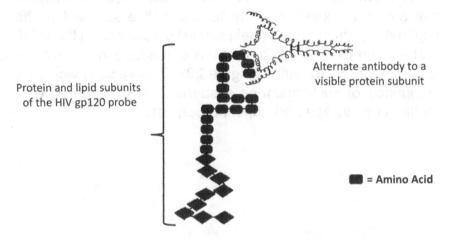

Protein and lipid subunits of the HIV gp120 probe

Alternate antibody to a visible protein subunit

■ = Amino Acid

Figure 29: An alternate antibody generated by the immune system in response to the vaccine shown attached to a smaller segment of the engagable portion of the protein subunit of the HIV gp120 probe

designed to latch onto by the B-cells of the immune system that created the antibody (Figure 29).

TESTING TO DEMONSTRATE A VACCINE'S EFFECTIVENESS

The selected portion of the protein subunit of the HIV gp120 probe is the key to the success of the vaccine. The reason a selected portion of the protein subunit being vital to the success of a HIV vaccine is that an antibody response to the protein subunit will produce antibodies that will latch onto the engagable protein portion of the HIV gp120 probe. Antibodies generated against the entire HIV gp120 molecule, that includes both a protein subunit and a lipid subunit, will be antibodies that will be physically too large in size to successfully engage a HIV gp120 probe embedded in the envelope of a HIV virion in the natural state and therefore such antibodies will be ineffective in preventing or treating an infection by HIV virions present inside a living body.

Antibodies are three dimensional structures as is the foreign substance the antibody is created to engage. An antibody needs to be able to successfully engage, attach and, at least for a period of time, adhere to the foreign substance in order to be able to exhibit the potential for acting as a neutralizing antibody. Further, the antibody needs to attach in such a manner to the foreign substance that the antibody, once attached, interferes with the potential disease causing function of the foreign substance.

A steel bullet fragment, the result of a firearms wound, may not be surgically removed from the body if the fragment resides in a location that is too dangerous to be surgically removed safely. The presence of a steel bullet fragment may or may not produce an antibody response. Antibodies generated in response to a steel bullet fragment may not produce any harmful effects to the bullet or the body's tissues and the steel bullet fragment may remain inside the person's body throughout the individual's remaining lifetime without generating any ill effect or altered state in response to the steel bullet fragment.

It has been suggested that the success of a vaccine is measured by the antibody response that can be measured following the administration of the vaccine. The human body's immune system often responds to any foreign substance that breaches the perimeter boundaries of the body. Silicon, a rather inert substance, sometimes used to coat medical devices that are inserted into the body, has been known to cause the human immune system to generate antibodies that can be measured. Antibodies to silicon used to coat medical devices, generated by the immune system, tend to represent a curiosity but are not known to exhibit any useful function, nor are such antibodies known to generally produce any deleterious effect with regards to the health of the body.

Any foreign antigen that is detected by the immune system will cause one or more antibodies to be generated, which will be antibodies unique to that antigen. The measurement of antibodies generated in relationship to the introduction of a vaccine only demonstrates that the immune system is able to detect one or more components of the antigens comprising the vaccine and if antibodies are generated, this occurrence is a statement by the immune system that one or more components of the vaccine are recognized as being a 'foreign substance' to the body. The introduction of a vaccine that produces an antibody response by the immune system does not guarantee that the vaccine will in any way neutralize the infectious threat of the entity that the vaccine is intended to act against.

The success of a vaccine to treat AIDS has been previously measured by administering the vaccine to human subjects and determining if the viral load significantly decreases or the T-Helper cell population significantly increases in number from baseline. The success of a vaccine in preventing an infection with HIV has been by vaccinating subjects, then infecting these subjects with virulent strain of HIV and determining over time, without further exposure to HIV, if the subjects develop evidence of an expanding population of HIV virions and/or a decline in the number of T-Helper cells.

An alternative means of testing the effectiveness of a vaccine is to demonstrate that the vaccine neutralizes the infectious nature of the HIV virion. To accomplish this, blood plasma containing antibodies would be combined with a population of HIV virions in vitro. Once the vaccine and HIV virions have been incubated together for a sufficient amount of time, the mixture would be passed through a filter system to investigate the vaccine's effectiveness.

The testing unit to evaluate a vaccine's effectiveness in neutralizing the infectious nature of HIV virions could be comprised of a one filter chamber (Figure 30). The filter chamber of the testing unit would contain a population of T-Helper cells that would act as a filter medium. If, without an effective vaccine present, HIV virions were allowed to incubate in such a filter chamber in their natural state, given sufficient time the majority of the HIV virions would engage the T-Helper cells comprising the filter medium. Thus when drained, the number of intact HIV virions present in the solution harvested from the filter chamber would be negligible.

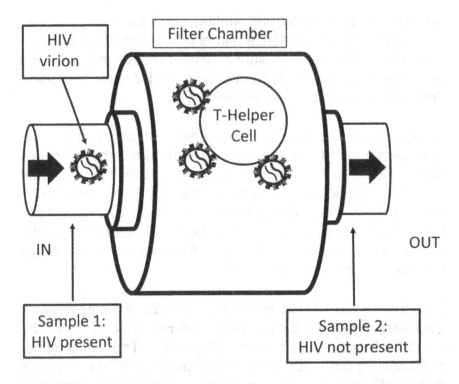

Figure 30: HIV attaches to T-Helper cells inside filter chamber and do not exit chamber

If a vaccine is introduced and is successful, the antibodies that the vaccine produces will adhere to the gp120 probes located on the surface of the HIV virion and prevent the HIV virions from attaching to T-Helper cells. If the HIV virions with antibodies attach to the gp120 probes of the HIV virions were incubated in a filter chamber containing T-Helper cells, the HIV virions with the antibody attached would pass through the filter and would be present in the blood plasma drained from the filter chamber because the HIV virions would not be able to attach to the T-Helper cells (Figure 31).

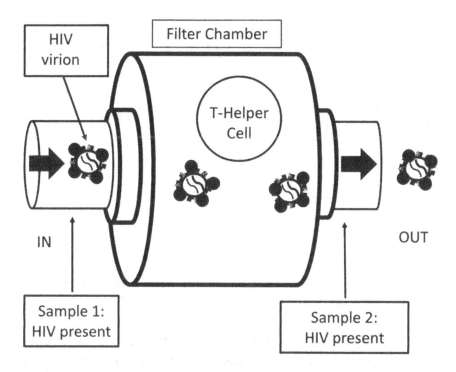

**Figure 31: HIV virions coated with antibodies cannot attach
to T-Helper cells inside the filter chamber and
exit the filter chamber**

To determine if a vaccine is indeed effective, without exposing a test subject to infectious HIV virions, a more elaborate testing unit could be constructed that consists of two filter chambers. The first filter chamber could have as its filter medium a collection of T-Helper cells. The second filter chamber could have as its filter medium a filter material that traps the Fc portion or tail portion of antibodies (Figure 32). The Fc portion of an IgG antibody is comprised of the constant region of two heavy chains (Figure 5).

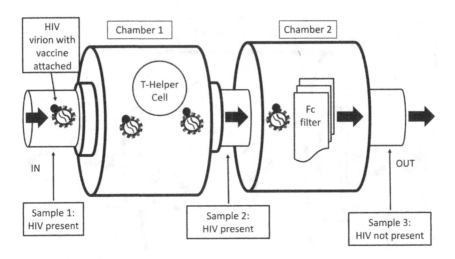

Figure 32: HIV Vaccine Testing Device demonstrates effective vaccine: HIV and vaccine captured in Fc filter

To now measure the extent of the effectiveness of a vaccine, a test subject could be inoculated with the antigen comprising the vaccine and representing an engagable portion of the protein subunit of the HIV gp120 probe. The antibody response to the antigen could be harvested from the test subject and reproduced. The antibody can be made in mass quantity to act as a test solution. A known quantity of antibody could then be mixed with a known quantity of infectious HIV virions. The mixture of antibody and HIV virions could then be passed through the two chamber HIV testing unit. The first chamber of the testing unit would be constructed with a filter medium comprised of T-Helper cells or a filter medium constructed in a manner where one or more sheets of lipid bilayer fashioned with a large quantity of CD4, CCR5 and CXCR4 cell-surface receptors. The second chamber of the testing device would possess a filter medium that would trap the Fc portion of IgG antibodies.

To demonstrate that a vaccine produces antibodies that are effective in adhering to HIV virions, following the mixture of antibodies and HIV virions being incubated in both filter chambers, the quantity of HIV virions trapped in the second filter mechanism is to be measured. Comparing the quantity of HIV virions trapped in the Fc filter medium of the second chamber to the known quantity that were introduced into the first chamber provides a ratio of effectiveness of a vaccine. The closer the ratio is to 'one' the more effective the vaccine is in neutralizing the infectious nature of HIV virions.

If following mixing HIV virions with a vaccine, the vaccine is ineffective, the HIV virions will be trapped in the first chamber and the quantity of ineffective antibodies will be trapped in the second chamber by the Fc filter medium (Figure 33).

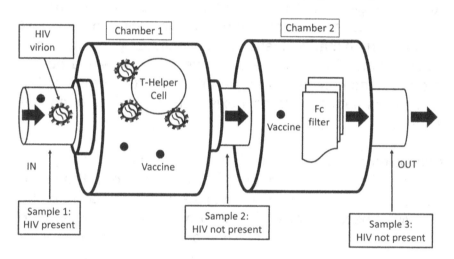

Figure 33: HIV Vaccine Testing Device demonstrates ineffective vaccine: HIV not present in sample 2 or 3, ineffective vaccine captured by Fc filter

Due to the fact that there may be an array of antibodies capable of latching to different binding sites on the engagable portion of the HIV gp120 protein subunit, being able to test for the effectiveness of a HIV vaccine allows for the determination of the most efficacious antigen to neutralize the infectious nature of HIV virions. If HIV's outer surface were to mutate, affecting the portion of the HIV gp120 probe that is engagable, this testing method would be able to dynamically insure that the most effective vaccine was being utilized to treat and prevent AIDS.

Conclusion:

Any foreign substance that breaches the perimeter of the body or is introduced into the body may evoke a response by the body's immune system such that an antibody is generated.

Not all antibodies that are generated by the immune system are neutralizing antibodies.

Antibodies generated by the immune system in response to the presence of an intact gp120 probe including the lipid and protein portion may be ineffective in neutralizing the infectious nature of the HIV virion because the antibody would be too large to attach effectively to the protein portion of the gp120 probe in its natural state as it exists on the surface of an HIV virion.

Antibodies generated by the immune system in response to the presence of the intact protein portion of the gp120 probe would be ineffective in neutralizing the infectious nature of the HIV virion because, again, the antibody would be too large to attach effectively to the protein portion of the gp120 probe in its natural state as it exists on the surface of an HIV virion.

A vaccine that would be effective in neutralizing the infectious nature of the HIV virion would generate an antibody capable of latching onto the entire engagable surface of the protein portion of the HIV gp120 probe or a section of the engagable surface of the protein portion of the HIV gp120 probe.

STRATEGY NUMBER FIVE: FUSION AND CHIMERIC ANTIBODIES AGAINST HIV

Vaccines may take time before a body's immune system is able to detect the antigen introduced in the vaccine and produce antibodies to the antigen in the vaccine. With regards to an HIV infection, time may be of the utmost importance given the manner in which HIV infects the body.

A critical opportunity to intervene and halt the infectious nature of the HIV virion may be immediately following exposure to the virus. As mentioned above, if a scavenger macrophage encounters an HIV virion, the macrophage may engulf the virus and then emit a chemical signal requesting T-Helper cells migrate to the region where HIV has breached the outer perimeter of the body. The action by the macrophage to send out a chemical message to draw T-Helper cells into the site of the initial infection may indeed simply make HIV's job much easier. HIV virions that have not been detected by an antigen presenting cell may lay in wait to ambush T-Helper cells. T-Helper cells that have yet to be activated by the antigen presenting cell may be particularly vulnerable to attack as they themselves may not be expecting to be the target of an infection. As the early response team of T-helper cells migrate into the area where the antigen presenting cell has emitted a chemoattractant signal, HIV virions may intercept and breach the outer membrane of these initial responders. By HIV virions infecting T-Helper cells responding to the antigen presenting cell's chemoattractant signal, the defensive response to the presence of HIV is delayed due to the T-Helper cells becoming dysfunctional by becoming infected with the HIV genome. In addition, HIV is allowed an effective means of evading detection by becoming cloaked inside the T-Helper cells initially responding to the antigen presenting cell's early signal that a breach has occurred. Planned or simply a twist of fate, HIV may sacrifice a few virions to the antigen presenting cells in order to alert the immune system to its presence, but in doing so HIV gains a strategic advantage against the immune system's defensive mechanisms.

This strategy exhibited by HIV, where the virus may intercept T-Helper cells, suggests that a critical time of action to treat a patient exposed to HIV, who have not been vaccinated or previously infected by the virus, is at the earliest opportune time following exposure to HIV virions. Antibodies provide a means by which an HIV infection may be halted and even possibly eradicated if the antibody were provided early enough following exposure to HIV virions.

Four forms of antibodies are possible which include (1) antibodies that the individual may generate on their own, (2) antibodies that are derived from the serum of another individual who has been exposed to an HIV infection, (3) fusion CD4 antibodies and (4) chimeric CD4 antibodies.

Antibodies that a patient may generate due to being provided a vaccine would need to be produced prior to the first exposure to an HIV infection in order to be effective. Antibodies that may be derived from an individual who has been exposed to HIV and produced neutralizing antibodies or has been exposed to an antigen such as a vaccine comprised of engagable protein subunits of the HIV gp120 probe may offer a successful means of combating the initial infection by HIV, if those antibodies produced by an individual can be replicated, tested for their effectiveness against HIV and distributed to others who have been exposed to HIV.

The HIV virion's gp120 probe is incessantly seeking to engage a T-Helper cell's CD4 cell-surface receptor. Fusion antibodies and chimeric antibodies represent hybrid protein structures where the protein portion of a CD4 receptor is attached or fused to the Fc portion of an IgG antibody. Fusion antibodies would be divided into two groups. One type of fusion antibody would be comprised of the protein portion of a human CD4 cell-surface receptor fused to the Fc portion of a human IgG antibody. The second form of fusion protein is comprised of a synthetic protein that acts in a similar manner as the human CD4 cell-surface receptor fused to the Fc portion of a human IgG antibody. A chimeric antibody refers to an antibody structure derived from two different animals. Chimeric antibodies may have part human components and part mouse components. A chimeric CD4 cell-surface receptor fused to the Fc portion of an IgG antibody might have portions of the structure taken from human protein design and a portion taken from mouse protein design, which such a structure would function similar to the fully human fusion antibody. Fusion CD4 antibodies or chimeric CD4 antibodies may provide an effective means of preventing HIV virions from infecting T-Helper cells in the early stage of an HIV infection (Figure 34). The protein subunit of the CD4 cell-surface receptor is the protein structure HIV's gp120 probe is designed to seek out and engage. Given today's state of technology, if found effective, such an antibody design would be readily producible and rapidly made available for use in clinics and hospitals.

HIV Fusion antibody or HIV Chimeric antibody

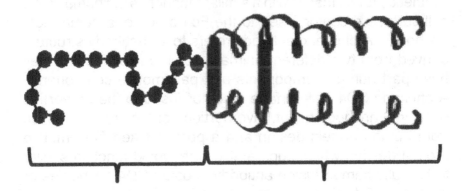

CD4 cell-surface
receptor protein

Fc portion IgG antibody

Figure 34: Fusion or chimeric HIV antibody comprised of a CD4 cell-surface receptor protein attached to the Fc portion of an IgG antibody

Fusion CD4 antibodies and chimeric CD4 antibodies may also be useful in preventing progressive infection by HIV virions in an individual who has been exposed to the virus. By providing an individual infected with HIV, regular dosing of either fusion CD4 antibodies or chimeric CD4 antibodies, copies of HIV virions exiting a host T-Helper cell could be aggressively engaged by such antibodies. If fusion CD4 antibodies or chimeric CD4 antibodies were to engage and neutralize copies of HIV virions circulating in the body and the treatment interval lasted long enough, eventually the number of infected T-Helper cells would be depleted and the presence of HIV would be eradicated, thus eliminating the threat of AIDS.

As mentioned previously, antibodies tend to be less effective in combating chronic viral infections then they are in eradicating bacterial infections. Bacteria reside outside animal cells and therefore render themselves readily available to being attacked and killed by antibodies circulating in an individual's blood and tissues. Since viruses shelter themselves inside host cells, a virus is only exposed as it traverses from the infected host cell that generated the virus virion to a noninfected host cell the virus might target. Circulating antibodies tend to have a limited window of opportunity to attach to and neutralize infectious virus virions.

Again, possibly the most successful opportunity for fusion CD4 antibodies or chimeric CD4 antibodies to treating the HIV infected individual is to intercede immediately following exposure to prevent HIV from infecting the individual beyond the initial stage of the virus having breached the skin or mucosal surfaces of the body. Used as what might be termed a 'morning after' therapy, where a quantity of fusion CD4 antibodies or chimeric CD4 antibodies is introduced into an individual as soon as possible following high risk exposure to a possible HIV infection either following a sexual encounter or a needle stick or a tainted blood transfusion, such fusion CD4 antibodies or chimeric CD4 antibodies may transiently flood an individual's system blocking HIV virions from being able to infect the T-Helper cells that initially respond to HIV's presence. By introducing into an individual a substantial dose of fusion antibodies or chimeric antibodies comprised of a CD4 receptor fused to the Fc portion of an IgG antibody, the gp120 probes affixed to the exterior envelope of HIV virions would be clogged with these fusion antibodies or chimeric antibodies, resulting in blocking HIV virions from being capable of engaging T-Helper cells (Figure 35). The impotent HIV virions could then be attacked by the body's immune defenses and eradicated in a similar manner as the body disposes of other viral infections.

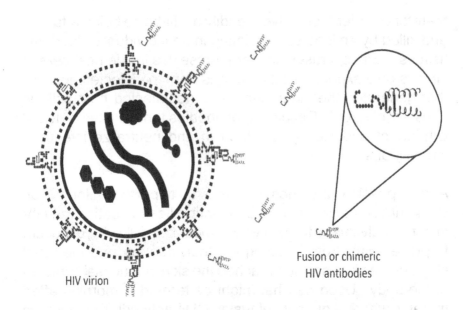

HIV virion

Fusion or chimeric
HIV antibodies

**Figure 35: Fusion or chimeric HIV antibodies
engage HIV virion**

The use of fusion antibodies and chimeric antibodies in general has been successfully utilized to treat other medical conditions. Rheumatoid arthritis, an inflammatory erosive joint disorder, has been successfully treated by providing patients with fusion antibodies or chimeric antibodies. The fusion antibodies or chimeric antibodies target circulating TNF alpha molecules to neutralize the effect of these molecules. The result of the presence of fusion antibodies or chimeric antibodies latching onto circulating TNF alpha molecules in active rheumatoid arthritis is a reduction in the biochemical signal that propagates inflammation, which in turn results in a reduction in the inflammation of joint tissues. Similar beneficial effects produced by fusion antibodies and chimeric antibodies are also seen in disease states such as inflammatory bowel disease and psoriatic arthritis.

If nothing else, an antibody synthesized from an antigen comprised the engagable portion of the HIV gp120 protein subunit or a fusion antibody or chimeric antibody comprised of the protein portion of the CD4 cell-surface receptor fused to the Fc portion of an IgG antibody should be developed to protect healthcare workers as well as other individuals at high risk of infection. Any healthcare worker who handles blood products, in any way, such as drawing blood, administering infusion therapy or any form of injection or who participates in surgical procedures could be protected from contracting HIV and developing AIDS if an antibody therapy were developed and made available to administer to any individual who became acutely exposed to blood products or body fluids that may contain infectious HIV virions. Having such a human antibody or fusion CD4 antibody or chimeric CD4 antibody available could save the lives of many dedicated healthcare workers as the worldwide battle to control HIV and treat its victims continues on each day.

STRATEGY NUMBER SIX: UTILIZING VIRUSES TO DELIVER DRUG THERAPY

The HIV virion already has the capacity to seek out, engage, and deliver a payload consisting of RNA genetic material to T-Helper cells in the body. The HIV virion could be modified to act as a vehicle and deliver an alternative payload. Modified HIV virions could deliver to T-Helper cells medications that would interfere with viral replication. The modified HIV virion could deliver directly to T-Helper cells a number of drug molecules to equip the T-Helper cell to resist infection by natural HIV virions (Patent Application A8). Such direct treatment of T-Helper cells by modified HIV virions would limit the potential side effects such medications might cause if the medication were administered systemically as a drug introduced into the body by itself.

STRATEGY NUMBER SEVEN: A CURE FOR AIDS

The results of the Black Death or Black Plague in the mid 14th century provide us with considerable knowledge regarding the virulence of bacteria and viruses. As Yersinia Pestis bacterium swept across Europe carried by rodents and transmitted to humans by fleas, natural forces led to the death of certain portions of the population and survival of a certain and ultimately the propagation of a particular subset of the population. As the Back Death killed a quarter of Europe's population, cats were removed due to superstitions that they were in allegiance with the cause of the menace. Removing cats, which naturally prey on rodents, unfortunately eliminated one of the best environmental defenses against the spread of the Black Death. There was also a grave lack of understanding that sanitary conditions in the cities and villages would reduce the spread of the disease.

The most effective resistance against the Black Death turned out to be a naturally occurring 'genetic flaw' rather than efforts orchestrated by humans. A mutation in the genes responsible for generating the CCR5 cell-surface receptor mounted the surface of T-Helper cells (Patent Application A9) created a resistance to infection by the Black Death. Yersinia pestis utilized the CCR5 cell-surface receptor as a means of accessing white blood cells. Using the CCR5 cell-surface receptor, Yersinia pestis paralyzed white cells, which resulted in a delay in the immune system's response to the presence of this deadly pathogen. The subset of the population that possessed the homologous genetic mutation survived, while those of the population that did not possess this flaw in their genes often succumbed to the fatal effects of the infection. Natural selection, as created by the Black Death, has caused the mutation of the CCR5 gene to become relatively prevalent in the European population. Seven centuries later, this genetic mutation results in a resistance to infection by HIV. Since HIV utilizes the CCR5 cell-surface receptor as a means of infecting T-Helper cells, those in the population that possess a faulty CCR5 receptor have T-Helper cells that HIV virions are unable to gain access to in order to deliver their viral genome.

Since up to 20% of the current European population possess one or two versions of the flawed CCR5 gene, it is obvious that expression of this particular genetic flaw has not led to any identifiable health issues; but possession of the flaw does condone resistance to HIV. Those individuals that possess two copies of the genetic mutation to the CCR5 gene exhibit the highest resistance to HIV.

Exploring this thought process further, if a genetic mutation, replicating that as seen naturally in the CCR5 gene, could be generated in persons at risk for contracting HIV, their T-Helper cells would become resistant to such an infection. If HIV could not properly engage the T–Helper cell population in a body, HIV would not be capable of replicating itself and the threat of AIDS would be eliminated for that individual.

The mutation of the CCR5 gene that resulted in immunity to contracting Yersinia pestis was a deletion of the last 32 base pairs of the genetic code associated with the CCR5 cell-surface receptor's gene. An approach would be to replicate this mutation in T-Helper cells that are either currently circulating in a body or precursor cells that are in the process of developing into mature T-Helper cells.

The T-Helper cell population begins as precursor cells in the bone marrow. Precursor T-Helper cells traverse the blood stream and migrate to the thymus, an organ located in the neck. In the thymus T-Helper cells undergo significant maturation. Many T-Helper cells fail in their effort to develop into mature T-Helper cells and are destroyed. T-Helper cells that complete the maturation process express the CD4 cell–surface receptor and leave the thymus to circulate the body to aid the immune system in defending the body from invading pathogens.

Thus, a strategy to prevent and cure AIDS would be to utilize a modified treatment virus to seek out precursor T-Helper cells and to strategically place one or more STOP codes in the portion of the precursor cell's DNA that codes for the CCR5 cell-surface receptor. STOP codes are segments of genetic information that cause genetic material to cease being decoded by biologic devices such as polymerase molecules that read genes. Thus, while in the early stages of a T-Helper cell's development, when it does not express CD4, CCR5 or CXCR4 cell-surface receptors, a medically therapeutic virus fashioned to deliver a STOP code to create a mutation in the CCR5 or CXCR4 cell-surface receptor gene in a precursor T-Helper cell, could be used to generate a modified CCR5 or CXCR4 cell-surface receptor when it is expressed by the mature T-Helper cell, resulting in the mature form of the T-helper cell being immune to HIV. That is in the case of the CCR5 cell-surface receptor gene, if a STOP code was inserted into the gene preventing the last 32 base pairs of the gene from being read, this would result in a flawed CCR5 cell-surface receptor to be expressed (Figure 36), likened to the naturally occurring genetic flaw that protected individuals from the fatal effects exhibited by Yersinia pestis. Utilizing a medically therapeutic virus, nature's genetic flaw could be mimicked. HIV would not be able to access these medically altered T-Helper cells when they reached maturity due to the gp41 probe on the surface of the HIV virions not being able to properly engage the flawed CCR5 cell-surface receptor. If HIV is incapable of accessing the T-Helper cells in a person's body the virus's virions becomes impotent and vulnerable to eradication by the immune system. Circulating the body, unable to gain a safe haven inside a T-Helper cell, the immune system's defenses would eventually spot the intruder and clear the HIV virions from the body. In effect, this action would cure the individual of AIDS.

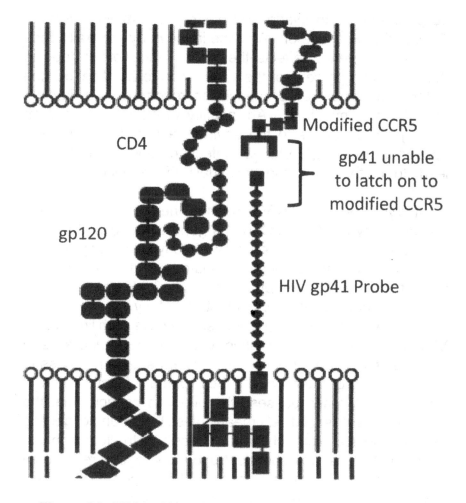

CD4

Modified CCR5

gp41 unable
to latch on to
modified CCR5

gp120

HIV gp41 Probe

**Figure 36: HIV gp41 probe unable to latch onto modified
CCR5 cell surface receptor**

While a mature T-Helper cell already expresses its receptors,
a similar approach may be effective in the event such a cell
divides.

CONCLUSION

Over the last 26 years HIV has provided us with a crucial
incentive to study and research viral infections. Deadly viruses
like HIV have taught us much about how a viral genome can

be programmed to evade and destroy the immune system. Though the presence of HIV alone in the body generally does not cause deleterious effects, the consequences of not stopping the replication process of the virus leads to a critical decline in the immune system's capacity to recognize and fight off opportunistic infections. An inability to effectively ward off pathogens ubiquitous to the environment leads to diseases caused by these opportunistic infections and this eventually leads to a fatal outcome in individuals afflicted with HIV.

A cataclysmic spread of HIV throughout the population has been hampered by the fact the virus is generally transmitted from one person to another by contact with body fluids. Unprotected sexual contact, the use of contaminated needles, or exposure to contaminated blood products or body fluids has led to the majority of new cases of HIV infection. Many viruses that co-exist in the environment don't necessarily have such limitations. Viruses are constantly mutating, changing their tactics as to how they may defeat the immune system and gain access to host cells in order to carry out their primary function, that of replication. Viruses possess the precious capacity that the passage of time is relatively meaningless to a strand of genetic material, since a segment of nucleotides constructed of genes, in and of itself, is not dependent upon any regular respiratory function to maintain its existence. It is important that new ideas regarding means to combat viral infections be generated and become readily available before HIV or another similar deadly virus mutates to a form that can be readily spread as an airborne or waterborne infection.

If HIV or some other deadly virus mutates to a form where it can be easily passed from one individual to another through the air or by water or through soil, such a deadly virus could put the lives of hundreds of millions or even billions of people at risk. Currently there exists no effective treatment to cure a patient infected with a lethal virus. In the case of a widespread outbreak of an aggressive pathologic virus every member of the world's population would be susceptible to infection and possibly a fatal outcome. Beyond isolation of infected individuals, every person will be at risk with the only hope being that an individual's native genes code for cell lines that express flawed cell-surface receptors that the virus is incapable of accessing. An infection by today's standards could be even more devastating than the Plague or the deadly influenza virus due to the overcrowding some portions of the world are experiencing. As the number of people inhabiting the world exponentially escalates, living conditions become increasingly congested in our cities, and the population becomes increasingly mobile, the population's risk of facing an aggressive and deadly virus that has mutated to the point that it can easily spread, increases dramatically as each day passes. Such a threat has occurred on a number of occasions in recorded history, and it is certain to recur again in the future.

It is imperative we develop the means to combat viral infections to the point where we are capable of completely eradicating a potentially deadly virus from the body. Incorporating blood-filtering techniques, actively developing scientifically modified viruses, generating innovative vaccines, and possibly creating cells that are genetically resistant to infection, in effect reflect strategies to combat viral infections on their own terms and provides a completely new arsenal of treatment options. The death toll that HIV is afflicting on the population around the world should serve as a wake-up call and makes it imperative that we dramatically improve the medical community's proficiency at combating viruses. If we wait until a deadly virus mutates and spreads by air or water or soil unimpeded through an unprotected population, we will have most certainly waited too long, and the entire population may be at risk with, by current standards, only the element of 'chance' dictating whether each person lives or dies. This is not acceptable.

II: Curing Diabetes, Eliminating Obesity and Fatigue, and Halting the Aging Process

'Studying the fundamentals of HIV and its behavior provides valuable insight in developing innovative treatments for a vast number of medical diseases that plague mankind.'

The process of aging and the medical conditions of diabetes, obesity and fatigue are all tied together by a common biophysiologic linkage. Aging and chronic fatigue represent a steady decline in the mechanisms necessary to convert the body's fuel sources into readily consumable units of energy that can be used to drive chemical reactions. A lack of optimum conversion of fuel to power results in a decrease in energy available to support the necessary biologic functions required by the demands of the body as a whole. The lack of energy everyone experiences as they age is often referred to as a reduction in the metabolism. Diabetes and obesity represent inefficient utilization, storage and conversion of the fuel the body has available to consume.

The fuel the body converts to energy is in the form of sugars, fats and carbohydrates. The fuel supplies available for consumption are generally derived from an individual's diet and quantities that have been stored in body tissues. Sugars, fats and carbohydrates are generally broken down to a single currency of potential energy known as glucose. Glucose is a six carbon sugar molecule. For each glucose molecule metabolized in the presence of an adequate oxygen supply, the yield may be as many as 38 energy molecules known as adenosine triphosphate (ATP) molecules. These ATP molecules provide the fundamental energy source for a wide variety of chemical reactions throughout the body.

Animal[5] cells have an outside boundary referred to as a cell membrane or plasma membrane. Cell surface receptors are fixed to the outside of the cell membrane and act as communication beacons for the cell to interact with the blood, other cells, and foreign substances. Contained inside the cell membrane is the cytoplasm, a nucleus and organelles. The cytoplasm is the fluid portion of the cell containing amino acids and nutrients. The nucleus contains the genetic information in the form of deoxyribonucleic acid (DNA). Organelles are structures that are suspended in the cytoplasm and exhibit specialized functions. There are a variety of organelles including the mitochondria, smooth endoplasmic reticulum, rough endoplasmic reticulum, Golgi apparatus, and storage vacuoles.

Glucose circulates in the fluid portion of the blood. The Beta cells in the Islets of Langerhans in the pancreas constantly monitor the level of glucose in the blood. When the blood glucose level rises above the normal level, the pancreas releases the protein insulin. When insulin is present in the blood, this protein stimulates cells to absorb glucose by interacting with the insulin cell-surface receptor on cells, thus lowering the level of circulating glucose. If the blood glucose level drops below the normal range, the pancreas releases glucagon, which stimulates the production of glucose by the liver and other cells to increase the amount of glucose available in the blood. Processing of blood glucose requires multiple biochemical steps. Glucose is transported into a cell by an insulin receptor (Figure 37).

---

5   Ibid.

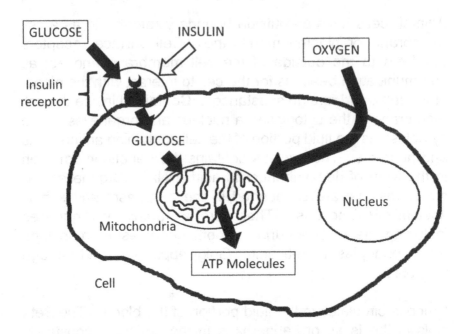

Figure 37: Insulin facilitates glucose entering into a cell so that the glucose can be utilized by the mitochondria to generate energy for the cell

Once inside a cell, glucose is broken down through three intricate multi-stepped biochemical pathways known as (1) glycolysis, (2) tricarboxylic acid cycle (TCA), and (3) oxidative phosphorylation. The majority of the metabolism of glucose occurs in the cell's organelle referred to as the mitochondria. Many specialized proteins, known as enzymes, participate in the breakdown of glucose and the conversion of stored energy in ATP molecules.

Mitochondria are therefore often referred to as the powerhouses of the cell (Figure 38). Mitochondria contain the majority of the biochemical processes required to convert glucose into ATP molecules. The initial steps of glycolysis may occur in the cytoplasm, but the remainder of the metabolism of glucose occurs in the mitochondrion including the final stages of glycolysis, the tricarboxylic acid cycle and oxidative phosphorylation. The number of mitochondria present in a cell may vary from a few of such organelles to several thousand. Liver cells may contain as many as 2200 mitochondria per cell.

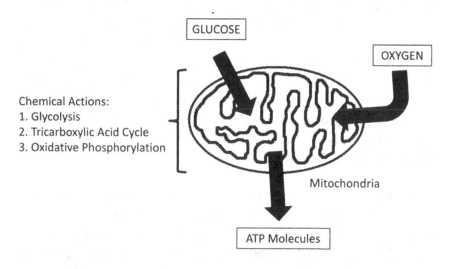

GLUCOSE

OXYGEN

Chemical Actions:
1. Glycolysis
2. Tricarboxylic Acid Cycle
3. Oxidative Phosphorylation

Mitochondria

ATP Molecules

Figure 38: Utilizing the processes of glycolysis, tricarboxylic acid cycle, and oxidative phosphorylation the mitochondria convert glucose into 36 ATP molecules

As the body ages, the function of the mitochondria significantly decreases. This reduction in energy production may be the direct result of a decline in the number or efficiency of the enzymes required to breakdown glucose molecules. The more mitochondria that become inactive, the greater the decline in energy production, which results in fewer energy molecules to participate in biochemical reactions required by cells. It is estimated that between ages 35-50 y.o. the energy production afforded by the mitochondria in the body decreases by half. Decline in energy production continues to occur as the body continues to age. By 90 years of age a body's energy production is estimated to have declined by nearly 87%. If the body lacks the proper supply of energy, the obvious result is a dramatic decline in the capacity for metabolism at the cellular level.

Diabetes mellitus, obesity, aging and chronic fatigue can all be linked to a dysfunctional conversion of glucose to ATP molecules. A cell is much like the engine of a motor vehicle. Provide the proper fuel supply and the engine runs; provide the proper amount of ATP molecules to a cell and cellular mechanisms will proceed. The difference between a car engine and the cell is the cell contains genetic material in the form of DNA and protein factories, such that the cell is capable of potentially repairing itself if required. Revitalizing the function of the mitochondria at the cellular level leads to optimal management of medical conditions such as diabetes and obesity, reversal of chronic fatigue and even halting or stalling of the aging process.

Insulin receptors and the enzymes that participate in glycolysis, tricarboxylic acid cycle and oxidative phosphorylation, are proteins generated under the direction of a cell's deoxyribonucleic acid (DNA). The DNA provides the genetic template to generate messenger ribonucleic acids (RNA). Messenger RNA travel from the nucleus of the cell to the cytoplasm. In the cytoplasm, ribosomes attach to messenger RNA. Ribosomes read the genetic code of the messenger RNA.   With the assistance of transport RNA that deliver amino acids to the ribosomes, ribosomes build protein molecules as dictated by the genetic code present in the messenger RNA. A number of ribosomes can be attached to one messenger RNA at the same time. Therefore numerous ribosomes can act to decipher the genetic code of a single messenger RNA to simultaneously construct identical copies of a particular protein molecule.

A virus is comprised of simply an outer shell, surface probes, genetic information and accessory proteins. In and of itself, a virus conducts no chemical processes. Naturally occurring viruses are in effect dormant until probes mounted on the surface of a virus's outer shell encounter the type of cell the virus can utilize to successfully create replicas of itself. Upon engaging the proper cell type to be used as a host, the virus injects its genetic material into the cell along with any accessory proteins that might be needed. Accessory proteins assist the genetic material in taking command of the host cell's functions and directing the host cell to make copies of the virus. Once replicas of the virus have been constructed, these copies exit the host cell and seek out other cells of the same type to commandeer and generate further copies of the virus.

Both the human immunodeficiency virus and the hepatitis C virus carry in their core ribonucleic acid (RNA) molecules as their genetic coding. These viral RNA molecules act as the blueprints for replication for these viruses. The human immunodeficiency virus, responsible for AIDS, injects its messenger RNA into its host, the T-Helper cell. Hepatitis C injects its messenger RNA into liver cells and in some individuals is responsible for producing a form of chronic active form of inflammation termed hepatitis. Utilizing the knowledge that viruses act as transport vehicles, that viruses are capable of carrying messenger RNA molecules and a virus's delivery target is dependent upon the type of probes mounted on the surface of the virus, a very powerful medical <u>treatment</u> tool can be devised.

In the natural state, a susceptible host cell, once infected with a virus's genetic material, acts as factory to produce replicas of the virus. The design of the viral replicas is dependent upon the genetic coding inserted into the host cell. Viral genetic coding dictates the construction parameters of the outside shell, the probes mounted on the surface of the virus, the inner core structures and the construction of the genetic material the viral replicas are intended to carry as a payload. It is generally understood that one or more changes that occur to a virus's genome during the replication process in a host cell that produce a mutation to a virus, will generate viral copies that may be more or less virulent than the original form of the virus. Mother Nature tends to alter the genome of viruses quite frequently during the replication phase of the virus's life-cycle.

A naturally occurring Hepatitis C virus (HCV) could be re-designed and through human ingenuity altered during the virus's copying process to have its native RNA deleted and instead be made to carry a medically therapeutic segment of ribonucleic acid to liver cells. Hybrid host liver cells could be fashioned to generate modified Hepatitis C virus virions to have mounted on their surface, specific probes that allow the modified virus to seek out specific cells in the body for medically therapeutic purposes (Figure 39). The payload a modified medically therapeutic virus carries can be fashioned to exert an effect inside specific cells in the body that require the assistance of certain messenger RNA to achieve a specific medical benefit.

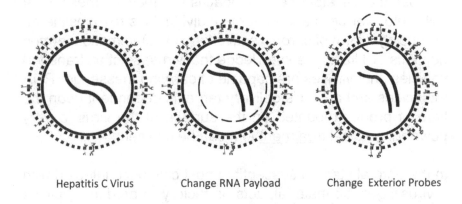

Hepatitis C Virus   Change RNA Payload   Change Exterior Probes

Figure 39: Re-configuration of HCV RNA payload and probes to create a medically therapeutic virus

Medically therapeutic viruses could be utilized to insert various messenger RNAs into cells (Figure 40). These medically therapeutic messenger RNAs would be decoded by ribosomes in a similar fashion as a cell's innate messenger RNAs. Medically therapeutic RNAs could be used to generate proteins structures such as insulin, insulin receptors, and enzymes. With regards to diabetes, providing Beta cells in the pancreas the capacity to up-regulate the generation of insulin or insulin receptors may represent a significant step forward in improving the control of this devastating disease.

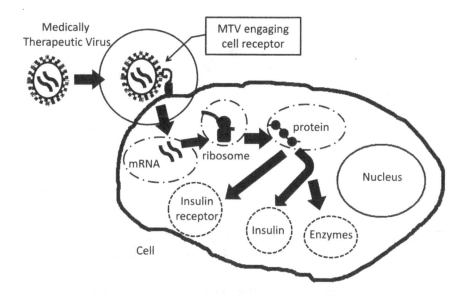

Figure 40: Medically Therapeutic Virus (MTV) delivers to a cell mRNA that are read by ribosomes to produce various proteins

Medically therapeutic RNA, carried and dispensed by medically therapeutic viruses, offers an entirely new approach to solving some of medicine's most challenging problems.

Utilizing hybrid host cells, a naturally occurring human immunodeficiency virus could be altered to have its native RNA deleted and instead the virus could be conscripted to carry a medically therapeutic segment of ribonucleic acid to a T-Helper cell. The exterior probes of the HIV virus could be altered to have the HIV virus transport medically therapeutic RNA to nearly any cell in the body (Figure 41). HIV offers an intriguing possibility as a medically therapeutic transport vehicle since it would seem HIV virions do not generate effective antibodies against their presence. Other viruses, including HCV, may after multiple doses generate neutralizing antibodies in an individual that may inhibit their use as a medical device.

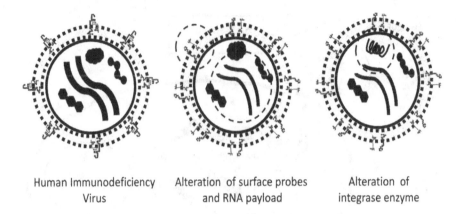

| Human Immunodeficiency Virus | Alteration of surface probes and RNA payload | Alteration of integrase enzyme |

Figure 41: Re-configuring HIV payload, probes and integrase to create medically therapeutic virus

Modified medically therapeutic viruses could therefore have the capability to deliver medically beneficial messenger RNA molecules to their host cell, to specific cells in the body or to potentially all cells in the body. There are at least twenty-three enzymes that participate in the biochemical processes of the conversion of glucose to ATP molecules. Each of these twenty-three enzymes is constructed by ribosomes deciphering genetic information from at least one unique messenger RNA molecule. In some cases the enzymes are a complex of proteins generated by more than one messenger RNA molecule.

The medical management of diabetes mellitus, obesity, chronic fatigue and aging could be enhanced by fashioning modified viruses to transport medically therapeutic messenger RNA molecules to cells in the body to re-vitalize the mitochondria in the cells of the body. The messenger RNA molecules transported to cells could code for the construction of insulin receptors or any of the over twenty three enzymes utilized in the aerobic respiration process to generate ATP energy molecules from glucose (Patent Applications B1, B2, and B3).

These medically therapeutic viruses would only be capable of acting as a transport vehicle and would not be capable of acting in any other manner. Such medically therapeutic viruses (MTVs) would not possess the capacity to evolve into an infectious entity because they would lack the genetic information that would make them capable of replicating themselves. These medically therapeutic viruses would only carry messenger RNA molecules that would generate a medically therapeutic beneficial effect inside the cells of the body.

Providing the mitochondria with a renewable supply of messenger RNA to allow cells to construct the enzymes needed to participate in the biochemical reactions constituting glycolysis, the TCA cycle and oxidative phosphorylation will help correct deficiencies in glucose metabolism at the cellular level (Figure 42). Such innovative medical treatments will lead to better health for those suffering from diabetes, obesity, chronic fatigue and aging.

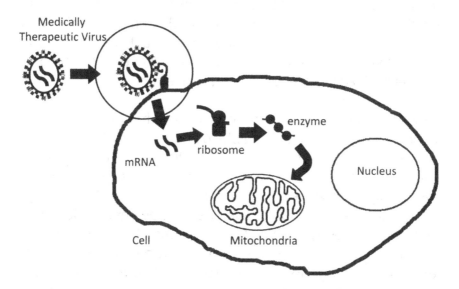

Figure 42: Medically Therapeutic Virus delivers to a cell mRNA that is used to produce enzymes to re-vitalize the mitochondria

III: Innovative Means for Intervention in Heart Attacks, Stroke, Diabetic Crisis, and Cancer

'The paradox: HIV virus offers an innovative alternative means to provide patients with critical nutrition in times of potentially fatal crisis.'

The common link between incurring a heart attack and suffering a stroke is a lack of readily available oxygen at the cellular level. Oxygen is the molecule that drives the aerobic respiration process inside the mitochondria of cells. Aerobic respiration is an efficient means of retrieving energy molecules from glucose. Where in the presence of oxygen the mitochondria in a cell is able to generate as many as 38 ATP energy molecules per glucose molecule consumed, in contrast, when there is a lack of sufficient oxygen the anaerobic process is limited to generating 2 ATP molecules per glucose molecule.

Without a constant supply of readily available oxygen certain essential body tissues are unable to keep up with the demands for energy molecule production. If a sufficient number of energy molecules are not being generated by a cell's mitochondria, vital biologic processes are unable to proceed and arrest of cell function, cell damage or even death may ensue. Sensitive portions of the body such as brain cells may have five minutes or less time before a lack of sufficient oxygen supply results in permanent damage to tissues. To this point, the only known means available to supply the cells of the body with oxygen has been red blood cells (RBCs) circulating in the blood stream.

One of the vital functions of blood is to act as the vehicle to transport red blood cells to all the tissues of the body. Inside red blood cells, hemoglobin is a protein structure in combination with iron that acts as the primary transport mechanism to carry oxygen molecules to the tissues where individual cells can utilize the oxygen for the purpose of aerobic respiration. Other important functions of blood include supplying the body's cells with nutrients such as glucose and the removal of waste products such as carbon dioxide from cells. Oxygen becomes critical, as demonstrated in the brain, where at a normal body temperature, brain cells cannot be without a sufficient supply of oxygen for more than five minutes before irreversible damage to brain cells begins to occur. Other tissues in the body besides the brain, including heart cells, demonstrate a chronic need for a persistently adequate supply of oxygen. If an ample amount of oxygen is unable to reach and nourish cells in the body in a timely fashion, cells die for lack of being able to generate a sufficient amount of energy to sustain the biochemical reactions that support life.

Oxygen and glucose are two necessary, vital consumable nutrients that provide all cells in the body the raw materials to generate ample energy in the form of adenosine triphosphate (ATP). Inside the cell, specifically inside the mitochondria, glucose is transformed by the biologic process of glycolysis into pyruvate. For generation of maximum number of ATP molecules from the parent molecule glucose, pyruvate is then metabolized by the tricarboxylic acid cycle and oxidative phosphorylation. Oxygen is a vital participant in the oxidative phosphorylation phase of glucose metabolism. When sufficient oxygen is available to the cell, by means of aerobic respiration one glucose molecule can yield 36 ATP molecules in nerve and muscle cells, and as many as 38 ATP molecules in liver and heart cells. In circumstances where an insufficient amount of oxygen is available to the cell, pyruvate is diverted to an anaerobic respiration process and is converted to lactic acid by the enzyme lactate dehydrogenase. The conversion of pyruvate to lactic acid yields only 2 ATP molecules. The production of only 2 ATP molecules per glucose molecule is not sufficient enough of an energy production to sustain cells in the body that require a high metabolism rate to sustain their survival. If such a low yield of ATP molecules persists, some of the vital tissues of the body will incur permanent damage.

The heart is comprised of muscle, valves, an electrical system, and a blood circulation system of arteries and veins. A heart attack generally occurs when one or more arteries in the heart become blocked and a sufficient volume of blood is unable to reach a portion of the heart muscle for a prolonged period of time. A stroke generally occurs when one or more arteries in the brain become blocked and a sufficient volume of blood is unable to reach a portion of the brain tissues for a prolonged period of time. An innovative solution to the problem of a lack of blood supply, which would normally result in a lack of adequate oxygenation of body tissues, is to develop an alternative means to supply endangered tissues with oxygen during crisis.

As mentioned earlier, viruses can be thought of as simply transport vehicles. A virus will transport whatever it carries to whatever cells its probes are fashioned to seek out and engage. In addition to transporting RNA and protein molecules, a virus, being relatively inert because it carries out no biologic functions, can be fashioned to carry drug molecules, oxygen molecules and ATP energy molecules (Figure 43).

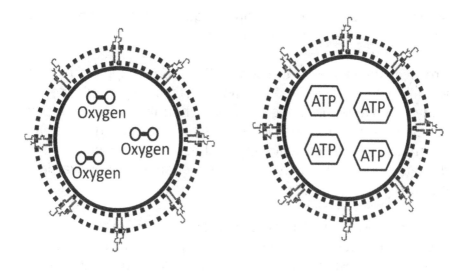

Payload: Oxygen   Payload: ATP molecules

Figure 43: SMART Viruses carrying therapeutic oxygen or ATP molecules

In times of crisis, where tissues are becoming irreversibly damaged due to a lack of adequate blood supply, appropriately formulated viruses could be introduced into the body to seek out specific cells and deliver to those cells drug molecules, oxygen molecules and/or ATP energy molecules. In the case of a stroke, where a portion of the brain is at risk of becoming permanently damaged, viruses could be introduced into the cerebral spinal fluid to transport to specific brain cells whatever the brain cells require to maintain their energy level at the point to insure survival of the tissues until an adequate blood supply is re-established to the tissues. In the case of a heart attack, where a portion of the heart's muscle tissue is at risk of becoming permanently damaged, viruses could be introduced through the chest wall by means of a needle designed to directly penetrate the heart muscle. Medically therapeutic viruses could transport to the heart muscle cells whatever the heart muscle cells require to maintain their energy level at the point to insure survival of the tissues until an adequate blood supply is re-introduced to the heart muscle at risk.

Providing the tissues of the body with a proper supply of oxygen will always be primarily a function of the blood circulating the body. However, in times of crisis, when the blood is unable to reach certain tissues of the body, viruses could act as an alternative means of delivering vital nutrients to tissues at risk during a critical time to extend the chance of survival in a person.

Diabetes mellitus (DM) is a medical condition where the pancreas is unable to adequately respond to the glucose level circulating in the blood. Beta cells present in the pancreas continuously monitor the blood glucose level. In an individual with normal blood glucose control, as the glucose level rises in the blood after a meal is consumed, Beta cells respond by delivering an adequate amount of insulin to match the rise in glucose to maintain the glucose level within the healthy physiologic range. Insulin circulating in the blood reacts with insulin receptors located on the surface of cells in the body and causes glucose to be transported from the blood into cells. In cases where the Beta cells are not able to adequately respond to rises in the glucose level in the blood this is considered diabetes mellitus. Cases of diabetes mellitus where the combination of diet control and oral medications are successful in properly regulating the blood sugar levels are considered to be cases termed non-insulin dependent diabetes. In cases were diet and oral medication are ineffective in maintaining adequate control of the blood sugar, the protein insulin is injected into the body at certain times of the day in an attempt to maintain an normal level of blood glucose. The circumstance requiring the use of insulin to control diabetes is referred to as insulin dependent diabetes mellitus (IDDM).

Diabetic crisis is related to a severe deficiency involving the proper metabolism of glucose. Blood sugar may rise several times above the normal range in the case of a crisis and therefore may interfere with how the blood functions as a transport mechanism of glucose, oxygen and other nutrients. During a diabetic crisis, even though the level of serum glucose is much greater than normal, glucose molecules may not be adequately transported into the cells of the body, due to adequate insulin level not being readily available. Therefore, paradoxically, though the glucose circulating in the blood is in excess, certain tissues in the body may be suffering from an inadequate amount of glucose present inside the cells themselves. Permanent damage may occur in cells when an inadequate amount of glucose or oxygen is not readily available. Utilizing medically therapeutic viruses to act as transport vehicles, in the event of a diabetic crisis, allows tissues to receive the glucose, oxygen or ATP molecules they require until the blood sugar can be decreased to the normal range by other means.

Providing an alternative means for brain cells and heart muscle cells to have access to proteins, nutrients such as glucose and oxygen, and energy molecules per modified viruses that carry these vital elements will greatly improve the survivability of individuals experiencing a heart attack, a stroke or a diabetic crisis.

Medically therapeutic drugs could be used to transport drugs directly to cells (Figure 44). In the case of cancer, medically therapeutic viruses could transport cytotoxic drugs directly to cancer cells. By utilizing medically therapeutic viruses to deliver and directly kill cancer cells many of the side effects of traditional systemic cancer fighting agents could be avoided.

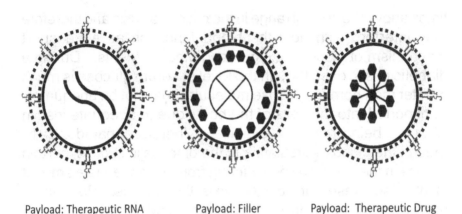

| Payload: Therapeutic RNA | Payload: Filler | Payload: Therapeutic Drug |

Figure 44: SMART Viruses carrying different payloads[6]

A wide variety of pharmaceutical products could be placed inside medically therapeutic viruses to achieve a vast array of medical treatment objectives. The possibilities are almost limitless.

---

6   SMART Viruses carrying different payloads including (a) therapeutic RNA to produce a calculated medical response, (b) inert filler when surface probes act to produce a desired medical effect, (c) therapeutic drugs to be delivered to certain target cells.

IV: Vision for the Future of Medicine

Where this effort is leading…

It is well known that the majority of the deoxyribonucleic acid (DNA) resides in the nucleus of animal cells. It is generally understood that the deoxyribonucleic acid is comprised of four different base pairs and that there exist in the order of 3 billion based pairs strung together and subdivided to form the 46 chromosomes that provide the instruction code to create, maintain, operate and propagate human life as we know it. It is further known that the 3 billion base pairs that make up the DNA are divided into subsets, some of which are recognized as genes. Genes provide the instruction code for the physical features of the body such as the color of a person's eyes, skin, hair, etc. Genes are generally responsible for all of the recognized physical attributes of the human body. Genes also code for the materials and enzymes a cell or the body as a whole requires to create various structures or perform various functions.

It is understood that a polymerase molecule maneuvering along the DNA, reads the instruction code on the DNA and produces a ribonucleic acid molecule (RNA). RNA is found in a variety of forms, three of which are generally recognized as messenger, ribosomal and transport RNA. Messenger RNAs are used as templates to produce proteins. Ribosomes attach to a messenger RNA in the cytoplasm and in the endoplasmic reticulum. The ribosomes decipher the genetic code and generate proteins in response to the genetic coding carried by a particular RNA molecule. Ribosomal RNA assists with the decoding of a messenger RNA. Transport RNAs carry amino acid molecules to the ribosomes so that proteins can be constructed as the messenger RNA is being decoded.

However, there are many questions left unanswered. For example, what is the mechanism that provides the intelligence to determine when and which messenger RNA molecules are to be generated by reading the DNA so that specific proteins can be manufactured when there exists a need to generate a specific protein? How do the polymerase molecules that read the DNA and produce RNA know where along the vast 3 billion base pair length of DNA to find the segment to read to produce the specific messenger RNA that is required? Something must orchestrate, in a timely and efficient manner, the process which reads the DNA and produces messenger RNAs and other elements the cell needs. There is the question that relates to how the more complex molecules the body requires are constructed? Discussed at numerous times in this text are glycoprotein structures that act as probes and cell-surface receptors. A glycoprotein is a molecule that possesses both a protein portion and a carbohydrate portion. Glycoprotein molecules are generally produced in the endoplasmic reticulum. The smooth endoplasmic reticulum is attached to the nucleus. Obviously the smooth endoplasmic reticulum produces proteins, carbohydrates and molecules that are a combination of these two elements, but it takes a certain level of intelligence to properly and consistently orchestrate the construction of such structures.

The patent applications described in this text are part of the preliminary effort to unlock the secrets of the elements of the true intelligence operating inside an animal cell that presides over and supports the healthy growth and maintenance of the cell. In addition, the effort seeks to provide an improved understanding of the intelligence needed to cause a cell to provide the body with specialized functions and that which is necessary to have each cell in a multi-cellular body operate and cooperate with one another to support the growth, general health, maintenance and survivability of the body as a whole.

Further, the future direction also includes efforts to understand the meaning of the biologic software instructions[7] comprising the DNA and RNA. By understanding the meaning behind the instruction code locked in the DNA and RNA, the intelligence behind growth and development of the cell and the body will be better understood.

Enhancing our knowledge of the biologic programming will allow us to understand:

1. The exact meaning of the arrangement of the 3 billion base pairs that comprise the DNA including not only the data files (genes), but also the main programs and the subroutines; deciphering the language that has been used to create these biologic data and programming instruction code files.

2. How the polymerase molecules are constructed and the manner by which they operate.

3. The filing system format code the polymerase molecules use to determine the exact location along the vast DNA to proceed to read the specific segment of DNA to produce the specific RNA molecule that is required.

4. The manner by which complex molecules are actually constructed by the endoplasmic reticulum and other structures such as the Golgi apparatus.

5. The root of the intelligence that runs the cell; the intelligence that determines when to manufacture proteins and other structures, the quantity required, and the exact function proteins and complex molecules will participate in once they have been manufactured.

---

7 Not to be confused with the Genetic Code.

As mentioned above, the smooth endoplasmic reticulum, which is attached to the nucleus of the cell, may in fact not only represent a protein and carbohydrate manufacturing center, but may represent a form of cellular computer processor. The nucleus may simply act as the storage center for instruction code. Polymerase molecules may be simply readers of the information stored in the physical nature of the DNA structure. The smooth endoplasmic reticulum being a manufacturing center attached to the nucleus may actually direct the polymerase molecular readers of the DNA where to fetch the next RNA molecule to continue the job of manufacturing proteins, carbohydrates or structures that represent a combination of these two elements.

Inside a desktop or laptop computer a similar function occurs. The central processing unit (CPU) interprets the instruction code sent to it by the device that stores a program in digital code. Present day computers generally utilize a hard drive to store computer programs in the form of lines of computer code and hard drives store the data to be used by computer programs. As a CPU reads sequential lines of computer programming, additional instruction codes and data are retrieved from the hard drive to allow the CPU to function at top speed. The CPU, RAM and hard drive actively communicate with each other to maintain peak performance and keep the computer operating to the satisfaction of the user.

In a similar manner the smooth endoplasmic reticulum may act as the central processing unit for sophisticated protein complex production and glycoprotein production. As the endoplasmic reticulum is constructing proteins and glycoproteins it may be actively accessing data and programming instructions from the chromosomes. As proteins and glycoproteins are being constructed biochemical signals may be being transmitted from the endoplasmic reticulum to the polymerase molecules reading the DNA to stimulate the polymerase molecules to retrieve further instructions. The DNA, which appears to be written in a base-four biologic computer language of A, C, T and G nucleotides, provides the instruction coding and data for the smooth endoplasmic reticulum to operate as a protein manufacturing center.

Looking at the structure of the DNA, the basic element is the 'nucleotide' which include the four nucleotides: adenine, cytosine, thymine, and guanine. The DNA is made up of a string of 3.2×10^9 base pairs of nucleotides (a base pair is two nucleotides joined together in a specific way). A 'nucleotide' is representative of a 'bit' in computer memory. A sequence of three nucleotides defines a codon. A codon is like a computer word. Codons identify amino acids used to construct proteins. Some genes define how to build specific proteins. Messenger RNA (mRNA) molecules are transcribed from DNA and carry the sequential codon code to construct a specific protein. Collections of genes are referred to as chromosomes. A collection of chromosomes in a living organism is referred to as its genome. The genome is stored in the nucleus of every cell in the organism such as the human body. The nucleus in a human cell contains 46 different chromosomes representing its DNA. The genes comprising the chromosomes are capable of generating an estimated 33,000 different proteins.

DNA functions somewhat like a hard drive or a memory chip. The chromosomes are directories with multiple data or programming file folders which are generally referred to as genes. The genes are programs which direct the manufacturing of a particular protein. Each gene most likely is tagged with a unique identifying code (UIC) that allows the polymerase molecules to find them and read them as required. When the cell requires manufacturing of a particular protein, the chromosome where the gene for the protein is stored is queried using the UIC and an RNA polymerase molecule (a protein complex that produces RNA) reads the DNA code dedicated to that gene and creates an mRNA of it. The mRNA then relocates to a processing area somewhat like in a computer where the program code on the hard drive is moved to Random Access Memory (RAM) for processing prior to the CPU reading the program code and executing the commands carried in the program code. Once moved to an area in the cell that its information can be utilized, the mRNA is read by one or more ribosomes in a process called translation to generate the protein defined by the biologic code contained in the mRNA. Deciphering the UIC system utilized by polymerase molecules to read the DNA would facilitate the ability to access genes and activate them in order to generate medically beneficial results.

While the Genetic Code is well documented and though to comprise 3% of the chromosomal material available in the nucleus of a human cell, the remaining 97 percent of the DNA's code is not yet understood. It is our intention to uncover the meaning of the remainder of the biologic code that comprises the DNA. We understand that there are chemical and biologic functions that occur due to chemical reactions assisted by enzymes that control some body functions. We seek to identify a higher order of intelligence governing the control processes. We would like to understand how simple computer instructions such as 'and', 'or', 'if' and 'go to' commands may be represented or at least are implied in the DNA and followed. We would like to identify how simple programming instructions are organized into more complex programs and subroutines. We intend to explore the workings of the intelligence that provides the foundation for cells to grow, to maintain themselves and to reproduce. By deciphering the exact meaning of the instruction code comprising the DNA we will be able to create a much more efficient interface between the technology available to manage medical diseases and prevent our patients from having to suffer due to serious medical conditions which are not satisfactorily treatable with today's technology. The more we understand about the technical aspects of the biologic programming of a cell, the better we can perform as clinicians for our patients.

Addendum:
Drafting an Entirely New Approach to Medicine & Technology

'It would seem a base four biologic computer language governs our genetics, is the fundamental format comprising the operating system inside our brains, and orchestrates, as well as coordinates, the existence between ourselves and all forms of life that exist in the ecosystem we call Earth--we have much to learn about this powerful universal quaternary code.'

Recently during a break in my schedule, I found myself outside under a bright blue sky admiring a black bird with a yellow vest standing atop of a concrete ledge. As this tiny creature effortlessly flapped its wings and descended from the ledge to the brick patio at my feet, it struck me that with a brain probably smaller than the size of a pea, in principle this bird could accomplish nearly as much as I, a human, could and in some respects possibly even more. As the bird stood scanning her environment I realized that this small creature, measuring only five inches high, a white stripe above the eye was indeed standing erect. Balanced expertly on two twig-like feet, this animal walked the ground in a similar fashion as I, a human. Walking upright is one of those attributes cherished by the human race as setting us apart from most of our cousins in the animal kingdom. Walking erect seems to have a righteous appeal to it, yet this tiny bird scurried across the brick patio as agile as any human I had ever seen.

Further, it struck me that without any formal education this delicate creature, weighing probably only a few ounces, knew how to forage for food, was alert for predators, and possessed a sense of direction. That all of the internal body works, similar to a human, including temperature control, respiration, digestion, blood circulation all worked on a smaller scale, but similar level of sophistication as my human body. This tiny creature knew to groom itself. Had a sense of community and by chirping did communicate with other members of her kind. When the timing was right, she could locate a mate and procreate her species. At a glance, as this bird scampered across the patio, I became amazed that with such a tiny brain, that for other than spoken and written words, this creature was accomplishing nearly everything that I could do (Figure 45). I realized that she, equipped with her tiny brain, indeed could arguably do more than I could with the massive brain sitting on my shoulders, because this bird had mastered the art of flight and all of the sophisticated aerodynamics that go along with soaring up and into a treacherous, ever windy environment existing above my head.

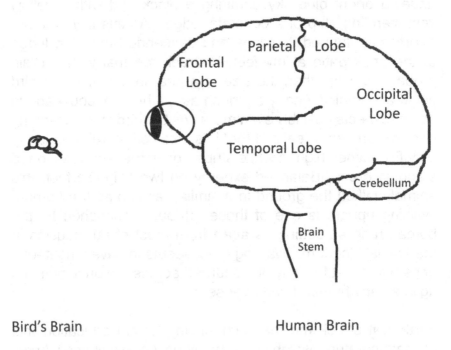

Bird's Brain   Human Brain

Figure 45: A bird's brain compared to the human brain

So what am I doing with a brain that, I would guess, is a thousand times larger than this winged mistress's brain? It is said that humans actively only utilize 25% of their brain capacity. After considering what a bird can accomplish with such a petite brain, possibly the initial approximation of our utilization of human brain power is markedly overestimating the portion we actually actively employ. It begs the question 'what is all that human gray matter doing between our ears?' Possibly, unlike my feathered friend, it is so we can make use of our upper extremities and legs jointly to do mundane chores such as mow the lawn, rake leaves, or drive a car. The notion that I need a brain that is physically 999 times the size of a bird's brain just to read words, speak a language and use my arms and legs in concert strikes me as a bit excessive. It would seem that there are other, better, uses for such a large cerebral cortex and all the gray matter that goes with it.

Computers are comprised of the basic elements of a central processing unit, a hard drive, RAM memory, a video card, power supply, a view screen and a keyboard. The hard drive stores computer programs and data files. The central processing unit (CPU) runs the programs stored on the hard drive. The RAM memory serves as the conduit between the CPU and the hard drive, as well as acts as a dynamic storage site for data and programming instructions. The power supply feeds life into the computer. The view screen and keyboard facilitate the user communicating with the CPU. Though I might see words on the view screen displayed in any of a hundred different fonts of my choosing, every detail of computer function and information storage is accomplished on the level of binary mathematics, otherwise referred to as the computer coding comprised of 'ones' and 'zeros'. The CPU of the most sophisticated computer on the planet can only crunch data streams that consist of this most elementary language of ones and zeros; that is a transistor is either 'on' or 'off' and previously this was referred to as machine language.

One would assume that the human brain is more sophisticated than a desk top or laptop computer that only responds to ones and zeros. If this were so, what mathematical language might act as the root basis of the human brain's programming power?... There must exist some form of universal control processing system language in our brains for all of us to be able to use our brains in a similar fashion. Since DNA, which comprises the forty-six chromosomes that reside in the nucleus in the cells of our bodies, is comprised of four nucleotides including thymine, guanine, adenine, and cytosine, it would seem reasonable to assume nature favors a base-four biologic programming language rather than a binary code.

Visible light is comprised of the three primary colors red, blue and yellow. White light represents all color and 'black' represents no color. It would seem if we assign black the definition of the 'null set', meaning absence of a signal, then the remaining parts of visible light including white, red, blue, and yellow make up a base-four code for our eyes to utilize as a means of communicating with the base-four programming language operating in our brain.

The term 'language' used in reference to speech and writing should not be confused with what this word represents in the computer world. The term 'computer language' is an expression that represents a format utilized to generate a set of instructions that run the core systems of a computer. Data strings that a computer language uses are where human speaking and writing symbols are often found. A single computer program could interface with people of differing human languages by changing the data strings to the language the computer's user is familiar with; this occurs on the internet all the time. Someone in China may be looking at a computer screen filled with Chinese characters, while someone in the United States may be peering at a computer screen with characters representative of the language they are most familiar with. On the other hand, a human language is simply a means accepted and utilized by a particular subset of people, to communicate amongst each other in a descriptive manner, the particulars of themselves and their surroundings. The human language with regards to the brain is somewhat likened to an operating system running a computer; both entities require an agreed upon set of symbols, semantics, instructions and rules to function properly. Our brains may have a deeper, more fundamental operating system, which acts as a core system that we subconsciously interface with using our expressive languages.

Most of us have experienced pulling a new computer from its box, setting it up, turning it on and watching the screen light up if all is running right. A computer is pre-loaded with a core program that runs the device. In the past such a core program was referred to as 'DOS' for disc operating system. More recently Microsoft's Windows or Apple's Mac's OS X are more familiar forms of a core operating system. To make computers 'user friendly', we tend to load onto our computers software that allows us to utilize the computer in the manner that we would like to use the device. We may load gaming software, music software, photo management software, word processing software, accounting software, and/ or internet browsing software to name but a few categories of useful programs. Each one of these computer programs is plugged into the computer's operating software system. The programming software we load onto our computers generally is intended to make our computers user friendly so that we can use our computers in a way that we wish to use them. Most computer users seldom have a need to directly interact with the core program that runs a computer.

The human brain may be constructed in a similar manner and that may be in part why it is so much larger than a bird's brain. There may be a core brain operating system software (BOSS). The languages of the world may simply be the software we load into our brains to make our brains user friendly to us so that we as individuals can use our brain in the manner we wish to use them. The BOSS may be responsible for organizing, filing, retrieving, and executing our thoughts on both a conscious and subconscious level. This core operating system and the core memory associated with it may not be generally apparent to us. The part of ourselves that may interact with this underlying BOSS is music. Music may indeed be a preset combination of sounds that interfaces with this core biologic software system running in our heads which stimulates our emotions, energizes our commitments and inspires our creativity.

A number of prominent figures throughout human history have expressed a sense of vision, insight and genius that was indeed well beyond the knowledge, technology and social structure of their time. Hippocrates broke free from the prevailing superstitions of his time and dramatically influenced the course of medicine, writing about illness being the result of disease rather than misfortune. Leonardo da Vinci jotted down in his notes his visions of flying machines, mechanized wheeled vehicles and underwater transport devices that were well ahead of the technology of his day. Einstein taught us the theories such as relativity and quantum mechanics at a time when peering out into the depths of space was crude and the dramatic pictures of the workings of the universe already captured by the Hubble telescope were but a dream.

The human brain has an immense capacity for problem solving and creativity. Our brains are indeed constructed not just as a computer, but as a network of computer processors all dedicated to multi-tasking at different high level functions simultaneously. With all of the processing power our brains have at their disposal, it would be bold, but not unreasonable to speculate that we also have at least one hard drive if not several hard drive memory areas residing in the cerebral cortex or the mid brain which are dedicated to file-like data storage. I would seem reasonable that humans have a functioning long-term and short-term memory storage areas, and the idea of a hard drive like memory area which helps us store such memories is an acceptable concept. The reason why people may think differently and thus have different aptitudes regarding brain function may be related to how the brain is hardwired between various processing units and the memory storage areas of the brain. An individual who is inclined to be proficient at music may have the pathways better developed between frontal cortex of the brain and the music center located in their temporal lobe with a memory area dedicated to merging imagery, emotion and musical notes together into scores of music (Figure 46). An individual who possesses an aptitude toward problem solving and engineering may have better developed pathways existing between the frontal cortex and the spacial processing center located in the back of the head between the occipital and parietal lobes of the brain with large areas of memory dedicated to conceptualizing and modifying three-dimensional color images.

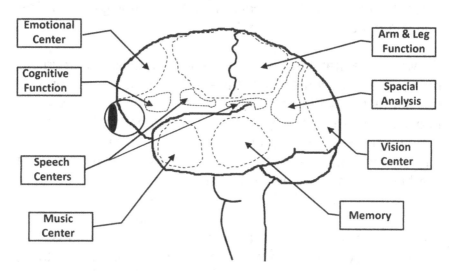

Figure 46: Different Areas of the Human Brain

The question is, in the deep recesses of the memory portion of the human brain does there exist a collection of data files that represent a permanent library of information that as time passes drives the progressive advancements in human technology? Is this such a farfetched concept? Is it really that hard to consider that within our expanded cortex that we don't have built into our memory circuits a library of data files that represent technologies that we are intended to develop and construct if the need is evident, the timing is right and the materials are attainable? If one returns to consider again the bird, which had gathered together a small clump of dried grass and took flight, how does this creature know how and where to build a nest to protect the eggs she will lay? The construction of a cup-shaped object built out of twigs, leaves, feathers, mud and saliva fixed in a tree or in a bush is a marvel in of itself. Some species of bird, such as Baltimore orioles construct elaborate nests that are hung from the bough of a tree. This represents a crude form of technology; but technology none the less. The means to construct a nest must be hardwired into the bird's brain; it is not a learned behavior passed on from generation to generation. Why then shouldn't it be acceptable to consider that the fundamental concepts of some technologies might be hardwired into human brains?

If it were true that there exist technology data files store in our brains, then every member of the human race carries around this same library of information inside their head; the capacity to access these files may in part be due to how an individual's brain is hardwired, level of education, and need to know. Such information could be very beneficial to the advancement of the human race if released in a regimented order. While, if this same technological information were released from the brain and introduced into mainstream society in a disorderly manner, this action could result in confusion and chaos. If such a library of wisdom is present in the human brain, there would need to exist a method of distributing this information in a timely and orderly fashion. Without some form of regimented release of information, ideas would never flourish to a point of being adequately developed. The concepts for constructing a spaceship to transport people across the galaxy need to be released after mankind has successfully mastered such methods of transportation as the boat, the car, and the plane. To have humans toiling to build an intergalactic space craft before they had developed he means to manufacture a motorized four-wheeled vehicle, would have resulted in a technological disaster.

In order to properly release information from technologic data files in an orderly fashion, that makes sense in a practical world, there needs to be a feed-back loop that stimulates the release of such information. Time in of itself does not offer a reliable means of judging the advancement of human technology. Setbacks to the advancement of technology may have come in the form of disease, natural disaster, or accidental occurrences that would have impacted key people in the population. War can act as a setback to the advancement of technology such as when the prestigious library at Alexandria of the ancient world was burned by barbarians. On the other hand, by virtue of necessity, war can act as a stimulus to the advancement of technology such as World War II having spawned the early development of rocket and jet plane technologies; which eventually launched the two dominant superpowers of the world into the race for the moon.

The 'means' to stimulate the timely and proficient dispersion of technological ideas from library files carried in the human brain would need to be termed a 'variable constant'. This element a 'variable constant' does not represent an oxymoron as might be expected, but instead a means of constructing a feedback loop that monitors the technological progress of humans. This concept 'variable constant' would vary constantly and linearly as technology changed and would provide the necessary signal to the brain, informing the library portion of the brain that the human race was ready for the details of the next technologic advancement to be revealed.

After considering numerous possibilities, the one element that infiltrates all of society and could be relied upon as a benchmark to signal the advancement of technology to the brain and fulfill the role of a 'variable constant' is 'music'. Music represents the one ubiquitous ingredient in our lives that weaves freely through our diverse cultures that could reliably be utilized as a means of revealing and dispersing technological ideas in a regimented manner. As technology advances, the construction of instruments advance, and thus the quality and quantity of diverse musical sounds advances and this provides the active feedback mechanism to the brain.

My children have much enjoyed the dramatic advancement of video games that evolved over the last two decades. In their incessant effort to continuously improve their skills at their favorite video games, my boys have explored various clues in how to best manipulate these games. A phenomenon that appeared in their speech nearly a decade ago was the phrase 'cheat codes'. To my sons, having access to a video game's 'cheat codes' that they could insert into the game's program, meant they could explore aspects of the game that the average player could not access. My boys tended to acquire these cheat codes for a specific game by either performing well in playing a particular game or from querying their friends or sometimes by accessing the game designer's website.

Different scores and styles of music might represent 'cheat codes' for the human brain. A 'musical key' might be a more appropriate term than 'cheat code'. A particular musical composition comprised of notes, tone, rhythm and dynamics, heard by a person, may unlock and open up a portion of the brain generally hidden from exploration by one's imagination. If one hundred people happen to hear a song containing a musical key embedded into the music, ninety nine of those people may simply appreciate the music for what it sounds like to them. One of the hundred people may someday be challenged to solve a problem and because at one time in the individual's life he or she was privied to hearing a particular segment of music that represented an advancement in music and therefore an advancement in technology, the individual's access to the technological library in their brain was upgraded and they can make constructive use of an expansion to their imagination (Figure 47).

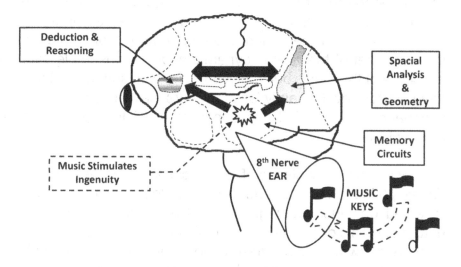

Figure 47: The music keys open memory circuits in the brain

There may be more than one category of musical keys. Musical keys may be present not only to assist with the advancement of technology but also for the progressive development of art, literature, medicine, and even socialization methodologies. Humans have resided on the planet for an estimated 2 million years, slowly spreading out and exploring the distant reaches of our land and oceans. It wasn't until the last five thousand years we have become civilized. It hasn't been until the last two hundred years that democracy truly flourished. In the last hundred years there has been a cataclysmic expansion in our technical prowess across the globe and much of that has gone hand-in-hand with a tremendous evolution in music from 'folk art' to 'symphony' to 'chamber music' to 'big band' to 'rhythm and blues' to 'jazz' to 'rock-n-roll' to 'disco' to 'heavy metal' to 'new age' to 'rap' to 'alternative rock' to name a few.

So why is it that high school jazz programs may be so vitally important to the fabric of our society? The music is endearing and even mesmerizing at times if it is your own child playing in the band; possibly a little less polished when listening to the band overall. Though I must say that the high school jazz band concerts that I have had the privilege of attending have provided me with immense entertainment, especially in trying to appreciate how the sound each instrument contributes to the sum total of the overall dynamic acoustic ensemble over the score of the music being played. The high school students have performed brilliantly and my ears have cherished the experience as my mind has pondered the intricacies of the music played.

History contains a multitude of references to the value of music. Greek philosopher and scientist Aristotle is known to have reflected on music stating, "It is not easy to determine the nature of music or why anyone should have a knowledge of it." Plato, a fellow legendary great Greek philosopher, apparently was a stern musical disciplinarian and he recognized a correspondence between the character of a man and the music that represented him. Confucius considered great music as being in harmony with the universe, restoring order to the physical world through that harmony. Music remains a puzzle as to why we value such an experience. More recently the value of music has been divided into two camps. One sect believes music to derive its value from the aesthetic quality or musical features of the experience, while the other sect believes music derives its value from the liberating expressive properties a musical composition provides the player as well as the audience.

Still, why of all things should the jazz program be a critical part of any high school agenda? In the construct of jazz, the jazz students are offered the opportunity to play solos. Often a solo in a jazz band is a brief piece of music that has been written for the song and the instrument playing the solo part. But at times, the conductor of the jazz band offers the students the opportunity to play impromptu music. Playing impromptu is the heart of jazz. Playing impromptu is the soul of jazz.

Playing impromptu is also where the fledgling musician has the opportunity to explore a new musical rhythm that might be beating in their head that they can express by way of the music they play with their instrument. It is by releasing this free flowing energy through music that we humans are able venture further down the hallways of the colossal library of knowledge that exists inside our heads. The feedback loop of the variable constant fused with the soul of music beating in the heart of a musician playing as a true artist of the craft, offers the change in rhythm by which the future of mankind marches (Figure 48).

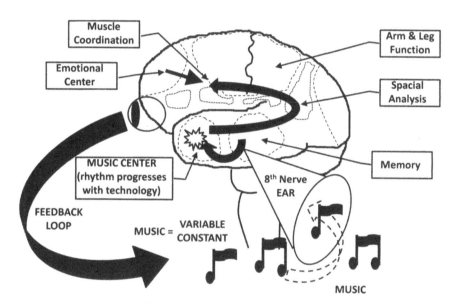

Figure 48: The musical rhythm in one's head helps develop further musical compositions that generates a feedback loop utilizing the variable constant

The day we fail to fund the jazz music program in our local high school is the day we shut the door to the library that inspires all of us to dream new and innovative thoughts. The day the excuses 'not to support high school jazz' outweigh our 'obligation' to fund this critically necessary program is also the day maybe I should trade in my brain for one that is 99.9%

smaller; but then I guess I would have to learn the art of flying as my winged friend has learned to master. On the other hand, the act of supporting the music programs in our schools may be one very vital way that we support all that is meant to be good, as well as insure the future of the human race for generations to come. Though each succeeding generation tends to covet the music of their era, Jazz and other dynamically creative genres of music such as New Age, Rock-N-Roll, and Pop-Rock may hold the secret to our continued ingenuity.

Epilogue

One of the deadliest menaces and greatest challenges mankind, as a collective, faces are viruses, for we have no medical tools to successfully eradicate their threat. Viruses are capable of widespread panepidemics potentially resulting in the loss of an epic numbers of lives. To some extent isolation protected our ancestors. As all parts of the globe become intimately interconnected with people traveling freely via air travel, a deadly outbreak could quickly spread to the majority of the dwellings around the planet. In evolutionary terms, if we fail in our mission to procure an effective means to successfully combat viral infections, these smallest and simplest of pathogens could eliminate the existence of the human race from the face of the planet in what could be considered an instant per the history of our world; and this desperate irony, the battle between the "highly intelligent" humans and robotic, insensate viruses, would represent the ultimate of tragedies. As humans, our survival is at stake and our honor of being considered intelligent beings is at grave risk. Successful solutions to minimize the impact of challenges created by the deadly viruses that currently exist on the planet, as well as the potentially fatal viruses that will evolve in the ensuing years, must be developed with great speed for the sake of the survival of future generations.

APPENDIX A:
Patent Applications to Eradicate AIDS

A1: ANTI-HUMAN IMMUNODEFICIENCY VIRUS SURRO-
GATE TARGET AGENT TECHNOLOGY FILTER INTENDED
TO NEUTRALIZE OR REMOVE HUMAN IMMUNODEFI-
CIENCY VIRUS VIRIONS FROM BLOOD

INDIVIDUALS REQUESTING PATENT: Dr. Lane B. Scheiber,
ScD and Dr. Lane B. Scheiber II, MD

NUMBER OF CLAIMS: 2 independent claims, 18 dependent
claims

ABSTRACT

The Human Immunodeficiency Virus poses a significant threat
to the world's population. Current strategies utilized to treat
infectious agents have not been adequate to contain and
eradicate this deadly viral infection. HIV seeks out its host, a
T–Helper cell, by utilizing glycoprotein 120 probes to engage a
CD4 cell-surface receptor located on the surface of a T-Helper
cell. Developing blood filtering techniques that incorporate
filter mediums that offer HIV virion's probes the opportunity to
engage the cell-surface receptors they are seeking offers a
means of neutralizing and removing HIV. Filtering the blood
of a patient with filter mediums comprised of T-Helper cells,

sheets of lipid bilayer or virus-like structures with each type of medium possessing cell-surface receptors intended to attract and engage HIV virions provides an effective strategy to prevent and treat AIDS.

BACKGROUND OF THE INVENTION

1. Field of the Invention

[0001]   This invention relates to any medical device that is utilized to filter the blood of a patient infected with the Human Immunodeficiency Virus with the intention of neutralizing or removing from the blood infectious Human Immunodeficiency Virus virions.

2. Description of Background Art

[0002]   It is estimated by the Center for Disease Control that in the United States 55,000 to 60,000 new cases of Human Immunodeficiency Virus (HIV) are occurring each year. It is thought that there are 900,000 people currently infected with HIV in the United States, with many victims not aware that they have contracted the virus. Further, it has been estimated that the Human Immunodeficiency Virus (HIV), the pathogen that causes Acquired Immune Deficiency Syndrome (AIDS), has infected as many as 30-60 million people around the globe.

[0003]   The presence of HIV first came to the general attention of those in the United States in 1981, when there appeared an outbreak of Kaposi's Sarcoma and Pneumocystis carinii pneumonia in gay men in New York and California. After over twenty-five years of research and investigation, eradicating the ever growing global humanitarian crisis posed by the HIV remains an elusive goal for the medical community. It is estimated the virus has already killed 25 million citizens of this planet.

[0004] The Human Immunodeficiency Virus has been previously referred to as human T-Lymphotrophic virus III (HTLV-III), lymphadenopathy-associated virus (LAV), and AIDS-associated retrovirus (ARV). Infection with HIV may occur by the virus being transferred by blood, semen, vaginal fluid, or breast milk. Four major means of transmission of HIV include unprotected sexual intercourse, contaminated needles, breast milk, and transmission from an infected mother to her baby at birth.

[0005] HIV is an ingeniously constructed very deadly virus, which represents the most challenging pathogen the medical community faces to date. Viruses in general, have been difficult to contain and eradicate due to the fact they are obligate parasites and tend not to carry out any biologic functions outside the cell the virus has targeted as its host. A virus when it exists outside the boundaries of a cell is generally referred to as a virion. HIV virions posses several attributes that make them very elusive and difficult to destroy.

[0006] Bacterial infections have posed an easier target for the medical community to eradicate from the body. Bacteria generally live and reproduce outside animal cells. Bacteria, like animal cells, carry out biologic functions. A large multi-celled organism such as the human body combats bacterial infections with a combined force of white cells, antibodies, complements and its lymphatic system. White cells circulate the body in search of bacteria. When a white cell encounters a bacterium, the white cell engulfs the bacterium, encapsulates the pathogen, processes the identification of the pathogen and kills the pathogen utilizing acids and destructive enzymes. The white cell then alerts the B-cells of the immune system as to the identity of the intruding bacterium. A subpopulation of B-cells is generated, dedicated to producing antibodies directed against the particular pathogen the circulating white cell encountered and identified. Antibodies, generated by B-cells, traverse the blood and body tissues in search of the bacteria they were

118

designed to repel. Once an antibody encounters a bacterium it is targeted to attack, the antibody attaches to the bacterium's outer wall. The effect antibodies have in coating the outside of a bacterium is to assist the white cells and the other components of the immune system in recognizing the bacterium, so that appropriate defensive action can be taken against the pathogen. Some antibodies, in addition to coating the bacterium, will act to punch holes through the bacterium's outer wall. If the integrity of the bacterium's cell wall is breached, this action generally leads to the death of the bacterium. Complements are primitive protein structures that circulate the blood stream in search of anything that appears consistent with a bacteria cell wall. Complements are indiscriminant. Once the complement proteins locate any form of bacterial cell wall, the complement proteins organize, and much like antibodies, act in concert to punch one or more holes though a bacterium's cell wall to compromise the viability of the bacterium. As part of the immune system lymphocytes in lymph nodes screen the lymph and cells in the spleen screen the blood in search of bacteria. When a bacterial pathogen is identified, such as by antibodies coating the surface, the bacterium is taken out of circulation and terminated.

[0007] Viruses pose a much different infectious vector to the body's defense system than either bacteria or cellular parasites. Since viruses do not carry out biologic processes outside their host cell, a virus can be destroyed, but they cannot be killed. A virus is simply comprised of one or more external shells and a portion of genetic material. The virus's genetic information is carried in the core of the virus. Antibodies can coat the exterior of a virus to make it easier for the white cells in the body to identify the viral pathogen, but the action of punching holes in the virus's external shell by antibodies or complement proteins does not necessarily kill the virus. Viruses also only briefly circulate in the blood and tissues of the body as an exposed entity. Using exterior probes, a virus hunts down a cell in the body that will act as an appropriate host so that the virus can replicate. Once the virus has found a proper host cell, the virus inserts its genome into the host cell. To complete its life-cycle, the virus's genetic material takes command of cellular functions and directs the host cell to make replicas of the virus.

[0008] Once the virus's genome has entered a host cell, the virus is in effect shielded from the body's immune system defense mechanisms. Inside a host cell, the presence of the virus is generally only represented as genetic information incorporated into the host cell's DNA. Once a virus has infected a cell in the body, the presence of the virus can only be eradicated if the host cell is destroyed. Antibodies and complements are generally designed not to attack the autologous tissues of the body. Circulating white cells and the immune cells which comprise lymph nodes and the spleen may or may not recognize that a cell, which has become a host for a virus, is infected with a virus's genome. If the immune system fails to identify a cell that has become infected with a virus, the virus's genetic material can proceed to force the infected cell to make copies of the virus. Since a virus is in essence simply a segment of genetic material, time is of no consequence to the life-cycle of the virus and a virus's genome may be carried for years by the host without a need to activate; such viruses are often termed latent viruses. A virus's genetic material may sit idle in a host cell for an extended period of time until the pathogen's programming senses the time is right to initiate the virus's replication process or an action of the host cell triggers the virus to replicate. The only opportunity for the immune system to destroy a latent virus is when copies of the virus leave the host cell and circulate in the blood or tissues in search of another perspective host cell.

[0009] The traditional medical approach to combating infectious agents such as bacteria and cellular parasites, therefore has limited value in managing or eradicating elusive or latent viral infections. Synthetic antibiotics, generally used to augment the body's capacity to produce naturally occurring antibodies against bacterial infections, have little success in combating latent viral infections. Stimulating the body's immune system's recognition of a virus by administering a vaccine also has had limited success in combating elusive viral infections. Vaccines generally are intended to introduce to the body pieces of a bacteria or virus, or an attenuated, noninfectious intact bacteria or virus so that the immune system is able to recognize and process the infectious agent and generate antibodies directed to assist in killing the pathogen. Once the immune system has been primed to recognize an intruder, antibodies will be produced by the immune system in great quantities in an effort to repel an invader. Over time, as the immune system down-regulates its antibody production in response to a lack of detecting the presence of the intruding pathogen, the quantity of antibodies circulating in the blood stream may decrease in number to a quantity that is insufficient to combat a pathogen. Since antibodies have limited value in combating some of the more elusive viruses that hibernate in host cells, vaccines have limited value in destroying latent viruses.

[0010] The Human Immunodeficiency Virus demonstrates four factors which make this pathogen particularly elusive and a difficult infectious agent to eradicate from the body. First: the host for HIV is the T-Helper cell. The T-Helper cell is a key element in the immune system's response since it helps coordinate the body's defensive actions against pathogens seeking to invade the body's tissues. In cases of a bacterial infection versus a viral infection, T-Helper cells actively direct which immune cells will rev-up in response to the infectious agent and engage the particular pathogen. Since HIV infects and disrupts T-Helper cells, coordination of the immune response against the virus is disrupted, thus limiting the body's capacity to mount a proper response against the presence of the virus and produce a sufficient action to successfully eradicate the virus.

[0011] Second: again, latent viruses such as HIV, have a strategic advantage. When the immune system first recognizes a pathogen and begins to generate antibodies against a particular pathogen, the response is generally robust. Once time has passed and the immune system fails to detect an active threat, the production of antibodies against the particular pathogen diminishes. When HIV infects a T-Helper cell, the viral genome may lay dormant, sometimes for years before taking command of the T-Helper cell's biologic functions. HIV may, therefore, generate a very active initial immune response to its presence, but if the virus sits dormant inside T-Helper cells for months or years, the antibody response to the virus will diminish over time. There may not be an adequate quantity of circulating antibodies to actively engage the HIV virions as they migrate from the T-Helper cell that generated the copies to uninfected T-Helper cells that will serve as a new host to support further replication. If the immune system's response is insufficient during the period while the virus is exposed and vulnerable, it becomes extremely difficult for the body to eradicate the virus.

[0012] Third, when replicas of the Human Immunodeficiency Virus are released from their host cell, during the budding process, the HIV virion coats itself with an exterior envelope comprised of a portion of the plasma membrane from the T-Helper cell that acted as the host for the virus. A T-Helper cell's plasma membrane is comprised of a lipid bilayer, a double layer of lipid molecules oriented with their polar ends at the outside of the membrane and the nonpolar ends in the membrane interior. The virus thus, in part, takes on an external appearance of a naturally occurring cell in the body. Since the exterior envelope of a HIV virion has the characteristics of a T-Helper cell it is more difficult for the immune system to recognize that it is a pathogen as it migrates through the body in search of another T-Helper cell to infect.

[0013] The Human Immunodeficiency Virus possesses a fourth, very elusive mode of action, which the virus readily utilizes to actively defeat the body's immune system. HIV carries in its genome a segment of genetic material that directs an infected T-Helper cell to create and mount on the surface the plasma membrane a FasL cell-surface receptor. Healthy T-Helper cells carry on the surface of their plasma membrane Fas cell-surface receptors. The Fas cell-surface receptor when engaged by a FasL cell-surface receptor on another cell, initiates apoptosis in the cell carrying the Fas cell-surface receptor. Apoptosis is a biologic process that causes a cell to terminate itself. A T-Helper cell infected with the HIV virus carrying a FasL cell-surface receptor is therefore capable of killing noninfected T-Helper cells that the infected T-Helper cell encounters as it circulates the body. The occurrence of AIDS is therefore propagated not only by the number of T-Helper cells that become incapacitated due to direct infection by HIV, but also by the number of noninfected T-Helper cells that are eliminated by coming in direct contact with infected T-Helper cells.

[0014]   Acquired Immune Deficiency Syndrome (AIDS) occurs as a result of the number of circulating T-Helper cells declining to a point where the immune system's capacity to mount a successful response against opportunistic infectious agents is significantly compromised. The number of viable T-Helper cells declines either because they become infected with the HIV virus or because they have been killed by encountering a T-Helper cell infected with HIV. When there is an insufficient population of non-HIV infected T-Helper cells to properly combat infectious agents such as Pneumocystis carinii or cytomegalo virus or other pathogens, the body becomes overwhelmed with the opportunistic infection and the patient becomes clinically ill. In cases where the combination of the patient's compromised immune system and medical assistance in terms of synthetic antibiotics intended to combat the opportunistic pathogens, fluids, intravenous nutrition and other treatments are not sufficient to sustain life, the body succumbs to the opportunistic infection and death ensues.

[0015] The Human Immunodeficiency Virus locates its host by utilizing probes located on its envelope. The HIV virion has two types of glycoprotein probes attached to the outer surface of its exterior envelope. A glycoprotein is a structure comprised of a protein component and a lipid component. HIV utilizes a glycoprotein 120 (gp 120) probe to locate a CD4 cell-surface receptor on the plasma membrane of a T-Helper cell. The plasma membrane of the T-Helper cell is comprised of a lipid bilayer. Cell-surface receptors are anchored in the lipid bilayer. Once an HIV gp 120 probe has successfully engaged a CD4 cell-surface receptor on a T-Helper cell a conformational change occurs in the gp 120 probe and a glycoprotein 41 (gp 41) probe is exposed. The gp 41 probe's intent is to engage a CXCR4 or CCR5 cell-surface receptor on the plasma membrane of the same T-Helper cell. Once a gp 41 probe on the HIV virion engages a CXCR4 or CCR5 cell-surface receptor, the HIV virion opens an access portal through the T-Helper cell's plasma membrane.

[0016] Once the virus has gained access to the T-Helper cell by opening a portal through the cell's outer membrane the virion inserts two positive strand RNA molecules approximately 9500 nucleotides in length. Inserted along with the RNA strands are the enzymes reverse transcriptase, protease and integrase. Once the virus's genome gains access to the interior of the T-Helper cell, in the cytoplasm the pair of RNA molecules are transformed to deoxyribonucleic acid by the reverse transcriptase enzyme. Following modification of the virus's genome to DNA, the virus's genetic information migrates to the host cell's nucleus. In the nucleus, with the assistance of the integrase protein, the virus's DNA becomes inserted into the T-Helper cell's native DNA. When the timing is appropriate, the now integrated viral DNA, becomes read by the host cell's polymerase molecules and the virus's genetic information commands certain cell functions to carry out the replication process to construct copies of the human deficiency virus.

[0017]   Present anti-viral therapy has been designed to target the enzymes that assist the HIV genome with the replication process.   Anti-viral therapy is intended to interfere with the action of these replication enzymes.   Part of the challenge of eradicating HIV is that once the virus inserts its genome into a T-Helper cell host, the viral genome may lay dormant until the proper circumstances evolve.   The virus's genome may sit idle inside a T-Helper cell for years before becoming activated, causing drugs that interfere with HIV's life cycle to have limited effect on eliminating the virus from the body.   Arresting the replication process does not insure that T-Helper cells infected with HIV do not continue to circulate the body killing noninfected T-Helper cells thus causing the patient to progress to a clinically apparent state of Acquired Immune Deficiency Syndrome and eventually succumbing to an opportunistic infection which eventually results in the death of the individual.

[0018]   The outer layer of the HIV virion is comprised of a portion of the T-Helper cell's outer cell membrane.   In the final stage of the replication process, as a copy of the HIV capsid, carrying the HIV genome, buds through the host cell's plasma membrane, the capsid acquires as its outermost shell a wrapping of lipid bilayer from the host cell's plasma membrane. Vaccines are generally comprised of pieces of a virus or bacterium, or copies of the entire virus or bacterium weakened to the point the pathogen is incapable of causing an infection. These pieces of a pathogen or copies of a nonvirulent pathogen prime the immune system such that a vaccine intent is to cause B-cells to produce antibodies that are programmed to seek out the surface characteristics of the pathogen comprising the vaccine. In the case of HIV, since the surface of the pathogen is an envelope comprised of lipid bilayer taken from the host T-Helper cell's plasma membrane, a vaccine comprised of portions of the exterior envelope of the HIV virions might not only target HIV virions, but might also have deleterious effects on the T-Helper cell population.   Some antibodies produced to combat HIV infections may not be able to tell the difference between an HIV virion and a T-Helper cell, and such antibodies may act to coat and assist in the elimination of both targets. In such a scenario, since such a vaccine might cause a decline in the number of available T-Helper cells, it is conceivable that a vaccine comprised of portions of the external envelope of HIV virions might paradoxically induce clinically apparent AIDS in a patient that a vaccine has been administered.

[0019] It is clear that the traditional approach of utilizing antibiotics or providing vaccines to stimulate the immune system to produce endogenous antibodies, by themselves, is an ineffective strategy to manage a virus as elusive and deadly as HIV. Drugs that interfere with the replication process of HIV generally slow progression of the infection by the virus, but do not necessarily eliminate the virus from the body nor eliminate the threat of the clinical symptoms of AIDS. A new strategy is required in order to successfully combat the threat of HIV.

[0020] Dialysis is generally thought of as a means of removing waste products in patients whose kidneys are no longer capable of effectively filtering the blood and eliminating waste from the body. One option immediately available to reduce the load of HIV virions circulating in the blood would be to physically remove HIV virions from the blood by utilizing a surrogate target to engage HIV. Dialysis utilizes the fact that waste products in the blood are smaller in size than blood cells, therefore by passing blood by a porous filter, blood cells and large proteins can be retained while waste products are separated from the blood cells. Reducing the load of HIV virions circulating in the blood reduces the number of T-Helper cells becoming infected with HIV and forestalls the onset of AIDS.

[0021] HIV virions are much smaller in size than red blood cells and white blood cells that circulate in the blood. The blood cells, when removed from the blood, leave the fluid portion of the blood which is often referred to as plasma. Once the cells have been removed, the fluid portion of the blood could be filtered and HIV separated from the plasma. The gp120 and gp 41 probes located on the surface of HIV are seeking to engage the CD4 and CXCR4 or CCR5 cell-surface receptors located on T-Helper cells. A filter device could be fashioned to be comprised of a chamber of circulating exogenous T-Helper cells coalesced as a collection of T-Helpers previously removed from the patient or a collection of T-Helpers pooled from blood bank donors or a collection of T-Helper cells artificially cultured outside the human body. Blood plasma taken from a patient infected with HIV would be introduced into the filter chamber as simultaneously blood plasma would be removed from the filter chamber. As blood plasma passes through the filter chamber, HIV would come in contact with the collection of exogenous T-Helper cells. As HIV's glycoprotein probes engaged the cell-surface receptors mounted on the exogenous T-Helper cells present in the chamber, the HIV virions would adhere to the exogenous T-Helper cells and either become stuck to the T-Helper cells thus being retained in the filter chamber as the blood plasma exited the chamber, or by the action of the HIV probes engaging the T-Helper cell's cell-surface receptors HIV would eject its genome thus making it incapable of infecting an endogenous T-Helper cell in the patient. The patient's blood plasma, now cleared of infectious HIV virions, could be infused back into the patient.

[0022] The technology to make such filtering mechanisms is readably available and could be quickly implemented for worldwide use to treat patients infected with HIV.

[0023] A quantity of T-Helper cells has a limited life-span and requires special handling measures to insure the T-Helper cells do not become metabolically inactive and then deteriorate to a point where they are ineffective as a filtering mechanism. A method to accomplish the same task without having to incorporate healthy T-Helper cells would be construct a filter mechanism that houses a material comprised only of the surface materials of a naturally occurring T-Helper cell, since, specifically, it is the cell-surface receptors that HIV virions' probes are seeking. The surface or outer membrane, often referred to as the plasma membrane, of a T-Helper cell is a lipid bilayer. Sheets or strips or spheres of lipid bilayer constructed with a large quantity of CD4, CXCR4 and CCR5 cell-surface receptors affixed to the surface, could be utilized, in place of T-Helper cells, as a surrogate target to attract and engage HIV virions. Since such sheets or strips or spheres of lipid bilayer are not necessarily metabolically active, the storage time may be significantly lengthened in comparison to metabolically active T-Helper cells. Similar to the design of a cell, a sphere comprised of lipid bilayer surface, attached to this surface a large quantity of CD4, CXCR4 and CCR5 cell-surface receptors, could be used as a surrogate target for HIV virions. A sphere comprised of a lipid bilayer shell or surface, with cell-surface receptors attached to the outer surface could potentially be stored and retain their viability for a much longer period of time than metabolically active T-Helper cells.

[0024] A filter device comprised of a filter chamber could be constructed in a manner where one or more sheets of lipid bilayer, or one or more strips of lipid bilayer, or a quantity of lipid bilayer spheres, each form of lipid bilayer constructed with a large quantity of CD4, CXCR4 and CCR5 cell-surface receptors, would be placed inside a filter chamber. Blood or blood plasma could be caused to pass through the filter chamber. As the blood or blood plasma passes across the surface of a sheet of lipid bilayer or strip of lipid bilayer or a sphere comprised of lipid bilayer material HIV virions would come in contact with CD4, CXCR4 and CXR5 cell-surface receptors present on the surface of the lipid bilayer material and engage the cell-surface receptors. The HIV virions making contact with the lipid bilayer material would either permanently adhere to the lipid bilayer material or by engaging the cell-surface receptors on the lipid bilayer material the HIV virions would be caused to eject their genome, which would neutralize the infectious threat of the HIV virions. The blood or blood plasma exiting the filter chamber would be cleared of HIV virions capable of infecting a T-Helper cell. This blood or blood plasma would then be reintroduced back into a body.

[0025]   Since HIV virions are searching their environment for CD4, CXCR4 and CXR5 cell-surface receptors a filter material comprised of any hypoallergenic material with CD4, CXCR4 and CXR5 cell-surface receptors or the protein portion of these receptors attached to the surface of the material could be placed inside the filtering chamber and act as an effective filter medium. Blood or blood plasma could be caused to pass through the filter chamber. As the blood or blood plasma passes across the surface of the hypoallergenic filter medium, HIV virions would come in contact with CD4, CXCR4 and CXR5 cell-surface receptors present on the surface of the hypoallergenic medium and engage the cell-surface receptors. The HIV virions making contact with the cell-surface receptors would either permanently adhere to the hypoallergenic filter medium or by engaging the cell-surface receptors on the hypoallergenic filter medium the HIV virions would be caused to eject their genome, which would neutralize the infectious threat of the HIV virions. The blood or blood plasma exiting the filter chamber would be cleared of HIV virions capable of infecting a T-Helper cell. This blood or blood plasma would then be reintroduced back into a body.

[0026]   White blood cells are physically larger than red blood cells. Bacteria are generally much smaller than red blood cells. HIV virions are much smaller than bacteria. HIV is comprised of an outer envelope, an internal capsid and the viral genome. Because of its small size HIV can potentially maneuver into places in the tissues where mobile cells are unable to go.

[0027]   An approach to managing HIV would be to create a product that would be relatively the same size as HIV so that the product could penetrate into every location that HIV might migrate. HIV's probes are seeking the CD4 and CCR5 and

CXCR4 cell-surface receptors of a T-Helper cell, thus a product to challenge HIV could be equipped with the same cell-surface receptors as would be found on a naturally occurring T-Helper cell.

[0028]   Utilizing genetic machinery and a colony of T-Helper cells or a colony of hybrid T-Helper cells or a colony of host cells, a product approximately the size of a HIV virion could be manufactured in a similar manner as how HIV naturally replicates, except the product would carry T-Helper cell cell-surface receptors CD4, CXCR4 and/or CCR5 instead of the glycoprotein probes associated with a naturally occurring HIV virion. The product would be constructed either with no genetic information present inside the capsid or genetic material to act as a filler substance, this genetic material being inert such that it could not carry out any useful function except that of acting as a filler.   Such a filler material would help the structure retain a spherical shape.

[0029]   Constructing a virus-like structure, with the surface characteristics of a virus, that has affixed to its exterior cell-surface receptors intended to engage a virus, is referred to as a Scientifically Modulated And Reprogrammed Target (SMART) virus. Such a structure could be simply a sphere of lipid bilayer material will cell-surface receptors attached to the outer surface as described previously, or such structures may carry a filler substance in order to maintain and retain the integrity of the shape of the structure.   Spheres comprised of lipid bilayer material may require a filler substance to retain their spherical shape if the size of the structure becomes very large. Copies of such a SMART virus could be placed in a filter chamber. The diameter of the SMART virus could be increased to a size larger than the naturally occurring HIV virion to facilitate containing the SMART virus inside the filter chamber as the blood or blood plasma passes through the filter chamber. Blood or blood plasma could be passed through the filter chamber containing a quantity of SMART virus. The SMART virus would be available within the walls of the chamber to engage HIV virions as the blood or blood plasma passed through the filter chamber. As HIV virions made contact with SMART viruses the HIV virions would engage the SMART viruses and become permanently attached and become trapped inside the chamber, or a HIV virion, upon engaging a SMART virus, would harmlessly eject the genetic material the HIV virion carries. Either trapping the HIV virion inside the filter chamber or causing the HIV virion to eject the genetic material that it carries, would neutralize the virulence of HIV and assist in managing the threat of AIDS.

BRIEF SUMMARY OF THE INVENTION

[0030]   Initially the Human Immunodeficiency Virus is attracted to its host, the T-Helper cell, by having its surface probes seek out a CD4 cell-surface receptor. Once a HIV virion's gp 120 probe successfully engages a CD4 cell-surface receptor a conformation change occurs in the gp 120 probe and a gp 41 probe attempts to engage either a CXCR4 or a CCR5 cell-surface receptor located on the target T-Helper cell. Described here is a device that simulates the target the HIV virions are seeking. It is a device intended to remove infectious Human Immunodeficiency Virus virions from a fluid such as blood or blood plasma. Blood is removed from a patient and this blood enters a filter chamber that contains a filter medium. As the blood transits through the filter chamber the blood makes contact with the filter medium present in the filter chamber. As the blood transits the filter chamber any HIV virions present in the blood have the opportunity to engage the three cell-surface receptors including the CD4 cell-surface receptor, the CCR5 cell-surface receptor and the CXCR4 cell-surface receptor which are well known to the medical and scientific community due to the fact they appear naturally on the surface of the Human T-Helper cell. Since the HIV virion engaged cell-surface receptors located on the surface of the filter medium rather than located on the surface of an endogenous T-Helper cell inside the body, the infectious nature of the HIV virions is neutralized by either the HIV virion becoming trapped inside the filter chamber by being attached the filter medium or the HIV virion is caused to harmlessly eject its genome. When HIV virions become trapped inside the filter chamber they are incapable of successfully engaging endogenous T-Helper cells inside the body. When a HIV virion is caused to eject its genome, the HIV virion is incapable of infecting T-Helper cell inside the body with its genome an endogenous. Trapping the HIV virion or causing the HIV virion to harmlessly eject its genome leads to neutralizing the infectious threat of HIV, which leads to effectively averting AIDS.

DETAILED DESCRIPTION OF THE INVENTION

[0031] The invention described herein is intended to filter infectious Human Immunodeficiency Virus virions from a fluid such as blood or blood plasma. The filtering process may be dynamic such as blood is actively removed from an individual, the blood transits through one or more filtering devices and the cleansed blood is then returned to the same individual. The filtering process may be more static in how it is conducted, where a specific quantity of blood is removed from one individual, the blood products are filtered through one or more filtering devices and this blood or separate blood products now cleansed of infectious HIV virions are, at a later time, infused into one or more individuals in need of such blood products.

[0032] Three cell-surface receptors CD4, CCR5 and CXCR4 are well known to the medical and scientific community and appear naturally on the surface of the Human T-Helper cells. The HIV virion expresses glycoprotein 120 (gp 120) probes and glycoprotein 41 (gp 41) probes on its outer envelope. HIV utilizes the T-Helper cell as its host cell for the purposes of replication.

[0033] In completing the virus's natural reproductive-cycle, HIV utilizes gp 120 probes positioned on the exterior envelope of a HIV virion to locate and engage a T-Helper cell's CD4 exterior cell-surface receptor. Once a HIV's gp 120 probe has successfully engaged a CD4 cell-surface receptor, a HIV virion's gp 41 probe engages either a CCR5 or CXCR4 exterior cell-surface receptor located on the T-Helper cell. A filter medium present inside the chamber of a filter device, expressing CD4, CCR5 and CXCR4 cell-surface receptors offers the target cell-surface receptors the HIV virions are seeking to engage. When a HIV virion's probes encounter a filter medium expressing CD4, CCR5 and CXCR4 cell-surface receptors, HIV's gp 120 probes would engage CD4 exterior surface receptors, then a HIV's gp 41 probe will engage either a CCR5 or CXCR4 exterior cell-surface receptor. Once the HIV gp 120 and gp 41 probes have engaged their respective receptors on the filter medium's exterior surface, the HIV is fixed to the surface of the filter medium and the HIV virion may eject its RNA genome payload. Since the HIV engaged a filter medium inside the filtering device the HIV virion becomes trapped inside the filter device and if the HIV virion ejects its RNA genome, the threat of the HIV virion being able to infect an endogenous T-Helper cell inside a body is effectively neutralized. The fluid, such as blood plasma, passing through such a filter becomes cleared of infectious HIV virions.

[0034] The medical device described herein, intended to remove infectious HIV virions from blood plasma, is comprised of a chamber, where blood plasma is introduced into the chamber at one location, the blood plasma comes into contact with a filter medium, the blood plasma exits the chamber at a different location than where the blood plasma entered the chamber. The filter medium inside the filter chamber may be comprised of several different materials and designs. The filter medium is intended to make available cell-surface receptors including CD4, CCR5 and CXCR4 for HIV virions to engage. The filter medium may be comprised of a quantity of exogenous T-Helper cells. The filter medium may be comprised of a quantity of lipid bilayer sheets which are comprised of similar materials as found existing as the outer membrane of a T-Helper cell, and affixed to the said lipid bilayer sheets are glycoprotein cell-surface receptors including a quantity of CD4 cell-surface receptors, CXCR4 cell-surface receptors, CCR5 cell-surface receptors. Such bilayer sheets may be of any suitable shape which might include such shapes as the shape of a square, the shape of a rectangle, the sheet may be attached to itself to be the shape of a cylinder. The filter medium may be comprised of a quantity of lipid bilayer strips which are comprised of similar materials as found existing as the outer membrane of a T-Helper cell, and affixed to the said lipid bilayer strips are cell-surface receptors including a quantity of CD4 cell-surface receptors, CXCR4 cell-surface receptors, CCR5 cell-surface receptors. Such strips may be long and thin with the dimension of the length greater than the dimension of the width, and may include any suitable shape such as a long thin strand or the shape of a coil or one end may be attached to another end to form the shape of a ring or circle. The filter medium may be comprised of a quantity of lipid bilayer spheres which are comprised of similar materials as found existing as the outer membrane of a T-Helper cell, and affixed to the said lipid bilayer spheres are cell-surface receptors including a quantity of CD4 cell-surface receptors, CXCR4 cell-surface receptors, CCR5 cell-surface receptors. The shapes of the spheres may include any suitable shape such as the shape of a ball, the shape of cylinder, the shape of an ellipsoid. The filter medium may be comprised of a quantity of modified viruses or virus-like structures with cell-surface receptors to include a quantity of CD4 cell-surface receptors, CXCR4 cell-surface receptors, CCR5 cell-surface receptors. The filter medium may be comprised of any suitable hypoallergenic material, which can be affixed to the surface a quantity of CD4 cell-surface receptors, CXCR4 cell-surface receptors, CCR5 cell-surface receptors or simply the protein portion of the CD4 cell-surface receptors, CXCR4 cell-surface receptors, CCR5 cell-surface receptors. The shape of the hypoallergenic material may include a variety of suitable shapes including the shape of a sheet, shape of a strip or shape of a sphere.

[0035]   The material to be used to create the walls of such a filter chamber may include any suitable material such as glass, rigid plastic, a flexible plastic, latex, steel, aluminum or other metal or metal alloy. A tube to carry blood or blood plasma to the filter chamber would be attached to the portal where the blood or blood plasma would enter the filter chamber. A tube would be attached to the portal of the filter chamber where the blood or blood plasma would exit the chamber to carry the filtered blood or blood plasma away from the chamber. The tubing carrying blood or blood plasma to the filter chamber and the tubing carrying blood or blood plasma away from the filter chamber would be comprised of materials such as a flexible plastic, rigid plastic, a flexible metal or a rigid metal or latex. A porous barrier located at the portal where the blood or blood plasma enters the filter chamber and a porous barrier located at the portal where the blood or blood plasma exits the filter chamber would be comprised of materials such as a flexible plastic, a rigid plastic, a flexible metal or a rigid metal or latex. The said porous barriers are comprised of a quantity of holes, said holes large enough to allow said blood or blood plasma to freely enter and exit said chamber, but said holes are restrictive enough so as to retain said filter medium inside the inner boundaries of said chamber as said blood or blood plasma transits through said chamber.

[0036]   To carry out the process to manufacture a modified medically therapeutic virus or virus-like structure, DNA or RNA code that would provide the necessary biologic instructions to generate the general physical outer structures of the modified virus or virus-like structure, would be inserted into a host. The host may include devices such as a host cell or a hybrid host cell. The host may utilize DNA or RNA or a combination of genetic instructions in order to accomplish the construction of medically therapeutic modified virus virions or virus-like structures. In some cases DNA or messenger RNA would be inserted into the host that would be coded to cause the production of cell-surface receptors that would be affixed to the surface of the modified virus virion or virus-like structure that would target the glycoprotein probes affixed to the surface of an HIV virion. The copies of the medically therapeutic modified viruses or medically therapeutic virus-like structures, upon exiting the host, would be collected, stored and utilized as a filter medium in the described filter chamber as necessary.

[0037] The medically therapeutic version of the modified virus and virus-like structures would be incapable of replication on its own due to the fact that the messenger RNA that would code for the replication process to produce copies of the virus or virus-like structure would not be present in the modified form of a virus or virus-like structure.

[0038] Lipid bilayer sheets, strips, spheres can be manufactured and combinations of CD4 cell-surface receptors, CXCR4 cell-surface receptors, and CCR5 cell-surface receptors can be affixed to the surface with the structure acting as a filter medium. Sheets of any suitable hypoallergenic material can be manufactured and combinations of CD4 cell-surface receptors, CXCR4 cell-surface receptors, and CCR5 cell-surface receptors can be affixed to the surface with the structure acting as a filter medium. Sheets of any suitable hypoallergenic material can be manufactured and combinations of the protein portion of the CD4 cell-surface receptors, CXCR4 cell-surface receptors, and CCR5 cell-surface receptors attached to the surface of the hypoallergenic surface and made available to engage the glycoprotein probes affixed to the surface of HIV virions with the structure acting as a filter medium.

[0039] The invention described herein is intended to filter infectious Human Immunodeficiency Virus virions from a fluid such as blood or blood plasma. The filtering process may be dynamic such as blood that is actively removed from an individual, the blood transits through one or more filtering devices and the cleansed blood is then returned to the same individual. In the filtering process as the blood from the individual makes contact with the filter medium inside the filter chamber to filter out or neutralize HIV virions present in blood or blood plasma. Blood cleansed of infectious HIV virions is returned to the same individual.

[0040]   The filter device may be used in a more static process, where a specific quantity of blood is removed from one individual, the blood products transit through one or more filtering devices and this now cleansed blood or separate blood products are, at a later time, infused into one or more other individuals in need of such cleansed blood products. The blood permanently removed from the first individual makes contact with the filter medium inside the filter chamber which filters out or neutralizes HIV virions present in blood or blood plasma. Blood removed from the first individual, now cleansed of infectious HIV virions, is then provided to one or more other individuals requiring such blood products.

CLAIMS: Reserved.

A2: ANTI-HUMAN IMMUNODEFICIENCY VIRUS SURRO-GATE TARGET AGENT TECHNOLOGY FILTER INTENDED TO TERMINATE T-HELPER CELLS INFECTED WITH THE HUMAN IMMUNODEFICIENCY VIRUS CIRCULATING IN BLOOD

INDIVIDUALS REQUESTING PATENT: Dr. Lane B. Scheiber, ScD and Dr. Lane B. Scheiber II, MD

NUMBER OF CLAIMS: 3 independent claims, 20 dependent claims

ABSTRACT

The Human Immunodeficiency Virus poses a significant threat to the world's population. Current strategies have not been adequate to contain and eradicate this deadly viral infection. HIV utilizes a T–Helper cell as a host to generate replicas of itself. Reversing HIV's own biologically deadly tactics and developing blood filtering techniques that incorporate filter mediums that engage the cell-surface receptors uniquely located on the surface of a T-Helper cell infected with the HIV genome can lead to terminating the infected T-Helper cells. Filter mediums possessing cell-surface receptors intended to terminate infected T-Helper cells by triggering apoptosis, is an effective means to eliminate HIV's host cells and thus provides a valuable strategy to prevent and treat AIDS. Similar techniques can be utilized to terminate other types of cells that act as hosts for pathogens as well as terminating cancer cells.

BACKGROUND OF THE INVENTION

1. Field of the Invention

[0001] This invention relates to any medical device that is utilized to filter the blood of a patient infected with the Human Immunodeficiency Virus with the intention of terminating T-Helper cells infected with the Human Immunodeficiency Virus genome.

2. Description of Background Art

[0002] It is estimated by the Center for Disease Control that in the United States 55,000 to 60,000 new cases of Human Immunodeficiency Virus (HIV) are occurring each year. It is thought that there are 900,000 people currently infected with HIV in the United States, with many victims not aware that they have contracted the virus. Further, it has been estimated that the Human Immunodeficiency Virus (HIV), the pathogen that causes Acquired Immune Deficiency Syndrome (AIDS), has infected as many as 30-60 million people around the globe.

[0003] The presence of HIV was first came to the attention of those in the United States in 1981, when there appeared an outbreak of Kaposi's Sarcoma and Pneumocystis carinii pneumonia in gay men in New York and California. After over twenty-five years of research and investigation, eradicating the ever growing global humanitarian crisis posed by the HIV remains an elusive goal for the medical community. It is estimated the virus has already killed 25 million citizens of this planet.

[0004] The Human Immunodeficiency Virus has been previously referred to as human T-Lymphotrophic virus III (HTLV-III), lymphadenopathy-associated virus (LAV), and AIDS-associated retrovirus (ARV). Infection with HIV may occur by the virus being transferred by blood, semen, vaginal fluid, or breast milk. Four major means of transmission of HIV include unprotected sexual intercourse, contaminated needles, breast milk, and transmission from an infected mother to her baby at birth.

[0005] HIV is an ingeniously constructed very deadly virus, which represents the most challenging pathogen the worldwide medical community faces to date. Viruses in general, have been difficult to contain and eradicate due to the fact they are obligate parasites and tend not to carry out any biologic functions outside the cell the virus has targeted as its host. A virus when it exists outside the boundaries of a cell is generally referred to as a virion. HIV virions posses several attributes that make them very elusive and difficult to destroy.

[0006] Bacterial infections have posed an easier target for the medical community to eradicate from the body. Bacteria generally live and reproduce outside animal cells. Bacteria, like animal cells, carryout biologic functions. A large multi-celled organism such as the human body combats bacterial infections with a combined force of white cells, antibodies, complements and its lymphatic system. White cells circulate the body in search of bacteria. When a white cell encounters a bacterium, the white cell engulfs the bacterium, encapsulates the pathogen, processes the identification of the pathogen and kills the pathogen utilizing acids and destructive enzymes. The white cell then alerts the B-cells of the immune system as to the identity of the intruding bacterium. A subpopulation of B-cells is generated, dedicated to producing antibodies directed against the particular pathogen the circulating white cell encountered and identified. Antibodies, generated by B-cells, traverse the blood and body tissues in search of the bacteria they were designed to repel. Once an antibody encounters a bacterium it is targeted to attack, the antibody attaches to the bacterium's outer wall. The effect antibodies have in coating the outside of a bacterium is to assist the white cells and the other components of the immune system in recognizing the bacterium, so that appropriate defensive action can be taken against the pathogen. Some antibodies, in addition to coating the bacterium, will act to punch holes through the bacterium's outer wall. If the integrity of the bacterium's cell wall is breached, this action generally leads to the death of the bacterium. Complements are primitive protein structures that circulate the blood stream in search of anything that appears consistent with a bacteria cell wall. Complements are indiscriminant. Once the complement proteins locate any form of bacterial cell wall, the complement proteins organize, and much like antibodies, act in concert to punch one or more holes though a bacterium's cell wall to compromise the viability of the bacterium. The lymphatic system is a diffuse network of thin walled vessels that drain excess water from extracellular fluids and join to form the thoracic duct and right lymph duct, which empty into the venous system near the heart. Lymph nodes are present at different locations in the body and screen the fluid transiting the lymphatic system, called lymph, to remove pathogens. Cells in the spleen screen the blood in search of bacteria. When a bacterial pathogen is identified, such as by antibodies coating the surface, the bacterium is taken out of circulation and terminated.

[0007] Viruses pose a much different infectious vector to the body's defense system than either bacteria or cellular parasites. Since viruses do not carry out biologic processes outside their host cell, a virus can be destroyed, but they cannot be killed. A virus is simply comprised of one or more external shells and a portion of genetic material. The virus's genetic information is carried in the core of the virus. Antibodies can coat the exterior of a virus to make it easier for the white cells in the body to identify the viral pathogen, but the action of punching holes in the virus's external shell by antibodies or complement proteins does not necessarily kill the virus. Viruses also only briefly circulate in the blood and tissues of the body as an exposed entity. Using exterior probes, a virus hunts down a cell in the body that will act as an appropriate host so that the virus can replicate. Once the virus has found a proper host cell, the virus inserts its genome into the host cell. To complete its life-cycle, the virus's genetic material takes command of cellular functions and directs the host cell to make replicas of the virus.

[0008] Once the virus's genome has entered a host cell, the virus is in effect shielded from the body's immune system defense mechanisms. Inside a host cell, the presence of the virus is generally only represented as genetic information incorporated into the host cell's DNA. Once a virus has infected a cell in the body, the presence of the virus can only be eradicated if the host cell is destroyed. Antibodies and complements are generally designed not to attack the autologous tissues of the body. Circulating white cells and the immune cells which comprise lymph nodes and the spleen may or may not recognize that a cell, which has become a host for a virus, is infected with a virus's genome. If the immune system fails to identify a cell that has become infected with a virus, the virus's genetic material can proceed to force the infected cell to make copies of the virus. Since a virus is in essence simply a segment of genetic material, time is of no consequence to the life-cycle of the virus and a virus's genome may be carried for years by the host without a need to activate; such viruses are often termed latent viruses. A virus's genetic material may sit idle in a host cell for an extended period of time until the pathogen's programming senses the time is right to initiate the virus's replication process or an action of the host cell triggers the virus to replicate. The only opportunity for the immune system to destroy a latent virus is when copies of the virus leave the host cell and circulate in the blood or tissues in search of another perspective host cell.

[0009] The traditional medical approach to combating infectious agents such as bacteria and cellular parasites, therefore has limited value in managing or eradicating elusive or latent viral infections. Synthetic antibiotics, generally used to augment the body's capacity to produce naturally occurring antibodies against bacterial infections, have little success in combating latent viral infections. Stimulating the body's immune system's recognition of a virus by administering a vaccine also has had limited success in combating elusive viral infections. Vaccines generally are intended to introduce to the body pieces of a bacteria or virus, or an attenuated, noninfectious intact bacteria or virus so that the immune system is able to recognize and process the infectious agent and generate antibodies directed to assist in killing the pathogen. Once the immune system has been primed to recognize an intruder, antibodies will be produced by the immune system in great quantities in an effort to repel an invader. Over time, as the immune system down-regulates its antibody production in response to a lack of detecting the presence of the intruding pathogen, the quantity of antibodies circulating in the blood stream may decrease in number to a quantity that is insufficient to combat a pathogen. Since antibodies have limited value in combating some of the more elusive viruses that hibernate in host cells, vaccines have limited value in destroying latent viruses.

[0010]   The Human Immunodeficiency Virus demonstrates four factors which make this pathogen particularly elusive and a difficult infectious agent to eradicate from the body. First: the host for HIV is the T-Helper cell. The T-Helper cell is a key element in the immune system's response since it helps coordinate the body's defensive actions against pathogens seeking to invade the body's tissues. In cases of a bacterial infection versus a viral infection, T-Helper cells actively direct which immune cells will rev-up in response to the infectious agent and engage the particular pathogen. Since HIV infects and disrupts T-Helper cells, coordination of the immune response against the virus is disrupted, thus limiting the body's capacity to mount a proper response against the presence of the virus and produce a sufficient action to successfully eradicate the virus.

[0011]   Second: again, latent viruses such as HIV, have a strategic advantage. When the immune system first recognizes a pathogen and begins to generate antibodies against a particular pathogen, the response is generally robust. Once time has passed and the immune system fails to detect an active threat, the production of antibodies against the particular pathogen diminishes. When HIV infects a T-Helper cell, the viral genome may lay dormant, sometimes for years before taking command of the T-Helper cell's biologic functions. HIV may, therefore, generate a very active initial immune response to its presence, but if the virus sits dormant inside T-Helper cells for months or years, the antibody response to the virus will diminish over time. There may not be an adequate quantity of circulating antibodies to actively engage the HIV virions as they migrate from the T-Helper cell that generated the copies to uninfected T-Helper cells that will serve as a new host to support further replication. If the immune system's response is insufficient during the period while the virus is exposed and vulnerable, it becomes extremely difficult for the body to eradicate the virus.

[0012] Third, when replicas of the Human Immunodeficiency Virus are released from their host cell, during the budding process the HIV virion coats itself with an exterior envelope comprised of a portion of the plasma membrane from the T-Helper cell that acted as the host for the virus. A T-Helper cell's plasma membrane is comprised of a lipid bilayer, a double layer of lipid molecules oriented with their polar ends at the outside of the membrane and the nonpolar ends in the membrane interior. The virus thus, in part, takes on an external appearance of a naturally occurring cell in the body. Since the exterior envelope of a HIV virion has the characteristics of a T-Helper cell it is more difficult for the immune system to recognize that it is a pathogen as it migrates through the body in search of another T-Helper cell to infect.

[0013] Fourth, the Human Immunodeficiency Virus exhibits a very elusive mode of action which the virus readily utilizes to actively defeat the body's immune system. HIV carries in its genome a segment of genetic material that directs an infected T-Helper cell to create and mount on the surface the plasma membrane a FasL cell-surface receptor. Healthy T-Helper cells carry on the surface of their plasma membrane Fas cell-surface receptors. The Fas cell-surface receptor when engaged by a FasL cell-surface receptor on another cell, initiates apoptosis in the cell carrying the Fas cell-surface receptor. Apoptosis is a biologic process that causes a cell to terminate itself. A T-Helper cell infected with the HIV virus carrying a FasL cell-surface receptor is therefore capable of killing noninfected T-Helper cells that the infected T-Helper cell encounters as it circulates the body. The occurrence of AIDS is therefore propagated not only by the number of T-Helper cells that become incapacitated due to direct infection by HIV, but also by the number of noninfected T-Helper cells that are eliminated by coming in direct contact with infected T-Helper cells.

[0014] Acquired Immune Deficiency Syndrome (AIDS) occurs as a result of the number of circulating T-Helper cells declining to a point where the immune system's capacity to mount a successful response against opportunistic infectious agents is significantly compromised. The number of viable T-Helper cells declines either because they become infected with the HIV virus or because they have been killed by encountering a T-Helper cell infected with HIV. When there is an insufficient population of non-HIV infected T-Helper cells to properly combat infectious agents such as Pneumocystis carinii or cytomegalo virus or other pathogens, the body becomes overwhelmed with the opportunistic infection and the patient becomes clinically ill. In cases where the combination of the patient's compromised immune system and medical assistance in terms of synthetic antibiotics intended to combat the opportunistic pathogens, fluids, intravenous nutrition and other treatments are not sufficient to sustain life, the body succumbs to the opportunistic infection and death ensues.

[0015] The Human Immunodeficiency Virus locates its host by utilizing probes located on its envelope. The HIV virion has two types of glycoprotein probes attached to the outer surface of its exterior envelope. A glycoprotein is a structure comprised of a protein component and a lipid component. HIV utilizes a glycoprotein 120 (gp 120) probe to locate a CD4 cell-surface receptor on the plasma membrane of a T-Helper cell. The plasma membrane of the T-Helper cell is comprised of a lipid bilayer. Cell-surface receptors are anchored in the lipid bilayer. Once an HIV gp 120 probe has successfully engaged a CD4 cell-surface receptor on a T-Helper cell a conformational change occurs in the gp 120 probe and a glycoprotein 41 (gp 41) probe is exposed. The gp 41 probe's intent is to engage a CXCR4 or CCR5 cell-surface receptor on the plasma membrane of the same T-Helper cell. Once a gp 41 probe on the HIV virion engages a CXCR4 or CCR5 cell-surface receptor, the HIV virion opens an access portal through the T-Helper cell's plasma membrane.

[0016] Once the virus has gained access to the T-Helper cell by opening a portal through the cell's outer membrane the virion inserts two positive strand RNA molecules approximately 9500 nucleotides in length. Inserted along with the RNA strands are the enzymes reverse transcriptase, protease and integrase. Once the virus's genome gains access to the interior of the T-Helper cell, in the cytoplasm the pair of RNA molecules are transformed to deoxyribonucleic acid by the reverse transcriptase enzyme. Following modification of the virus's genome to DNA, the virus's genetic information migrates to the host cell's nucleus. In the nucleus, with the assistance of the integrase protein, the virus's DNA becomes inserted into the T-Helper cell's native DNA. When the timing is appropriate, the now integrated viral DNA, becomes read by the host cell's polymerase molecules and the virus's genetic information commands certain cell functions to carry out the replication process to construct copies of the human deficiency virus.

[0017]   Present anti-viral therapy has been designed to target the enzymes that assist the HIV genome with the replication process.   Anti-viral therapy is intended to interfere with the action of these replication enzymes.   Part of the challenge of eradicating HIV is that once the virus inserts its genome into a T-Helper cell host, the viral genome may lay dormant until the proper circumstances evolve.   The virus's genome may sit idle inside a T-Helper cell for years before becoming activated, causing drugs that interfere with HIV's life cycle to have limited effect on eliminating the virus from the body.   Arresting the replication process does not insure that T-Helper cells infected with HIV do not continue to circulate the body killing noninfected T-Helper cells thus causing the patient to progress to a clinically apparent state of Acquired Immune Deficiency Syndrome and eventually succumbing to an opportunistic infection which eventually results in the death of the individual.

[0018]   The outer layer of the HIV virion is comprised of a portion of the T-Helper cell's outer cell membrane.   In the final stage of the replication process, as a copy of the HIV capsid, carrying the HIV genome, buds through the host cell's plasma membrane, the capsid acquires as its outermost shell a wrapping of lipid bilayer from the host cell's plasma membrane. Vaccines are generally comprised of pieces of a virus or bacterium, or copies of the entire virus or bacterium weakened to the point the pathogen is incapable of causing an infection. These pieces of a pathogen or copies of a nonvirulent pathogen prime the immune system such that a vaccine intent is to cause B-cells to produce antibodies that are programmed to seek out the surface characteristics of the pathogen comprising the vaccine. In the case of HIV, since the surface of the pathogen is an envelope comprised of lipid bilayer taken from the host T-Helper cell's plasma membrane, a vaccine comprised of portions of the exterior envelope of the HIV virions might not only target HIV virions, but might also have deleterious effects on the T-Helper cell population.   Some antibodies produced to combat HIV infections may not be able to tell the difference between an HIV virion and a T-Helper cell, and such antibodies may act to coat and assist in the elimination of both targets. In such a scenario, since such a vaccine might cause a decline in the number of available T-Helper cells, it is conceivable that a vaccine comprised of portions of the external envelope of HIV virions might paradoxically induce clinically apparent AIDS in a patient that a vaccine has been administered.

[0019]   It is clear that the traditional approach of utilizing antibiotics or providing vaccines to stimulate the immune system to produce endogenous antibodies, by themselves, is an ineffective strategy to manage a virus as elusive and deadly as HIV. Drugs that interfere with the replication process of HIV generally slow progression of the infection by the virus, but do not necessarily eliminate the virus from the body nor eliminate the threat of the clinical symptoms of AIDS. A new strategy is required in order to successfully combat the threat of HIV.

[0020]   Dialysis is generally thought of as a means of removing waste products in patients whose kidneys are no longer capable of effectively filtering the blood and eliminating waste from the body. One option immediately available to reduce the load of T-Helper cells infected with the HIV genome circulating in the blood is by engaging them in a filter chamber with a specially constructed filter medium utilizing a reverse logic with regards to how an infected T-Helper cell would engage and kill a non-infected T-Helper cell, and use this action utilized by an infected T-Helper cell to identify T-Helper cells infected by HIV and terminate them.   Reducing the number of HIV infected T-Helper cells would forestall, if not prevent, the onset of AIDS by eliminating T-Helper cells acting as hosts for the virus and eliminating the population of T-Helper cells that act to kill healthy T-Helper cells.

[0021]   As mentioned earlier, HIV carries in its genome a segment of genetic material that directs an infected T-Helper cell to create and mount on its surface a FasL receptor. T-Helper cells carry, on the surface of their cell plasma membrane a Fas receptor. The Fas receptor, when triggered, initiates apoptosis in the cell. Apoptosis is a biologic process that causes a cell to terminate itself. A T-Helper cell infected with the HIV virus is therefore capable of killing noninfected T-Helper cells that the infected T-Helper cell encounters as it circulates the body. The occurrence of AIDS is therefore enhanced not only by the number of T-Helper cells that become incapacitated due to direct infection by the HIV virus, but also by the number of noninfected T-Helper cells that are eliminated by coming in contact with infected T-Helper cells.

[0022]   Fas receptors and FasL receptors could be affixed to a filter medium composed of lipid bilayer material or any hypoallergenic material that cell-surface receptors could be affixed to the outer surface. The lipid bilayer material or the hypoallergenic surface material could be in the shape of a sheet, a strip or a sphere. A sheet could take the shape of a square, a rectangle, or the ends could be attached and the sheet could take the shape of a cylinder. A strip could take the shape of a long thin strand where the length is much greater in dimension than the width, or the shape of a coil, or if the ends are attached the strip could take the shape of a ring or circle. The sphere could take the shape of a ball or a cylinder or an ellipsoid.

[0023]   A lipid bilayer filter medium or a hypoallergenic filter medium with Fas and FasL cell-surface receptors could be used as a filter medium in the filter chamber described in this text. Inside a filter chamber, as blood passed through the chamber, a Fas receptor affixed to the surface of the filter medium would engage a FasL receptor located on an infected T-Helper cell. Once the FasL receptor on the infected T-Helper cell has been engaged by a Fas receptor affixed to the filter medium, a FasL receptor affixed to the same filter medium would then engage a Fas cell-surface receptor on the same infected T-Helper cell. When the filter medium's FasL receptor engages a Fas cell-surface receptor on an infected T-Helper cell this action would cause apoptosis to be triggered in the infected T-Helper cell. Triggering apoptosis in an HIV infected T-Helper cell will cause the cell to kill itself. By terminating HIV infected T-Helper cells, the HIV infection could be prevented from proceeding because by terminating the host cells utilized by HIV, HIV would not be able to replicate itself and HIV virions would no longer emerge to infect additional T-Helper cells.

[0024]   Constructing a virus-like structure, with the surface characteristics of a virus, that has affixed to its exterior cell-surface receptors intended to engage a T-Helper cell, is referred to as a Scientifically Modulated And Reprogrammed Target (SMART) virus. Such a structure could be simply a sphere of lipid bilayer material with cell-surface receptors attached to the outer surface as described previously, or such structures may carry a filler substance in order to maintain the integrity of the shape of the structure. As the size of the spheres comprised of lipid bilayer material is increased, as needed to be utilized as a filter medium, an inert filler substance may be needed to be placed inside the sphere in order for the sphere to retain their spherical shape. Copies of such a SMART virus could be placed in a filter chamber. Such a filler substance inside the virus-like structure may be represented by a protein or a genetic material that would serve no useful purpose other than acting as a filler. The diameter of the SMART virus could be increased to a size larger than the naturally occurring T-Helper cell to facilitate containing the SMART virus inside the filter chamber as the blood passes through the filter chamber. The SMART virus would be available and remain within the walls of the chamber to engage T-Helper cells as the blood transits through the filter chamber.

[0025] Bilayer lipid sheets, hypoallergenic surfaces, scientifically modified and reprogrammed treatment (SMART) viruses otherwise known as virus-like structures, can all be created to act as a filter medium and possess on their surface both Fas and FasL cell-surface receptors. These filter mediums can be fashioned such that the Fas receptor could be physically more prominent than the FasL receptor. The Fas receptor on the surface of a filter medium can be physically mounted further out from the FasL receptor, or in a manner likened as to how HIV is constructed with the gp 120 and gp 41 probes, the Fas receptor may hide the FasL receptor. On the surface of the naturally occurring HIV virion the gp 120 probe covers the gp 41 probe. When the gp 120 probe engages a CD4 cell-surface receptor a conformation change occurs in the gp 120 probe such that the gp 41 probe becomes exposed so that the gp 41 probe can engage either a CXCR4 or CCR5 cell-surface receptor located on the surface of a healthy T-Helper cell. On the surface of a filter medium the Fas receptor would be constructed to be engaged first by an infected T-Helper cell, and once engaged, the FasL receptor affixed to the filter medium would become available to engage a Fas receptor located on an infected T-Helper cell.

[0026] Cell-surface receptors are comprised of a protein portion and a lipid portion. The protein portion acts as the receptor. The lipid portion acts as the anchor to fix the cell-surface receptor into the lipid bilayer on the surface of a cell or on the surface of a HIV virion. The lipid portion of the cell-surface receptor could be altered to adjust the distance the protein portion of the cell-surface receptor is physically from the surface of the lipid bilayer. By adjusting the construction, thereby increasing the length of the lipid portion of the Fas cell-surface receptor, the Fas cell-surface receptor affixed to the filter medium could be fashioned to be engaged before a FasL cell-surface receptor affixed to the filter medium is engaged. Alternately the protein portion of the cell-surface receptor closest to the lipid portion of the cell-surface receptor could be lengthened such that increasing the length of the protein portion of the Fas cell-surface receptor, the Fas cell-surface receptor affixed to the filter medium could be fashioned to be engaged before a FasL cell-surface receptor affixed to the filter medium is engaged. Alternatively, the lipid or protein portion of the FasL cell-surface receptor affixed to the surface of a filter medium could be shortened such that the Fas cell-surface receptor affixed to the filter medium is engaged before a FasL cell-surface receptor affixed to the filter medium could be engaged. The intention of positioning the Fas and FasL cell-surface receptors as described is to evoke the action of the T-Helper cells infected with Human Immunodeficiency Virus genome engaging said cell-surface receptors found on the surface of said filter medium in the manner described will trigger apoptosis inside the T-Helper cells infected with the Human Immunodeficiency Virus genome for the purpose of terminating T-Helper cells infected with the Human Immunodeficiency Virus genome, but because the Fas cell-surface receptor affixed to the filter medium must be engaged before a FasL cell-surface receptor affixed to the filter medium can be engaged, T-Helper cells not infected with HIV and other cells expressing a Fas cell-surface receptor will not be harmed by transiting through the described medical filter device.

[0027] This technology has a much broader range of beneficial medical treatment uses beyond simply eliminating T-Helper cells infected with the HIV genome from the blood. All cells have cell-surface receptors. Many cells in the body have affixed to their surface cell-surface receptors that are unique to the specific type of cell. By utilizing the concept of mounting on a filter medium specialized cell-surface receptors that engage a unique cell-surface receptor located on the surface of a specific target cell circulating in the blood, specific target cells which also express a Fas cell-surface receptor on their surface can be caused to be terminated, with such action resulting a beneficial medical outcome. To accomplish this, on a filter medium would be affixed specialized cell surface receptors and FasL cell-surface receptors. The specialized cell-surface receptors would be constructed to be more prominent than the FasL cell-surface receptors, such that the specialized cell-surface receptors would be engage before a FasL cell-surface receptor could be engaged. As blood transits through a filter chamber with the above-mentioned filter medium contained inside, specific target cells would come in contact with the filter medium. Once the unique cell-surface receptor located on the specific target cell engaged a specialized cell-surface receptor affixed to the filter medium, then the FasL cell-surface receptor affixed to the filter medium would engage a Fas cell-surface receptor on the specific target cell. By the action of the FasL cell-surface receptor affixed to the filter medium engaging the Fas cell-surface receptor located on the specific target cell, the signal of apoptosis would be triggered in the specific target cell and the specific target cell would terminate itself. By physically constructing the cell-surface receptors on the filter medium such that the specialized cell-surface receptor must be engaged before the FasL cell-surface receptors can be engaged, facilitates that cells that do not carry the unique cell-surface receptor such as affixed to the surface of the specific target cell, will not be harmed by transiting through the medical filter device.

[0028] Such a filter device could be used to treat patients with cancers such as various forms of leukemia. Forms of leukemia flood the circulating blood with numerous leukemic cells. The presence of this abundance of leukemic cells interferes with the function of normal blood cells and blood plasma. For several forms of leukemia such as chronic lymphocytic Leukemia (CLL), the medical treatment approach has provided very limited benefit. Often for CLL patients, available chemotherapy treatment produces side effects that are worse than the effects of the CLL on the patient. Patients with CLL often suffer for years with the leukemia adversely affecting their bodies. A filter medium designed to utilize specialized cell-surface receptors to engage one or more unique cell-surface receptors on a leukemic cell, which once a leukemic cell would be engaged, then FasL receptors on the filter medium could engage one or more Fas cell-surface receptors on the leukemic cell, the result of which would be the leukemic cell would receive the signal that would tell the leukemic cell to terminate itself. Successfully terminating leukemic cells would reduce the quantity of circulating leukemic cells. A reduction in the quantity of circulating leukemic cells would improve beneficial performance of blood in such patients.

[0029] Other medical conditions such as parasitic infections, where a parasite has infected a blood cell and the infected blood cell expresses a unique cell-surface receptor and a Fas cell-surface receptor, such an infected cell could be terminated by a similar strategy as described above.

[0030] Any cell that is harmful to the body that circulated in the blood, that carries a unique cell-surface receptor and carries a Fas cell-surface receptor could be terminated by the above-mentioned strategy and thus eliminated from the body, to produce a medically beneficial effect.

[0031] A filter device could be fashioned to be placed inside the body to act to continuously filter the blood and terminate cancer cells of a particular type that transit the blood stream. Concerns regarding metastatic cancer could be treated by such a device. Metastatic cancer occurs when cells from a primary cancer site in the body leave the primary site and migrate through the blood and develop one or more secondary or satellite sites of cancer in the body. Once a person is found to have a cancer, or in an individual who is at high risk for developing metastatic cancer, a filter could be placed in a blood vessel, a vein or an artery, and such a filter would continuously filter the blood and engage only the cancer cells that transit through the filter allowing all other blood cells to pass through unharmed. Knowing the type of cancer the filter was created to engage, the filter medium could be created to have fixed to its surface specialized cell-surface receptors that engage unique cell-surface receptors on the surface of the specific type of targeted cancer cell. A cancer cell of a specific type that transits through the filter would be engaged by the specialized cell-surface receptor affixed to the filter medium. Once the specific type of cancer cell is engaged, a FasL cell-surface receptor located on the filter medium would engage a Fas cell-surface receptor located on the cancer cell and such an action would trigger apoptosis in the cancer cell and the cancer cell would terminate itself. The filter device would not need to be renewed and the filter device would not clog blood flow because the cancer cells would exit the filter chamber, cell death would ensue at a later time and such cells would then eventually be removed from circulation and re-absorb by the body. Such a device could be fashioned to be inserted in a vessel of the lymphatic system to constantly filter lymph and engage and terminate infected T-Helper cells or other specific target cells as they transit through the filter device. Cancers often spread locally from a primary site through the lymphatic system and such a filter device could be inserted into a vessel of the lymphatic system downstream to a primary site of cancer to screen and terminate any cancer cells that had migrated from the primary site of the cancer.

[0032]   Similarly, a patient infected with HIV or patient at high risk for infection with HIV, could have a small filter placed inside their body. Such a filter could continuously screen the blood with the intention that any T-Helper cell infected with the HIV genome that is expressing both FasL and Fas cell-surface receptors that transit though the filter device will be engaged.   Once a Fas cell-surface receptor affixed to the filter medium inside the filter device has been engaged by a FasL cell-surface receptor located on an infected T-Helper cell, a FasL cell-surface receptor affixed to the filter medium would then engage a Fas cell-surface receptor on the infected T-Helper cell. When the filter medium's FasL cell-surface receptor engages a Fas cell-surface receptor located on an infected T-Helper cell this action will cause apoptosis to be triggered in the infected T-Helper cell. Triggering apoptosis in a cell will cause the cell to kill itself. By this means infected T-Helpers, the host cell of HIV, can be continuously eliminated from the body. Such a filter would not need to be renewed and the filter would not clog blood flow because the infected T-Helper cells would exit the filter chamber, cell death would ensue at a later time and such cells would be removed from circulation and be re-absorb by the body.

BRIEF SUMMARY OF THE INVENTION

[0033] A T-Helper cell infected with the Human Immunodeficiency Virus genome express FasL cell-surface receptors and Fas cell-surface receptors on its exterior surface. This medical filter device is intended to engage T-Helper cells circulating in the blood. The filter medium contained inside the filter device has affixed to its surface Fas and FasL cell-surface receptors. The Fas cell-surface receptors affixed to the surface of the filter medium located inside the device are more prominent than the FasL cell-surface receptors located on the surface of the filter medium. As infected T-Helper cells transit the filter device, the FasL cell-surface receptors they carry will engage Fas cell-surface receptors affixed to the filter medium. Once a FasL cell-surface receptor on an infected T-Helper cell has engaged a Fas cell-surface receptor affixed to the filter medium, a FasL cell-surface receptor affixed to the filter medium will engage a Fas cell-surface receptor located on the surface of the infected T-Helper cell. By having a FasL cell-surface receptor affixed to the filter medium engage a Fas cell-surface receptor located on an infected T-Helper cell, the process of apoptosis is triggered in the T-Helper cell carrying the Fas cell-surface receptor. Activating the process of apoptosis in a cell leads to cell death. By terminating T-Helper cells that are infected with the Human Immunodeficiency Virus genome leads to an effective means for averting AIDS. A similar strategy utilizing specialized cell-surface receptors and FasL cell-surface receptors can be employed to terminate specific target cells such as cancer cells and cells harboring parasites for the purpose of achieving a beneficial medically therapeutic outcome. A medical device constructed with a filter medium can be fashioned to be placed in a vessel of the lymphatic system which would continuously screen lymph and terminate cancer cells or other target cells to result in a medically beneficial outcome.

DETAILED DESCRIPTION OF THE INVENTION

[0034] The invention described herein is intended to terminate T-Helper cells infected with Human Immunodeficiency Virus and other specific target cells such as cancer cells and host cells harboring parasites, as they circulate in fluid such as blood or lymph. The medical device may be used in an intermittent dynamic process such as where blood is actively removed from an individual, the blood transits through one or more filtering devices and the cleansed blood is then returned to the same individual. The medical device may be used in a process which is more static, where a specific quantity of blood is removed from one individual, the blood products transit through one or more filtering devices and this now cleansed blood or separate blood products are, at a later time, infused into one or more individuals in need of such blood products. The medical device may be used in a continuous dynamic process, where a filter device is inserted in a blood vessel or a lymphatic vessel inside the body, which such a medical device constantly acts to filter the blood or lymph and engage and terminate infected T-Helper cells or other specific target cells as they transit through the filter device.

[0035] The medical device described herein, intended to terminate T-Helper cells infected with HIV genome as they exist in blood, is comprised of a chamber, where blood is introduced into the chamber at one location, the blood comes into contact with a filter medium, the blood exits the chamber at a different location than where the blood plasma entered the chamber. The filter medium inside the filter chamber may be comprised of several different materials and designs. The filter medium is intended to make available cell-surface receptors including Fas and FasL for T-Helper cells infected with HIV genome to engage. The filter medium may be comprised of a quantity of lipid bilayer sheets which are comprised of similar materials as found existing as the outer membrane of a T-Helper cell, and affixed to the said lipid bilayer sheets are glycoprotein cell-surface receptors including a quantity of Fas cell-surface receptors and FasL cell-surface receptors. Such bilayer sheets may be of any suitable shape which might include such shapes as the shape of a square, the shape of a rectangle, the sheet may be attached to itself to be the shape of a cylinder. The filter medium may be comprised of a quantity of lipid bilayer strips which are comprised of similar materials as found existing as the outer membrane of a T-Helper cell, and affixed to the said lipid bilayer strips are glycoprotein cell-surface receptors including a quantity of Fas cell-surface receptors and FasL cell-surface receptors. Such strips may be long and thin and may include any suitable shape such as a long thin strand, or the shape of a coil or one end may be attached to another end to form the shape of a ring or circle. The filter medium may be comprised of a quantity of lipid bilayer spheres which are comprised of similar materials as found existing as the outer membrane of a T-Helper cell, and affixed to the said lipid bilayer spheres are glycoprotein cell-surface receptors including a quantity of Fas cell-surface receptors and FasL cell-surface receptors. The shapes of the spheres may include any suitable shape such as the shape of a ball, the shape of cylinder, the shape of an ellipsoid. The filter medium may be comprised of a quantity of virus-like structures with cell-surface receptors to include a quantity of Fas cell-surface receptors and FasL cell-surface receptors. The filter medium may be comprised of any suitable hypoallergenic material, which can be affixed to the surface a quantity of Fas cell-surface receptors and FasL cell-surface receptors or simply the protein portion of the Fas cell-surface receptors and FasL cell-surface receptors. The shape of the hypoallergenic material may include a variety of suitable shapes including the shape of a sheet, shape of a strip or shape of a sphere.

[0036] The material to be used to create the walls of such a filter chamber may include any suitable hypoallergenic material such as glass, rigid plastic, a flexible plastic, latex, steel, aluminum or other metal or metal alloy. A tube to carry blood or blood plasma to the filter chamber would be attached to the portal where the blood or blood plasma would enter the filter chamber. A tube would be attached to the portal of the filter chamber where the blood or blood plasma would exit the chamber to carry the filtered blood or blood plasma away from the chamber. The tubing carrying blood or blood plasma to the filter chamber and the tubing carrying blood or blood plasma away from the filter chamber would be comprised of any hypoallergenic material such as a flexible plastic, rigid plastic, a flexible metal or a rigid metal or latex. A porous barrier located at the portal where the blood or blood plasma enters the filter chamber and a porous barrier located at the portal where the blood or blood plasma exits the filter chamber would be comprised of materials such as a flexible plastic, a rigid plastic, a flexible metal or a rigid metal or latex. The said porous barriers are comprised of a quantity of holes, said holes large enough to allow said blood or blood plasma to freely exit said chamber, but said holes are restrictive enough so as to retain said filter medium inside the inner boundaries of said chamber as said blood or blood plasma transits through said chamber. The filter medium contained inside the filter chamber may be free-floating within the inner boundaries of the filter chamber or may be physically fixed to the chamber such that the filter medium does not move freely inside the filter chamber and cannot exit the filter chamber.

[0037] Lipid bilayer sheets, strips, spheres can be manufactured and combinations of Fas cell-surface receptors and FasL cell-surface receptors can be affixed to the surface with the entire structure acting as a filter medium. Sheets of any suitable hypoallergenic material can be manufactured and combinations of Fas cell-surface receptors and FasL cell-surface receptors can be affixed to the surface with the structure acting as a filter medium. Sheets of any suitable hypoallergenic material can be manufactured and combinations of the protein portion of the Fas cell-surface receptors and FasL cell-surface receptors attached to the surface of the hypoallergenic surface and made available to engage either glycoprotein probes on HIV or cell-surface receptors on a T-Helper cell, with the structure acting as a filter medium.

[0038] To carry out the process to manufacture a virus-like structure, DNA or RNA code that would provide the necessary biologic instructions to generate the general physical outer structures of the virus-like structure, would be inserted into a host. The host may include devices such as a host cell or a hybrid host cell. The host may utilize DNA or RNA or a combination of genetic instructions in order to accomplish the construction of medically therapeutic virus-like structures. In some cases DNA or messenger RNA would be inserted into the host that would be coded to cause the production of cell-surface receptors that would be affixed to the surface of the virus-like structure that would target the glycoprotein probes affixed to the surface of an HIV virion or the FasL and Fas cell-surface receptors on infected T-Helper cells. The copies of the medically therapeutic virus-like structures, upon exiting the host, would be collected, stored and utilized as a filter medium in the described filter chamber as necessary.

[0039] The medically therapeutic version of the virus-like structures would be incapable of replication on its own due to the fact that the messenger RNA or DNA that would code for the replication process to produce copies of the virus-like structure would not be present in the virus-like structures.

[0040] The medical device intended to terminate T-Helper cells infected with the HIV genome is comprised of a chamber, where blood is introduced into the chamber at one location, the blood comes into contact with a filter medium, the blood exits the chamber at a different location than where the blood entered the chamber. The filter medium inside the filter chamber is fashioned to express on its surface a quantity of Fas cell-surface receptors and FasL cell-surface receptors. The Fas cell-surface receptors are mounted on the surface of the filter medium in a manner that they are to be engaged before the FasL cell-surface receptors can be engaged.

[0041] The invention described herein is intended to terminate T-Helper cells infected with the HIV genome from a fluid such as blood. The filtering process may be intermittently dynamic such as blood that is actively removed from an individual, the blood transits through one or more filtering devices and the cleansed blood is then returned to the same individual. In the filtering process as the blood from the individual makes contact with the filter medium inside the filter device terminates T-Helper cells infected with the HIV virus. Blood cleansed of HIV is returned to the same individual.

[0042] The filter device may be used in a more static process, where a specific quantity of blood is removed from one individual, the blood products transit through one or more filtering devices and this now cleansed blood or separate blood products are, at a later time, infused into one or more other individuals in need of such cleansed blood products. The blood permanently removed from the first individual makes contact with the filter medium inside the filter device terminates T-Helper cells infected with the HIV virus. Blood removed from the first individual, now cleansed of HIV infected T-Helper cells, is then provided to one or more other individuals requiring such blood.

[0043] The medical device may be used in a continuous dynamic process, where a filter device is inserted in a blood vessel inside the body, which constantly acts to constantly filter the blood and engage and terminate infected T-Helper cells as they transit through the filter device.

[0044] This technology has a much broader range of beneficial uses beyond just eliminating T-Helper cells infected with the HIV genome from the blood. All cells have surface cell receptors. Many cells in the body have affixed to their surface cell-surface receptors that are unique to the specific type of cell. By utilizing the concept of mounting on a filter medium specialized cell-surface receptors that engage a unique cell-surface receptor located on the surface of a specific target cell circulating in the blood, specific target cells can be caused to be terminated, with such action resulting a beneficial medical outcome. To accomplish this, on a filter medium would be affixed specialized cell surface receptors and FasL cell-surface receptors. The specialized cell-surface receptors would be constructed to be more prominent than the FasL cell-surface receptors, such that the specialized cell-surface receptors would be engaged before a FasL cell-surface receptor could be engaged. As blood transited through a filter chamber with the above-mentioned filter medium contained inside, specific target cells would come in contact with the filter medium. Once the unique cell-surface receptor on the specific target cell engaged a specialized cell-surface receptor on the filter medium, then the FasL cell-surface receptor on the filter medium would engage a Fas cell-surface receptor on the specific target cell. By the action of the FasL cell-surface receptor affixed to the filter medium engaging the Fas cell-surface receptor located on the specific target cell, the signal of apoptosis would be triggered in the specific target cell and the specific target cell would terminate itself. By constructing the cell-surface receptors on the filter medium such that the specialized cell-surface receptor must be engaged before the FasL cell-surface receptor can be engaged, facilitates that cells that do not carry the unique cell-surface receptor such as affixed to the surface of the specific target cell will not be harmed by transiting through the filter device.

[0045] Such a filter device could be used to treat patients with cancers such as various forms of leukemia. Forms of leukemia flood the circulating blood with numerous leukemic cells. The presence of this abundance of leukemic cells interferes with the function of normal blood cells and blood plasma. For several forms of leukemia such as chronic lymphocytic Leukemia (CLL), the medical treatment approach has provided very limited benefit. Often for CLL patients, available chemotherapy treatment produces side effects that are worse than the effects of the CLL on the patient. Patients with CLL often suffer for years with the leukemia adversely affecting their bodies. A filter medium designed to utilize specialized cell-surface receptors to engage one or more unique cell-surface receptors on a leukemic cell, which once a leukemic cell would be engaged, then FasL receptors on the filter medium could engage one or more Fas cell-surface receptors on the leukemic cell, the result of which would be the leukemic cell would receive the signal that would tell it to terminate itself. Successfully terminating leukemic cells would reduce the quantity of circulating leukemic cells. A reduction in the quantity of circulating leukemic cells would improve beneficial performance of blood.

[0046] Other medical conditions such as parasitic infections, where a parasite has infected a blood cell and the infected blood cell expresses a unique cell-surface receptor and a Fas cell-surface receptor, such an infected cell could be terminated by a similar strategy as described above.

[0047] Any cell that is harmful to the body that circulated in the blood, that carries a unique cell-surface receptor and carries a Fas cell-surface receptor could be terminated by the above-mentioned strategy and thus eliminated from the body, to produce a medically beneficial effect.

[0048] The medical device may be constructed to exist outside the body and engage in an intermittent dynamic process where blood is actively removed from an individual, the blood transits through one or more filtering devices and the cleansed blood is then returned to the same individual. The medical device may be constructed to exist outside the body and engage in a more static process where a specific quantity of blood is removed from one individual, the blood products transit through one or more filtering chambers and this now cleansed blood or separate blood products are, at a later time, is infused into one or more individuals in need of such blood products. The medical device may be constructed as a device to be inserted in a blood vessel inside the body, which the medical device constantly acts to filter the blood and engage and terminate specific target cells such as infected T-Helper cells, cancer cells, host cells infected by a parasite, as such cells transit through the filter device.

[0049] Portions of the lymphatic system can be continuously filtered with such a medical device. Utilizing the concept of mounting on a filter medium specialized cell-surface receptors that engage a unique cell-surface receptor located on the surface of a specific target cell transiting the lymph, specific target cells can be caused to be terminated, with such action resulting a beneficial medical outcome. To accomplish this, on a filter medium would be affixed specialized cell surface receptors and FasL cell-surface receptors. The specialized cell-surface receptors would be constructed to be more prominent than the FasL cell-surface receptors, such that the specialized cell-surface receptors would be engage before a FasL cell-surface receptor could be engaged. As lymph transits through a filter chamber with the above-mentioned filter medium contained inside, specific target cells would come in contact with the filter medium. Once the unique cell-surface receptor on the specific target cell engages a specialized cell-surface receptor on the filter medium, then the FasL cell-surface receptor on the filter medium would engage a Fas cell-surface receptor on the specific target cell. By the action of the FasL cell-surface receptor affixed to the filter medium engaging the Fas cell-surface receptor located on the specific target cell, the signal of apoptosis would be triggered in the specific target cell and the specific target cell would terminate itself. By constructing the cell-surface receptors on the filter medium such that the specialized cell-surface receptor must be engaged before the FasL cell-surface receptor can be engaged, facilitates that cells that do not carry the unique cell-surface receptor such as affixed to the surface of the specific target cell will not be harmed by transiting through the filter device. Such a medical device could be fashioned to be inserted in a vessel of the lymphatic system to constantly filter lymph to engage and terminate infected T-Helper cells or other specific target cells as they transit through the medical device.

CLAIMS: Reserved.

A3: SCIENTIFICALLY MODULATED AND REPROGRAMMED TREATMENT (SMART) VIRUS TECHNOLOGY INTENDED TO NEUTRALIZE THE HUMAN IMMUNODEFICIENCY VIRUS

INDIVIDUALS REQUESTING PATENT: Dr. Lane B. Scheiber, ScD and Dr. Lane B. Scheiber II, MD

NUMBER OF CLAIMS: 18

ABSTRACT

The concept is to combat one of the deadliest infectious diseases known by fighting fire with fire. Scientifically Modulated And Reprogrammed Treatment (SMART) Virus technology is intended to neutralize the Human Immunodeficiency Virus. The SMART Virus carrying combinations of CD4, CCR5 and CXCR4 cell-surface receptors is capable of engaging the HIV's gp 120 and gp 41 exterior probes in an identical manner as would HIV's host, a T-Helper cell. When HIV encounters a SMART Virus the HIV virion would either adhere to the SMART Virus unable to further migrate in search of a T-Helper cell, harmlessly eject its RNA genetic payload or inject its RNA genome into the SMART Virus. Given HIV engaged a SMART Virus rather than a T-Helper cell, the HIV RNA genome becomes unable to infect a T-Helper cell, therefore the threat of Acquired Immunodeficiency Syndrome caused by HIV is averted.

BACKGROUND OF THE INVENTION

Field of the Invention

This invention relates to any medical device intended to physically interact directly with the Human Immunodeficiency Virus (HIV) or other virus to neutralize the capacity of the virus to properly infect its target host cell.

Description of the Background Art

[0001] The Human Immunodeficiency Virus (HIV), which is responsible for Acquired Immunodeficiency Disease Syndrome (AIDS), threatens the lives of approximately 170 millions of people worldwide. There are different strains of HIV that exist around the world. Most predominantly HIV-1 exists worldwide and HIV-2 is generally found in Western Africa, the western coastal regions of India and in Europe. Amongst HIV-1 and HIV-2 they can be further subdivided into different strains including an 'R5' strain which uses a CCR5 cell-surface receptor on a T-Helper cell to identify its host and an 'X4' strain which uses a CXCR4 cell-surface receptor located on a T-Helper cell to identify its host. The approach to controlling this disease has been the application of drugs directed at interfering with the replication process, in an attempt to slow down the rate of replication of the virus. Millions of people continue to die and the virus continues to pose an escalating threat despite current treatment strategies. The virus is generally communicated between individuals by contact with body fluids carrying intact HIV.

[0002] Though there are recognized differences between HIV-1 and HIV-2, for purposes of further discussion the term 'HIV' will refer to both HIV-1 and HIV-2, unless otherwise noted. HIV is a retrovirus with its genetic material in the form of two identical copies of a positive sense single stranded ribonucleic acid (RNA) molecule, each approximately 9500 nucleotides long. HIV is approximately 50 nm in diameter, about one seventieth the size of a white cell carrying the marker Cluster Designation 4 (CD4) exterior cell-surface receptor.

[0003] A eukaryote cell is a nucleated cell. Animal cells generally are comprised of a cell membrane, cytoplasm, a nucleus and organelles. The cell membrane consists of a lipid bilayer where two layers of lipid molecules oriented with their polar ends pointed outside of the membrane and their nonpolar ends points toward the inside of the membrane. Polarized ends of the lipid molecules are hydrophobic, therefore the lipid bilayer functions to control the movement of water, nutrients and hormones in and out of the cell. A variety of receptors affixed to the exterior of the lipid bilayer membrane assist in the cell communicating with its environment. The cytoplasm inside a cell is comprised of amino acids and nutrients, and forms the interior fluid matrix of the cell. The nucleus is surrounded by a double membrane and contains the majority of the cell's genetic material. Organelles are structures generally found in the cytoplasm that perform specialized functions of the cells. Organelles found inside a cell may include the mitochondria, endoplasmic reticulum, Golgi complex, lysosomes, vacuoles.

[0004] Genetic material in a eukaryote is generally in the form of deoxyribonucleic acid (DNA) with the majority located in the nucleus of the cell, but DNA may also be found in the mitochondria of cells. By the process of transcription, a section of the DNA is read by a polymerase and a molecule of ribonucleic acid (RNA) is generated. DNA is comprised of sections of combinations of four nucleotides: adenine, cytosine, guanine, and thymine. When two strands of nucleotides are arranged together, such as in the double helix configuration of chromosomal DNA, adenine on one strand is always matched to thymine in the opposing strand and cytosine on one strand is always matched to guanine in the opposing strand. RNAs that are generated are usually single stranded chains of nucleotides, constructed of similar adenine, cytosine and guanine nucleotides as DNA, but instead of 'thymine', RNAs are constructed with the nucleotide 'uracil'. RNAs are generally divided into three categories including messenger RNA (mRNA), ribosomal RNA (rRNA) and transfer RNA (tRNA). Messenger RNA are considered positive sense and interact with ribosomes to generate protein molecules. Ribosomes read the code physically built into the messenger RNAs, and with the aid of rRNA and tRNA, generate protein molecules by bonding together amino acids in linear configurations as directed by the code on the messenger RNA.

[0005] HIV is approximately spherical in shape and comprised of an outer lipid bilayer envelope, a matrix protein, a capsid, two strands of RNA, nucleocapsid protein and proteins to assist in the replication process. The virus's core or capsid is icosahedral in shape and acts as a protective shell to carry the genetic payload. The capsid is comprised of numerous copies of the capsid protein (p24), the number and arrangement of the capsid proteins determines the overall dimensions of the capsid shell; HIV uses approximately 2,000 p24 to construct its capsid. The capsid carries the two single strands of RNA each containing a copy of the virus's nine genes, the nucleocapsid protein, reverse transcriptase, protease and integrase. The nucleocapsid protein causes the RNA to coil up so that it can fit inside the capsid. The protein matrix consisting of protein 17 (p17) covers the capsid. The HIV envelope is derived from the plasma membrane as the virus buds or pushes through the host cell's plasma membrane as it exits and migrates from the host cell. Anchored in and projecting out from the HIV's lipid bilayer outer membrane, otherwise referred to as an envelope, are exterior probes well known to the medical and scientific community as glycoprotein 120 (gp 120) and glycoprotein 41 (gp 41). The term glycoprotein refers to a protein with a carbohydrate attached. The gp 41 probe is anchored to the outer envelope and is in close proximity to the gp 120 probe. The probes can be found arranged together into protein complexes, which may contain up to three gp 120 probes and three gp 41 probes. Protein complexes have been described as 'spikes'. It has been reported that an HIV outer envelope may project from ten to seventy-two said spikes.

[0006] Viruses are obligate intracellular parasites designed to infect cells often with great specificity to a particular cell type it uses as a host. Viruses do not carry out any biologically active processes on their own when outside a host cell. A virus requires a host in order to reproduce itself. Viruses circulate the environment without the need for nutrition or energy production through respiration. Viruses are in essence a vehicle that carries the genetic programming instructions necessary to cause an appropriate host cell to generate identical copies of the same virus. Some viruses do introduce to their host cells programming instructions that result in toxic effects to the body that has been infected by the virus. HIV transits the environment at large with its surface probes seeking to engage its host, a human T-Helper cell. Human T-Helper cells express a number of receptors on their outer plasma membrane including Cluster Designation 4 (CD4), Chemotactic Chemokine Receptor 5 (CCR5) and CX Chemokine Receptor 4 (CXCR4).

[0007] HIV utilizes the Human T-Helper cell as its host for the purpose of replicating copies of itself. To initiate its reproductive-cycle, the gp 120 probe on a HIV virion makes initial contact with a T-Helper cell's CD4 cell-surface receptor. Virion is a term that refers to a complete structure of a virus as it exists outside of a host cell. Following the engagement of the gp 120 probe with the CD 4 cell-surface receptor, the gp 120 alters its configuration to allow the HIV gp 41 probe to engage a second receptor on the surface of the T-Helper cell, either a CCR5 cell-surface receptor or a CXCR4 cell-surface receptor. Once the HIV virion's gp 120 probe has successfully engaged a T-Helper cell's CD4 and the HIV's gp 41 probe has successfully engaged the T-Helper cell's CCR5 or CXCR4 cell-surface receptor, then the HIV virion is able to transfer its capsid containing the two strands of ribonucleic acid (RNA) and the support proteins including as reverse transcriptase, protease, and integrase into the T-Helper cell. Once the capsid has gained access to the interior of the T-Helper cell, utilizing the transferred HIV enzyme 'reverse transcriptase', the RNA molecules undergo reverse transcription to deoxyribonucleic acid (DNA). Protease helps modify HIV's genome. Aided by the integrase, the virus's RNA transcribed into DNA migrates to the T-Helper cell's nucleus and is inserted into the T-Helper cell's native DNA. The HIV genetic material then redirects the resources of the T-Helper cell to facilitate the manufacture of copies of HIV.

[0008] Most predominantly HIV-1 exists worldwide and HIV-2 is generally found in Western Africa, the western coastal regions of India and Europe. Amongst HIV-1 and HIV-2 that use CD4 as the initial cell-surface receptor to gain entry into a T-Helper cell, they can be further divided by an 'R5' strain which uses a CCR5 cell-surface receptor on a T-Helper cell to identify its host; an 'X4' strain which uses a CXCR4 cell-surface receptor located on a T-Helper cell to identify its host. It is also believed at least one strain of HIV-2 may infect a T-Helper cell without engaging a CD4 cell-surface receptor, but uses either a CCR5 or a CXCR4 cell-surface receptor on a T-Helper cell host. There has also been identified at least one strain of HIV-2 believed not utilize the CD4, CCR5 or the CXCR4 cell-surface receptors to engage a T-Helper cell host, the mode of entry unknown at this time.

[0009] Naturally occurring T-Helper cells, not infected with HIV, help orchestrate the human body's immune response to infectious agents that threaten the health and integrity of the body. The HIV virus, by taking control and altering the function of the T-Helper cells in the body, creates a state of ill health. By redirecting the T-Helper cell's function to produce copies of the HIV virus rather than coordinate appropriate immune responses against potentially infectious agents leaves the body as a whole vulnerable to attack by other infectious agents that can do harm to the tissues of the body. In addition, the HIV genome carries a 'nef' gene. Once the HIV's DNA is inserted into the host cell's native DNA, the nef gene provides instructions for a Fas ligand (FasL) cell-surface marker to be manufactured and expressed on the surface of the infected T-Helper cell. Noninfected T-Helper cells (meaning not infected with HIV) express a Fas cell-surface marker. When a HIV infected T-Helper cell expressing the Fas ligand (FasL) cell-surface marker encounters a Fas cell-surface marker (also referred to as CD95 cell-surface receptor) on a noninfected T-Helper cell, a lethal signal is passed to the noninfected t-Helper cell. When the FasL cell-surface marker engages a Fas cell-surface marker, the process of apoptosis is triggered in the noninfected T-Helper cell. Apoptosis is the natural process of programmed cell death. By triggering apoptosis in noninfected T-Helper cells, HIV infected T-Helper cells are capable of killing the noninfected T-Helper cells they encounter. The clinical ramifications of Acquired Immunodeficiency Syndrome (AIDS) occur when the number of noninfected T-Helper cells declines to the point the immune system is unable to defend the body as a whole from dangerous infectious agents.

[0010] The Scientifically Modulated And Reprogrammed Treatment (SMART) Virus represents a surrogate target for HIV. SMART viruses would engage HIV directly to negate the infectivity of HIV and therefore neutralize the threat of HIV. It appears the HIV infected T-Helper cells pose the threat to a body's immune system by terminating noninfected T-Helper cells, which a critical number are needed to defend the body from infectious agents. Since the clinical characteristics of AIDS appears to coincide more with the decline of non-infected T-Helper cells below a critical number and not necessarily with the number of HIV infected T-Helper cells, controlling the population of HIV infected T-Helper cells or ridding the environment of HIV infected T-Helper cells would be a successful approach to managing AIDS.

BRIEF SUMMARY OF THE INVENTION

[0011] A Scientifically Modulated And Reprogrammed Treatment (SMART) Virus is comprised of an inner capsid similar to the naturally occurring HIV icosahedral capsid. The SMART Virus capsid would be encapsulated with a protein matrix similar to the protein matrix that encapsulates the HIV's capsid. A lipid bilayer envelope would then encapsulate the matrix protein coat and capsid similar to the lipid bilayer than encapsulates the matrix protein of HIV. Up to three different types of cell-surface receptors are mounted on the outside of the outer envelope, referred to as: CD 4, CCR5 and CXCR4. The three cell-surface receptors CD 4, CCR5 and CXCR4 are identical in construction, arrangement and function to the CD 4, CCR5 and CXCR4 receptors that appear naturally on the surface of noninfected human T-Helper cells. The capsid of the therapeutic version of the SMART Virus would carry either no genetic payload or would carry RNA molecules that would not be capable of replicating the virus-like structure in the natural environment. The amount of genetic payload or filler would relate to the intended stability of the SMART virus once released into the environment. SMART viruses are intended to act as surrogate T-Helper cells by mimicking the T-Helper cell target and engaging HIV's external surface probes in a manner to negate HIV's capability to infect T-Helper cells.

DETAILED DESCRIPTION

[0012] Scientifically Modulated And Reprogrammed Treatment (SMART) Virus technology is intended to neutralize the Human Immunodeficiency Virus wherever the virus might be found. SMART Virus technology is comprised of a lipid bilayer envelope identical in construct to the naturally occurring HIV outer envelope, and mounted to the SMART virus's outer envelope are up to three different types of cell-surface receptors referred to as Cluster Designation 4 (CD4), Chemotactic Chemokine Receptor 5 (CCR5) and CX Chemokine Receptor 4 (CXCR4).

The three cell-surface receptors, the CD 4 receptor, the CCR5 receptor and the CXCR4 receptor are well known to the medical and scientific community due to the fact they appear naturally on the surface of the Human T-Helper cell. Within the SMART virus's outer envelope are matrix protein and a capsid to act as the interior conformational structure to provide the appropriate size and shape to the outer envelope as needed. The size of the SMART virus ranges from 7 nanometer (nm) in width (the diameter of HIV is approximately 50 nm) to a diameter in the order of the size of a naturally occurring noninfected T-Helper cell, and up to the diameter of one meter. T-Helper cells are mobile structures and constantly alter their shape and size, but are approximately 3500 nm in diameter. The range in size of the SMART Virus is dependent upon the type of application for which the SMART Virus is required to be utilized.

[0013]   To initiate its natural reproductive cycle, HIV engages a T-Helper cell by a glycoprotein 120 (gp 120) probe engaging a T-Helper cell's CD4 exterior cell-surface receptor; once this occurs HIV's glycoprotein 41 (gp 41) probe engages the T-Helper cell's CCR5 or CXCR4 exterior cell-surface receptor. The SMART Virus, carrying CD 4, CCR5 and CXCR4 surface receptors, is capable of traveling anywhere HIV virions are likely to travel and engage HIV. When HIV encounters a SMART Virus, the HIV's gp 120 probe would engage the SMART Virus's CD 4 exterior cell-surface receptor, then the HIV's gp 41 probe would engage either the CCR5 or the CXCR4 exterior cell-surface receptor on the SMART Virus. Once HIV's gp 120 and gp 41 probes have engaged their respective receptors on the SMART Virus, HIV would either eject into the surrounding environment the capsid carrying the RNA payload or HIV would inject its capsid and RNA genetic payload into the SMART Virus or the HIV would permanently adhere to the SMART Virus making the HIV virion incapable of being able to interact and infect a T-Helper cell. Since HIV engaged a SMART Virus rather than a T-Helper cell, the HIV RNA genome is rendered harmless and the threat of HIV's infectivity is effectively neutralized. In the event HIV is unable to create additional copies of itself and unable to further threaten T-Helper cells, the threat of Acquired Immunodeficiency Disease Syndrome is successfully neutralized.

[0014]　SMART Virus technology can be used as a cleaning device to neutralize and rid a surface or a fluid environment of HIV. Since the SMART virus is similar in construction to HIV, the SMART Virus is intended to traverse and survive in any environment where HIV might exist. SMART Virus is intended to engage HIV where ever it may exist.

[0015]　HIV utilizes T-Helper cells as a natural factory for generating copies of HIV.　HIV utilizes a fusion technique where the virion envelope fuses with the cellular membrane of the host cell and directly releases the capsid containing the RNA genome and replicating enzymes into the cytoplasm of the host cell. HIV utilizes enzymes created by its own genome and enzymes native to the T-Helper cell to generate the proteins it requires to construct copies of HIV. Once the appropriate copies of the RNA, nucleocapsid protein, integrase, protease, reverse transcriptase enzyme, capsid proteins, matrix protein and external probes have been manufactured and collected together, the capsid carrying the RNA genetic payload is enveloped by the matrix protein and pushes through the host cell's plasma membrane in a process called budding. The HIV copy becomes encapsulated in an envelope comprised of a lipid bilayer as it separates from the host cell and becomes an independent entity termed a virion. Probes stick out through the lipid bilayer envelope of the virion to seek the receptors located on an appropriate host cell.

[0016]　To produce copies of the SMART Virus a T-Helper cell can be utilized, bacteria with a lipid bilayer membrane could be utilized or other appropriate host cell could be utilized. The technology to manufacture viruses carrying a therapeutic DNA gene has already been worked out and implemented.　The process to generate a medically therapeutic virus to target a particular cell and deliver a specific genetic payload to a specific target cell is a matter of placing inside a host cell the appropriate genetic instructions and enzymes to facilitate the host cell to manufacture the intended 'medically therapeutic' virus.

[0017]   In the case of the SMART Virus, the construction of the final medically therapeutic copies of the SMART Virus include the appropriate instructions and biologic machinery necessary to generate the capsid proteins, matrix proteins, external cell-surface receptors C4, CCR5 and CXCR4, any filling material to be placed inside the capsid and stimulate the budding process. The size of the capsid is dependent upon the capsid proteins used to construct the capsid. For descriptive purposes the use of the term 'capsid' is interchangeable with the term 'capsid shell'. Different naturally occurring viruses are constructed with a different size capsid depending upon the number and arrangement of capsid proteins utilized to construct a virus's capsid. The diameter of the SMART Virus is in part dependent upon the number and arrangement of capsid proteins used to construct the capsid. A genetic payload to act as a filler, incapable of stimulating a disease state in any life form, may be required to fill the inside the capsid of some of the larger diameter SMART Viruses in order to support the successful construction of a particular size of SMART Virus and to facilitate the SMART virus remaining sturdy enough and thus intact once released into the environment to enable it to successfully carry out its intended function.

[0018]   SMART Virus technology can be used as a cleaning device to neutralize and rid a surface or a fluid environment of HIV by one of three manners. HIV's probes gp 120 and gp 41 are intended to engage a native T-Helper cell's CD4, and the CCR5 or the CXCR4 exterior cell-surface receptor. Once HIV's probes have successfully made contact and functionally engaged a T-Helper cell's receptors HIV injects its capsid into the T-Helper cell. The SMART Virus's receptors would function in the identical manner as a T-Helper cell's receptors. The action of a SMART Virus is to attract and engage HIV. Following the SMART Virus's receptors engaging HIV's probes the SMART Virus would neutralize HIV by: (1) adhering to HIV preventing contact of HIV with a T-Helper cell, (2) causing HIV to eject its capsid into the environment outside HIV's envelope making the HIV genetic payload incapable of infecting a T-Helper cell, (3) causing HIV to inject its capsid into the SMART Virus thus capturing the HIV genetic payload and preventing it from infecting a T-Helper cell. Any of these three actions would interfere with HIV's functional capacity to infect a T-Helper cell. If HIV is unable to infect a T-Helper cell, HIV is unable to replicate and it is unable to further influence T-Helper cells to kill noninfected T-Helper cells by the FasL apoptosis triggering mechanism, and therefore the infectious threat HIV poses is effectively neutralized.

[0019] The diameter of the SMART virus is between 7 nm in diameter (the size of the diameter of HIV is approximately 50 nm) to a diameter in the order of the size of a naturally occurring noninfected T-Helper cell, to a diameter of one meter. T-Helper cells are mobile and constantly alter their shape and size, but are approximately 3500 nm in diameter. The range in size of the SMART Virus is dependent upon the type of application for which the SMART Virus is required to be utilized. One or more smaller sized SMART Viruses may simply adhere to a single HIV virion, and thus by adhering to the HIV and engaging the virus's probes make the HIV virion incapable of successfully engaging a T-Helper cell. Larger diameter SMART Viruses might engage one or more HIV virions preventing the HIV virions from further migrating through the environment in search of a T-Helper cell to infect. A SMART Virus may engage a HIV virion and by successfully attaching to the virion's probes in the same manner as a T-Helper cell would engage the virion's probes, cause the HIV virion to eject its capsid into the environment outside the virion's outer envelope. SMART Viruses may also engage a HIV virion and by successfully attaching to the virion's probes in the same manner as a T-Helper cell would engage the virion's probes, cause the HIV virion to inject its capsid into the SMART Virus as if the SMART Virus were a T-Helper cell. The diameter of the SMART Virus would depend upon the size of the reservoir the SMART Virus would be intended to contain to collect one or more HIV capsids. The SMART Virus intended to collect more than one HIV capsid may be best designed not to permanently adhere to HIV once it has accepted the HIV's capsid so that it can functionally engage additional HIV virions to collect additional HIV capsids.

CLAIMS: Reserved.

A4: UNIVERSAL BARRIER TO PREVENT INFECTIONS FROM HUMAN IMMUNODEFICIENCY VIRUS

INDIVIDUALS REQUESTING PATENT: Dr. Lane B. Scheiber, ScD and Dr. Lane B. Scheiber II, MD

NUMBER OF CLAIMS: 2 independent claims, 18 dependent claims

ABSTRACT

The Human Immunodeficiency Virus poses a significant threat to the world's population. Current strategies to treat infectious agents have not been adequate to eradicate such deadly viral infections. HIV seeks out its host, a T–Helper cell, by utilizing glycoprotein 120 probes to engage a CD4 cell-surface receptor located on the surface of a T-Helper cell. Developing devices to offer HIV virions' probes the opportunity to engage the cell-surface receptors they are seeking offers a means of neutralizing the infectious threat of HIV. A device in the form of a solution containing a filter medium comprised of sheets or strips or spheres of lipid bilayer or virus-like structures or hypoallergenic surfaces to carry cell-surface receptors, each type of medium having affixed to its surface cell-surface receptors intended to engage and neutralize the infectious nature of HIV virions provides an effective strategy to avert AIDS.

BACKGROUND OF THE INVENTION

1. Field of the Invention

[0001] This invention relates to any medical device that is utilized to act as a barrier to protect a person from contracting the Human Immunodeficiency Virus by neutralizing the infectious nature of Human Immunodeficiency Virus virions.

2. Description of Background Art

[0002] It has been estimated by the Center for Disease Control that in the United States 55,000 to 60,000 new cases of Human Immunodeficiency Virus (HIV) are occurring each year. It is thought that there are 900,000 people currently infected with HIV in the United States, with many victims not aware that they have contracted the virus. Further, it has been estimated that the Human Immunodeficiency Virus (HIV), the pathogen that causes Acquired Immune Deficiency Syndrome (AIDS), has infected as many as 30-60 million people around the globe.

[0003] The presence of HIV was first came to the attention of those in the United States in 1981, when there appeared an outbreak of Kaposi's Sarcoma and Pneumocystis carinii pneumonia in gay men in New York and California. After over twenty-five years of research and investigation, eradicating the ever growing global humanitarian crisis posed by the HIV remains an elusive goal for the medical community. It is estimated the virus has already killed 25 million citizens of this planet.

[0004] The Human Immunodeficiency Virus has been previously referred to as human T-Lymphotrophic virus III (HTLV-III), lymphadenopathy-associated virus (LAV), and AIDS-associated retrovirus (ARV). Infection with HIV may occur by the virus being transferred by blood, semen, vaginal fluid, or breast milk. Four major means of transmission of HIV include unprotected sexual intercourse, contaminated needles, breast milk, and transmission from an infected mother to her baby at birth.

[0005] HIV is an ingeniously constructed very deadly virus, which represents the most challenging pathogen the worldwide medical community faces to date. Viruses in general, have been difficult to contain and eradicate due to the fact they are obligate parasites and tend not to carry out any biologic functions outside the cell the virus has targeted as its host. A virus when it exists outside the boundaries of a cell is generally referred to as a virion. HIV virions posses several attributes that make them very elusive and difficult to destroy.

[0006] For purposes of this text, the term 'body' refers to the material part of a man or a woman, generally including the head, neck, trunk, extremities and all usual internal structures. For the purposes of this text, the term 'vagina' refers to the genital canal in a woman extending from the uterus to the vulva.

[0007] Bacterial infections have posed an easier target for the medical community to eradicate from the body. Bacteria generally live and reproduce outside animal cells. Bacteria, like animal cells, carryout biologic functions. A large multi-celled organism such as the human body combats bacterial infections with a combined force of white cells, antibodies, complements and its lymphatic system. White cells circulate the body in search of bacteria. When a white cell encounters a bacterium, the white cell engulfs the bacterium, encapsulates the pathogen, processes the identification of the pathogen and kills the pathogen utilizing acids and destructive enzymes. The white cell then alerts the B-cells of the immune system as to the identity of the intruding bacterium. A subpopulation of B-cells is generated, dedicated to producing antibodies directed against the particular pathogen the circulating white cell encountered and identified. Antibodies, generated by B-cells, traverse the

·

blood and body tissues in search of the bacteria they were designed to repel. Once an antibody encounters a bacterium it is targeted to attack, the antibody attaches to the bacterium's outer wall. The effect antibodies have in coating the outside of a bacterium is to assist the white cells and the other components of the immune system in recognizing the bacterium, so that appropriate defensive action can be taken against the pathogen. Some antibodies, in addition to coating the bacterium, will act to punch holes through the bacterium's outer wall. If the integrity of the bacterium's cell wall is breached, this action generally leads to the death of the bacterium. Complements are primitive protein structures that circulate the blood stream in search of anything that appears consistent with a bacteria cell wall. Complements are indiscriminant. Once the complement proteins locate any form of bacterial cell wall, the complement proteins organize, and much like antibodies, act in concert to punch one or more holes though a bacterium's cell wall to compromise the viability of the bacterium. The lymphatic system is a diffuse network of thin walled vessels that drain excess water from extracellular fluids and join to form the thoracic duct and right lymph duct, which empty into the venous system near the heart. Lymph nodes are present at different locations in the body and screen the fluid transiting the lymphatic system, called lymph, to remove pathogens. Cells in the spleen screen the blood in search of bacteria. When a bacterial pathogen is identified, such as by antibodies coating the surface, the bacterium is taken out of circulation and terminated.

[0008] Viruses pose a much different infectious vector to the body's defense system than either bacteria or cellular parasites. Since viruses do not carry out biologic processes outside their host cell, a virus can be destroyed, but they cannot be killed. A virus is simply comprised of one or more external shells and a portion of genetic material. The virus's genetic information is carried in the core of the virus. Antibodies can coat the exterior of a virus to make it easier for the white cells in the body to identify the viral pathogen, but the action of punching holes in the virus's external shell by antibodies or complement proteins does not necessarily kill the virus. Viruses also only briefly circulate in the blood and tissues of the body as an exposed entity. Using exterior probes, a virus hunts down a cell in the body that will act as an appropriate host so that the virus can replicate. Once the virus has found a proper host cell, the virus inserts its genome into the host cell. To complete its life-cycle, the virus's genetic material takes command of cellular functions and directs the host cell to make replicas of the virus.

[0009] Once the virus's genome has entered a host cell, the virus is in effect shielded from the body's immune system defense mechanisms. Inside a host cell, the presence of the virus is generally only represented as genetic information incorporated into the host cell's DNA. Once a virus has infected a cell in the body, the presence of the virus can only be eradicated if the host cell is destroyed. Antibodies and complements are generally designed not to attack the autologous tissues of the body. Circulating white cells and the immune cells which comprise lymph nodes and the spleen may or may not recognize that a cell, which has become a host for a virus, is infected with a virus's genome. If the immune system fails to identify a cell that has become infected with a virus, the virus's genetic material can proceed to force the infected cell to make copies of the virus. Since a virus is in essence simply a segment of genetic material, time is of no consequence to the life-cycle of the virus and a virus's genome may be carried for years by the host without a need to activate; such viruses are often termed latent viruses. A virus's genetic material may sit idle in a host cell for an extended period of time until the pathogen's programming senses the time is right to initiate the virus's replication process or an action of the host cell triggers the virus to replicate. The only opportunity for the immune system to destroy a latent virus is when copies of the virus leave the host cell and circulate in the blood or tissues in search of another perspective host cell.

[0010] The traditional medical approach to combating infectious agents such as bacteria and cellular parasites, therefore has limited value in managing or eradicating elusive or latent viral infections. Synthetic antibiotics, generally used to augment the body's capacity to produce naturally occurring antibodies against bacterial infections, have little success in combating latent viral infections. Stimulating the body's immune system's recognition of a virus by administering a vaccine also has had limited success in combating elusive viral infections. Vaccines generally are intended to introduce to the body pieces of a bacteria or virus, or an attenuated, noninfectious intact bacteria or virus so that the immune system is able to recognize and process the infectious agent and generate antibodies directed to assist in killing the pathogen. Once the immune system has been primed to recognize an intruder, antibodies will be produced by the immune system in great quantities in an effort to repel an invader. Over time, as the immune system down-regulates its antibody production in response to a lack of detecting the presence of the intruding pathogen, the quantity of antibodies circulating in the blood stream may decrease in number to a quantity that is insufficient to combat a pathogen. Since antibodies have limited value in combating some of the more elusive viruses that hibernate in host cells, vaccines have limited value in destroying latent viruses.

[0011] The Human Immunodeficiency Virus demonstrates four factors which make this pathogen particularly elusive and a difficult infectious agent to eradicate from the body. First: the host for HIV is the T-Helper cell. The T-Helper cell is a key element in the immune system's response since it helps coordinate the body's defensive actions against pathogens seeking to invade the body's tissues. In cases of a bacterial infection versus a viral infection, T-Helper cells actively direct which immune cells will rev-up in response to the infectious agent and engage the particular pathogen. Since HIV infects and disrupts T-Helper cells, coordination of the immune response against the virus is disrupted, thus limiting the body's capacity to mount a proper response against the presence of the virus and produce a sufficient action to successfully eradicate the virus.

[0012] Second: again, latent viruses such as HIV, have a strategic advantage. When the immune system first recognizes a pathogen and begins to generate antibodies against a particular pathogen, the response is generally robust. Once time has passed and the immune system fails to detect an active threat, the production of antibodies against the particular pathogen diminishes. When HIV infects a T-Helper cell, the viral genome may lay dormant, sometimes for years before taking command of the T-Helper cell's biologic functions. HIV may, therefore, generate a very active initial immune response to its presence, but if the virus sits dormant inside T-Helper cells for months or years, the antibody response to the virus will diminish over time. There may not be an adequate quantity of circulating antibodies to actively engage the HIV virions as they migrate from the T-Helper cell that generated the copies to uninfected T-Helper cells that will serve as a new host to support further replication. If the immune system's response is insufficient during the period while the virus is exposed and vulnerable, it becomes extremely difficult for the body to eradicate the virus.

[0013] Third, when replicas of the Human Immunodeficiency Virus are released from their host cell, during the budding process the HIV virion coats itself with an exterior envelope comprised of a portion of the plasma membrane from the T-Helper cell that acted as the host for the virus. A T-Helper cell's plasma membrane is comprised of a lipid bilayer, a double layer of lipid molecules oriented with their polar ends at the outside of the membrane and the nonpolar ends in the membrane interior. The virus thus, in part, takes on an external appearance of a naturally occurring cell in the body. Since the exterior envelope of a HIV virion has the characteristics of a T-Helper cell it is more difficult for the immune system to recognize that it is a pathogen as it migrates through the body in search of another T-Helper cell to infect.

[0014]   Fourth, the Human Immunodeficiency Virus exhibits a very elusive mode of action which the virus readily utilizes to actively defeat the body's immune system. HIV carries in its genome a segment of genetic material that directs an infected T-Helper cell to create and mount on the surface the plasma membrane a FasL cell-surface receptor. Healthy T-Helper cells carry on the surface of their plasma membrane Fas cell-surface receptors. The Fas cell-surface receptor when engaged by a FasL cell-surface receptor on another cell, initiates apoptosis in the cell carrying the Fas cell-surface receptor. Apoptosis is a biologic process that causes a cell to terminate itself. A T-Helper cell infected with the HIV virus carrying a FasL cell-surface receptor is therefore capable of killing noninfected T-Helper cells that the infected T-Helper cell encounters as it circulates the body. The occurrence of AIDS is therefore propagated not only by the number of T-Helper cells that become incapacitated due to direct infection by HIV, but also by the number of noninfected T-Helper cells that are eliminated by coming in direct contact with infected T-Helper cells.

[0015]   Acquired Immune Deficiency Syndrome (AIDS) occurs as a result of the number of circulating T-Helper cells declining to a point where the immune system's capacity to mount a successful response against opportunistic infectious agents is significantly compromised. The number of viable T-Helper cells declines either because they become infected with the HIV virus or because they have been killed by encountering a T-Helper cell infected with HIV. When there is an insufficient population of non-HIV infected T-Helper cells to properly combat infectious agents such as Pneumocystis carinii or cytomegalo virus or other pathogens, the body becomes overwhelmed with the opportunistic infection and the patient becomes clinically ill. In cases where the combination of the patient's compromised immune system and medical assistance in terms of synthetic antibiotics intended to combat the opportunistic pathogens, fluids, intravenous nutrition and other treatments are not sufficient to sustain life, the body succumbs to the opportunistic infection and death ensues.

[0016]   The Human Immunodeficiency Virus locates its host by utilizing probes located on its envelope. The HIV virion has two types of glycoprotein probes attached to the outer surface of its exterior envelope. A glycoprotein is a structure comprised of a protein component and a lipid component. HIV utilizes a glycoprotein 120 (gp 120) probe to locate a CD4 cell-surface receptor on the plasma membrane of a T-Helper cell. The plasma membrane of the T-Helper cell is comprised of a lipid bilayer. Cell-surface receptors are anchored in the lipid bilayer. Once an HIV gp 120 probe has successfully engaged a CD4 cell-surface receptor on a T-Helper cell a conformational change occurs in the gp 120 probe and a glycoprotein 41 (gp 41) probe is exposed. The gp 41 probe's intent is to engage a CXCR4 or CCR5 cell-surface receptor on the plasma membrane of the same T-Helper cell. Once a gp 41 probe on the HIV virion engages a CXCR4 or CCR5 cell-surface receptor, the HIV virion opens an access portal through the T-Helper cell's plasma membrane.

[0017]   Once the virus has gained access to the T-Helper cell by opening a portal through the cell's outer membrane the virion inserts two positive strand RNA molecules approximately 9500 nucleotides in length. Inserted along with the RNA strands are the enzymes reverse transcriptase, protease and integrase. Once the virus's genome gains access to the interior of the T-Helper cell, in the cytoplasm the pair of RNA molecules are transformed to deoxyribonucleic acid by the reverse transcriptase enzyme. Following modification of the virus's genome to DNA, the virus's genetic information migrates to the host cell's nucleus. In the nucleus, with the assistance of the integrase protein, the virus's DNA becomes inserted into the T-Helper cell's native DNA. When the timing is appropriate, the now integrated viral DNA, becomes read by the host cell's polymerase molecules and the virus's genetic information commands certain cell functions to carry out the replication process to construct copies of the human deficiency virus.

[0018] Present anti-viral therapy has been designed to target the enzymes that assist the HIV genome with the replication process. Anti-viral therapy is intended to interfere with the action of these replication enzymes. Part of the challenge of eradicating HIV is that once the virus inserts its genome into a T-Helper cell host, the viral genome may lay dormant until the proper circumstances evolve. The virus's genome may sit idle inside a T-Helper cell for years before becoming activated, causing drugs that interfere with HIV's life cycle to have limited effect on eliminating the virus from the body. Arresting the replication process does not insure that T-Helper cells infected with HIV do not continue to circulate the body killing noninfected T-Helper cells thus causing the patient to progress to a clinically apparent state of Acquired Immune Deficiency Syndrome and eventually succumbing to an opportunistic infection which eventually results in the death of the individual.

[0019] The outer layer of the HIV virion is comprised of a portion of the T-Helper cell's outer cell membrane. In the final stage of the replication process, as a copy of the HIV capsid, carrying the HIV genome, buds through the host cell's plasma membrane, the capsid acquires as its outermost shell a wrapping of lipid bilayer from the host cell's plasma membrane. Vaccines are generally comprised of pieces of a virus or bacterium, or copies of the entire virus or bacterium weakened to the point the pathogen is incapable of causing an infection. These pieces of a pathogen or copies of a nonvirulent pathogen prime the immune system such that a vaccine intent is to cause B-cells to produce antibodies that are programmed to seek out the surface characteristics of the pathogen comprising the vaccine. In the case of HIV, since the surface of the pathogen is an envelope comprised of lipid bilayer taken from the host

T-Helper cell's plasma membrane, a vaccine comprised of portions of the exterior envelope of the HIV virions might not only target HIV virions, but might also have deleterious effects on the T-Helper cell population. Some antibodies produced to combat HIV infections may not be able to tell the difference between an HIV virion and a T-Helper cell, and such antibodies may act to coat and assist in the elimination of both targets. In such a scenario, since such a vaccine might cause a decline in the number of available T-Helper cells, it is conceivable that a vaccine comprised of portions of the external envelope of HIV virions might paradoxically induce clinically apparent AIDS in a patient that a vaccine has been administered.

[0020] It is clear that the traditional approach of utilizing antibiotics or providing vaccines to stimulate the immune system to produce endogenous antibodies, by themselves, is an ineffective strategy to manage a virus as elusive and deadly as HIV. Drugs that interfere with the replication process of HIV generally slow progression of the infection by the virus, but do not necessarily eliminate the virus from the body nor eliminate the threat of the clinical symptoms of AIDS. A new strategy is required in order to successfully combat the threat of HIV.

[0021] The Human Immunodeficiency Virus virions are much smaller in size than the red blood cells and white blood cells. The gp120 and gp 41 probes located on the surface of HIV are seeking to engage the CD4 and CXCR4 or CCR5 cell-surface receptors located on T-Helper cells. A filter medium intended to engage HIV virions could be constructed such that body fluids which carry HIV virions would come in contact with the surface features of the filter medium. As HIV's glycoprotein probes, gp120 and gp 41, engage the CD4 and CXCR4 or CCR5 cell-surface receptors affixed to the surface of the filter medium in a similar manners as to how the CD4 and CXCR4 or CCR5 cell-surface receptors affixed to the surface of a naturally occurring T-Helper cell, the HIV virions would adhere to the filter medium and either become stuck to the filter medium or by the action of the HIV probes engaging the filter medium cell-surface receptors HIV virions would eject their genome rendering the HIV virion incapable of infecting an endogenous T-Helper cell in the woman.

[0022]   The technology to make such filter medium is readably available and could be quickly implemented for worldwide use to prevent infections by HIV virions.

[0023]   A device, to accomplish the task of acting as a barrier to neutralize Human Immunodeficiency Virus virions, would be to use a filter medium with constructed surface characteristics similar to the surface characteristics of a naturally occurring T-Helper cell, since, specifically, it is the cell-surface receptors affixed to the surface of a T-Helper cell that the HIV virion's probes are seeking.   T-Helper cells are constructed with the outer membrane being comprised of a lipid bilayer.   Cell-surface receptors are anchored into this lipid bilayer and the protein portion of the cell-surface receptor extends out and away from the surface of the T-Helper cell.   Sheets of lipid bilayer constructed with a generous quantity of CD4, CXCR4 and CCR5 cell-surface receptors affixed to the surface, would attract and engage HIV virions as a surrogate target in place of endogenous T-Helper cells the HIV virions are seeking as a host.

[0024]   A medical device could be constructed in a manner where a quantity of lipid bilayer fashioned in the shape of sheets or strips or spheres would be constructed with a generous quantity of CD4, CXCR4 and CCR5 cell-surface receptors affixed to the surface of the filter medium.   The filter medium would be fashioned to be a liquid or a cream.   As body fluids mix with the filter medium and pass across the surface of a sheet or strip or sphere of lipid bilayer, HIV virions would come in contact with CD4, CXCR4 and CXR5 cell-surface receptors present on the surface of the lipid bilayer and engage the cell-surface receptors.   The HIV virions making contact with the lipid bilayer would either permanently adhere to the lipid bilayer or by engaging the cell-surface receptors on the lipid bilayer the HIV virions would be caused to eject their genome, which would neutralize the infectious threat of the HIV virions. The body fluids would be cleared of HIV virions capable of infecting T-Helper cells endogenous to a body.

[0025] Since HIV virions are searching their environment for CD4, CXCR4 and CXR5 cell-surface receptors a filter material comprised of any hypoallergenic material suitable to attach CD4, CXCR4 and CXR5 cell-surface receptors or the protein portion of these receptors, to the surface of the material. As the body fluids mix with the filter medium and pass across the surface of a sheet or strips or spheres of a hypoallergenic material with CD4, CXCR4 and CXR5 cell-surface receptors, HIV virions would come in contact with CD4, CXCR4 and CXR5 cell-surface receptors present on the surface of the hypoallergenic material and engage the cell-surface receptors. The HIV virions making contact with the cell-surface receptors affixed to the hypoallergenic material would either permanently adhere to the hypoallergenic material or by engaging the cell-surface receptors affixed to the surface of the hypoallergenic material the HIV virions would be caused to eject their genome, which would neutralize the infectious threat of the HIV virions. The body fluids would be cleared of HIV virions capable of infecting T-Helper cells endogenous to a body.

[0026] White blood cells are physically larger than red blood cells. Bacteria are generally much smaller than red blood cells. HIV virions are much smaller than bacteria. HIV is comprised of an outer envelope, an internal capsid and the viral genome. Because of its small size HIV can potentially maneuver into places in the body's tissues or crevasses between tissues where mobile cells are unable to go.

[0027] An approach to managing HIV would be to create a product that would be relatively the same size as HIV so that the product could penetrate into every location that HIV might migrate. HIV's probes are seeking the CD4 and CCR5 and CXCR4 cell-surface receptors of a T-Helper cell, thus a product to challenge HIV could be equipped with the same cell-surface receptors as would be found on a naturally occurring T-Helper cell.

[0028] Utilizing genetic machinery and a colony of T-Helper cells or a colony of hybrid T-Helper cells or a colony of specially designed host cells, a medically therapeutic modified virus or virus-like product approximately the size of a HIV virion could be manufactured in a similar manner as how HIV naturally replicates, except the product would carry the T-Helper cell cell-surface receptors CD4, CXCR4 and/or CCR5 instead of the glycoprotein probes associated with a naturally occurring HIV virion. The virus-like product would be constructed either with no genetic information present inside the capsid or genetic material to act as a filler, this genetic material being inert such that it could not carry out any useful function.

[0029] Constructing a virus-like structure, that has affixed to its exterior cell-surface receptors intended to engage a virus, is referred to as a Scientifically Modulated And Reprogrammed Target (SMART) virus. The SMART virus would be available to engage Human Immunodeficiency Virus virions present in body fluids. As HIV virions make contact with SMART viruses the HIV virions would engage the SMART virus and become permanently attached and become trapped by the filter medium, or the HIV virions, upon engaging a SMART virus, would harmlessly eject the genetic material the HIV virion carries. Either engaging and trapping the HIV virion or causing the HIV virion to eject the genetic material that it carries, would neutralize the virulence of HIV and assist in managing the threat of AIDS.

BRIEF SUMMARY OF THE INVENTION

[0030]   Initially the Human Immunodeficiency Virus is attracted to its host, the T-helper cell, by having its surface probes seek out a CD4 cell-surface receptor. Once HIV virion's gp 120 probe successfully engages a CD4 cell-surface receptor a conformation change occurs in the gp 120 probe and a gp 41 probe attempts to engage either a CXCR4 or a CCR5 cell-surface receptor located on the target T-Helper cell. Described here is a device that offers a surrogate target HIV virions are seeking.   The device is intended to be applied to any surface that may contain Human Immunodeficiency Virus virions, including but not limited to the vagina in a woman, the oral cavity in a body, and the rectum in a body. It is a device intended to remove the threat of the infectious threat of Human Immunodeficiency Virus virions from body fluids. It is a device used to clean surfaces by removing the infectious threat of Human Immunodeficiency Virus present on such a surface or protect a body from becoming infected by the Human Immunodeficiency Virus carried by body fluids that might be deposited into the body by way of the vagina, the oral cavity, or the rectum. As the body fluids make contact with the filter medium any HIV virions present in the body fluids have the opportunity to engage the three cell surface receptors the CD 4 receptor, the CCR5 receptor and the CXCR4 receptor which are well known to the medical and scientific community due to the fact they appear naturally on the surface of the Human T-Helper cell. Since the HIV virion engaged cell-surface receptors located on the surface of the filter medium rather than located on the surface of an endogenous T-Helper cell inside the body, the infectious nature of the HIV virions is neutralized by either the HIV virion becoming trapped by the filter medium or the HIV virion is caused to harmlessly eject its genome. When HIV virions become trapped by the filter medium it is incapable of migrating further to successfully engaging endogenous T-Helper cells inside the body. When a HIV virion is caused to eject its genome, the HIV virion is incapable of infecting an endogenous T-Helper cell inside the body. Trapping the HIV virion or causing the HIV virion to harmlessly eject its genome leads to neutralizing the infectious threat of HIV, which leads to effectively averting AIDS.

DETAILED DESCRIPTION OF THE INVENTION

[0031] The invention described herein is intended to neutralize the infectious nature of Human Immunodeficiency Virus virions carried in body fluids. The medical device is comprised of a filter medium or a filter medium suspended in a hypoallergenic fluid or cream. The medical device is intended to be applied to surfaces where body fluids infected with the Human Immunodeficiency Virus may be. The mixing of the filter medium comprising the medical device with fluids that contain Human Immunodeficiency Virus virions is meant to result in the neutralization of the infectious nature of the Human Immunodeficiency Virus virions.

[0032] Three cell receptors CD4, CCR5 and CXCR4 are well known to the medical and scientific community and appear naturally on the surface of the Human T-Helper cells. The HIV virion expresses gp 120 glycoprotein probes and glycoprotein 41 probes on its outer envelope. HIV utilizes the T-Helper cell as its host cell for the purposes of replication.

[0033] In completing the virus's natural reproductive-cycle, HIV utilizes the gp 120 probe positioned on the exterior envelope of an HIV virion to locate and engage a T-Helper cell's CD4 exterior cell-surface receptor. Once the HIV's gp 120 has successfully engaged a CD 4 cell-surface receptor, the HIV virion's gp 41 probe engages either a CCR5 or CXCR4 exterior cell-surface receptor on the T-Helper cell. A filter medium expressing CD4, CCR5 and CXCR4 cell-surface receptors offers a surrogate target expressing the cell-surface receptors HIV virions are seeking to engage. When HIV virion's probes encounter a filter medium expressing CD4, CCR5 and CXCR4 cell-surface receptors, affixed to the surface of the filter medium similar to the manner these cell-surface receptors are affixed to the surface of naturally occurring T-Helper cells, HIV's gp 120 probes would engage CD 4 exterior surface receptors, followed then by HIV's gp 41 probes engaging either CCR5 or CXCR4 exterior cell-surface receptors. Once the HIV gp 120 probes and gp 41 probes have engaged their respective cell-surface receptors affixed to the filter medium's exterior surface, the HIV is fixed to the surface of the filter medium and the HIV virion may eject RNA genome it carries. Since the HIV engaged a filter medium the HIV virion becomes affixed and trapped by the filter device and if the HIV virion ejects its RNA genome, the threat of the HIV virion being able to infect an endogenous T-Helper cell inside a body is effectively neutralized. The body fluids passing through such a filter becomes cleared of infectious HIV virions.

[0034] The medical device described herein, intended to neutralize infectious HIV virions in body fluids that come into contact with the filter medium. The filter medium comprising this medical device may be fashioned from a variety of different materials and fashioned in a variety of different shapes. The filter medium is intended to make available cell-surface receptors including CD 4, CCR5 and CXCR4, affixed to the surface of the filter medium similar to the manner these cell-surface receptors are affixed to the surface of naturally occurring T-Helper cells, for HIV virions to engage. The filter medium may be comprised of a quantity of exogenous T-Helper cells. The filter medium may be comprised of a quantity of lipid bilayer sheets which are comprised of similar materials as found existing as the outer membrane of a T-Helper cell, and affixed to the said lipid bilayer sheets are glycoprotein cell-surface receptors including a quantity of CD4 cell-surface receptors, CXCR4 cell-surface receptors, CCR5 cell-surface receptors. The filter medium may be comprised of a quantity of modified viruses or virus-like structures with cell-surface receptors to include a quantity of CD4 cell-surface receptors, CXCR4 cell-surface receptors, CCR5 cell-surface receptors. The filter medium may be comprised of any appropriate hypoallergenic material, which can be affixed to the surface a quantity of CD4 cell-surface receptors, CXCR4 cell-surface receptors, CCR5 cell-surface receptors or simply the protein portion of the CD4 cell-surface receptors, CXCR4 cell-surface receptors, CCR5 cell-surface receptors.

[0035] To carry out the process to manufacture a modified medically therapeutic virus, messenger RNA that would code for the general physical outer structures of the modified virus, such as instruction code to generate a modified HIV virion or a modified Hepatitis C virus virion or other virus virion or other virus-like structure, would be inserted into a host. The host may include devices such as a host cell or a hybrid host cell. The host may utilize DNA or RNA or a combination of genetic instructions in order to accomplish the construction of medically therapeutic modified virus virions. In some cases DNA or messenger RNA would be inserted into the host that would be coded to cause the production of surface probes that would be affixed to the surface of the virus virion that would target the glycoprotein probes affixed to the surface of an HIV virion. The copies of the medically therapeutic modified viruses or medically therapeutic virus-like structures, upon exiting the host, would be collected, stored and utilized as a medical treatment as necessary.

[0036] The medically therapeutic version of the modified virus and virus-like structures would be incapable of replication on its own due to the fact that the messenger RNA that would code for the replication process to produce copies of the virus or virus-like structure would not be present in the modified form of a virus or virus-like structure.

[0037] Lipid bilayer sheets can be manufactured and combinations of CD 4 cell-surface receptors, CXCR4 cell-surface receptors, CCR5 cell-surface receptors can be affixed to the surface similar to the manner these cell-surface receptors are affixed to the surface of naturally occurring T-Helper cells, with the entire structure acting as a filter medium. Sheets of any appropriate hypoallergenic material can be manufactured and combinations of CD 4 cell-surface receptors, CXCR4 cell-surface receptors, CCR5 cell-surface receptors can be affixed to the surface with the entire structure acting as a filter medium. Sheets of any appropriate hypoallergenic material can be manufactured and combinations of the protein portion of the CD 4 cell-surface receptors, CXCR4 cell-surface receptors, CCR5 cell-surface receptors available to engage either glycoprotein probes on HIV or cell-surface receptors on a T-Helper cell, affixed to the surface of the hypoallergenic material with the entire structure acting as a filter medium.

[0038] The filter medium may be suspended in any suitable hypoallergenic fluid or cream.

[0039] The filter medium may be mixed with and coexist with a quantity of an agent that acts as a spermatocide to prevent sperm present in the vagina from being able to proceed from the vagina to fertilize an egg and cause the woman to become pregnant.

[0040] The filter medium can be mixed and coexist with a quantity of lubricant.

[0041] The filter medium can be mixed and coexist with a quantity of moisturizer.

CLAIMS: Reserved.

A5: FEMALE BARRIER TO PREVENT INFECTIONS FROM HUMAN IMMUNODEFICIENCY VIRUS

INDIVIDUALS REQUESTING PATENT: Dr. Lane B. Scheiber, ScD and Dr. Lane B. Scheiber II, MD

NUMBER OF CLAIMS: 2 independent claims, 18 dependent claims

ABSTRACT

The Human Immunodeficiency Virus poses a significant threat to the world's population. Current strategies utilized to treat infectious agents have not been adequate to eradicate such deadly viral infections. HIV seeks out its host, a T–Helper cell, by having utilizing glycoprotein 120 probes to engage CD4 cell-surface receptors located on the surface of a T-Helper cell. Development of protective barrier techniques for women to utilize during sex that incorporate filter mediums that offer HIV virions' probes the opportunity to engage the cell-surface receptors they are seeking offers a means of neutralizing the infectious threat of HIV. Providing barriers with filter mediums comprised of sheets, strips, or spheres of lipid bilayer or virus-like structures or hypoallergenic surfaces to carry cell-surface receptors, each type of medium having affixed cell-surface receptors intended to engage HIV virions provides an effective strategy to prevent AIDS in women.

BACKGROUND OF THE INVENTION

1. Field of the Invention

[0001] This invention relates to any medical device that is utilized to act as a barrier utilized by a woman to protect the woman from contracting the Human Immunodeficiency Virus as a result of engaging in sex with a man by neutralizing the infectious nature of Human Immunodeficiency Virus virions.

2. Description of Background Art

[0002] It has been estimated by the Center for Disease Control that in the United States 55,000 to 60,000 new cases of Human Immunodeficiency Virus (HIV) are occurring each year. It is thought that there are 900,000 people currently infected with HIV in the United States, with many victims not aware that they have contracted the virus. Further, it has been estimated that the Human Immunodeficiency Virus (HIV), the pathogen that causes Acquired Immune Deficiency Syndrome (AIDS), has infected as many as 30-60 million people around the globe.

[0003] The presence of HIV was first came to the attention of those in the United States in 1981, when there appeared an outbreak of Kaposi's Sarcoma and Pneumocystis carinii pneumonia in gay men in New York and California. After over twenty-five years of research and investigation, eradicating the ever growing global humanitarian crisis posed by the HIV remains an elusive goal for the medical community. It is estimated the virus has already killed 25 million citizens of this planet.

[0004] The Human Immunodeficiency Virus has been previously referred to as human T-Lymphotrophic virus III (HTLV-III), lymphadenopathy-associated virus (LAV), and AIDS-associated retrovirus (ARV). Infection with HIV may occur by the virus being transferred by blood, semen, vaginal fluid, or breast milk. Four major means of transmission of HIV include unprotected sexual intercourse, contaminated needles, breast milk, and transmission from an infected mother to her baby at birth.

[0005] HIV is an ingeniously constructed very deadly virus, which represents the most challenging pathogen the worldwide medical community faces to date. Viruses in general, have been difficult to contain and eradicate due to the fact they are obligate parasites and tend not to carry out any biologic functions outside the cell the virus has targeted as its host. A virus when it exists outside the boundaries of a cell is generally referred to as a virion. HIV virions posses several attributes that make them very elusive and difficult to destroy.

[0006] For purposes of this text, the term 'body' refers to the material part of a man or a woman, generally including the head, neck, trunk, extremities and all usual internal structures. For the purposes of this text, the term 'vagina' refers to the genital canal in a woman extending from the uterus to the vulva.

[0007] Bacterial infections have posed an easier target for the medical community to eradicate from the body. Bacteria generally live and reproduce outside animal cells. Bacteria, like animal cells, carryout biologic functions. A large multi-celled organism such as the human body combats bacterial infections with a combined force of white cells, antibodies, complements and its lymphatic system. White cells circulate the body in search of bacteria. When a white cell encounters a bacterium, the white cell engulfs the bacterium, encapsulates the pathogen, processes the identification of the pathogen and kills the pathogen utilizing acids and destructive enzymes. The white cell then alerts the B-cells of the immune system as to the identity of the intruding bacterium. A subpopulation of B-cells is generated, dedicated to producing antibodies directed against the particular pathogen the circulating white cell encountered and identified. Antibodies, generated by B-cells, traverse the blood and body tissues in search of the bacteria they were designed to repel. Once an antibody encounters a bacterium it is targeted to attack, the antibody attaches to the bacterium's outer wall. The effect antibodies have in coating the outside of a bacterium is to assist the white cells and the other components of the immune system in recognizing the bacterium, so that appropriate defensive action can be taken against the pathogen. Some antibodies, in addition to coating the bacterium, will act to punch holes through the bacterium's outer wall. If the integrity of the bacterium's cell wall is breached, this action generally leads to the death of the bacterium. Complements are primitive protein structures that circulate the blood stream in search of anything that appears consistent with a bacteria cell wall. Complements are indiscriminant. Once the complement proteins locate any form of bacterial cell wall, the complement proteins organize, and much like antibodies, act in concert to punch one or more holes though a bacterium's cell wall to compromise the viability of the bacterium. The lymphatic system is a diffuse network of thin walled vessels that drain excess water from extracellular fluids and join to form the thoracic duct and right lymph duct, which empty into the venous system near the heart. Lymph nodes are present at different locations in the body and screen the fluid transiting the lymphatic system, called lymph, to remove pathogens. Cells in the spleen screen the blood in search of bacteria. When a bacterial pathogen is identified, such as by antibodies coating the surface, the bacterium is taken out of circulation and terminated.

[0008] Viruses pose a much different infectious vector to the body's defense system than either bacteria or cellular parasites. Since viruses do not carry out biologic processes outside their host cell, a virus can be destroyed, but they cannot be killed. A virus is simply comprised of one or more external shells and a portion of genetic material. The virus's genetic information is carried in the core of the virus. Antibodies can coat the exterior of a virus to make it easier for the white cells in the body to identify the viral pathogen, but the action of punching holes in the virus's external shell by antibodies or complement proteins does not necessarily kill the virus. Viruses also only briefly circulate in the blood and tissues of the body as an exposed entity. Using exterior probes, a virus hunts down a cell in the body that will act as an appropriate host so that the virus can replicate. Once the virus has found a proper host cell, the virus inserts its genome into the host cell. To complete its life-cycle, the virus's genetic material takes command of cellular functions and directs the host cell to make replicas of the virus.

[0009] Once the virus's genome has entered a host cell, the virus is in effect shielded from the body's immune system defense mechanisms. Inside a host cell, the presence of the virus is generally only represented as genetic information incorporated into the host cell's DNA. Once a virus has infected a cell in the body, the presence of the virus can only be eradicated if the host cell is destroyed. Antibodies and complements are generally designed not to attack the autologous tissues of the body. Circulating white cells and the immune cells which comprise lymph nodes and the spleen may or may not recognize that a cell, which has become a host for a virus, is infected with a virus's genome. If the immune system fails to identify a cell that has become infected with a virus, the virus's genetic material can proceed to force the infected cell to make copies of the virus. Since a virus is in essence simply a segment of genetic material, time is of no consequence to the life-cycle of the virus and a virus's genome may be carried for years by the host without a need to activate; such viruses are often termed latent viruses. A virus's genetic material may sit idle in a host cell for an extended period of time until the pathogen's programming senses the time is right to initiate the virus's replication process or an action of the host cell triggers the virus to replicate. The only opportunity for the immune system to destroy a latent virus is when copies of the virus leave the host cell and circulate in the blood or tissues in search of another perspective host cell.

[0010] The traditional medical approach to combating infectious agents such as bacteria and cellular parasites, therefore has limited value in managing or eradicating elusive or latent viral infections. Synthetic antibiotics, generally used to augment the body's capacity to produce naturally occurring antibodies against bacterial infections, have little success in combating latent viral infections. Stimulating the body's immune system's recognition of a virus by administering a vaccine also has had limited success in combating elusive viral infections. Vaccines generally are intended to introduce to the body pieces of a bacteria or virus, or an attenuated, noninfectious intact bacteria or virus so that the immune system is able to recognize and process the infectious agent and generate antibodies directed to assist in killing the pathogen. Once the immune system has been primed to recognize an intruder, antibodies will be produced by the immune system in great quantities in an effort to repel an invader. Over time, as the immune system down-regulates its antibody production in response to a lack of detecting the presence of the intruding pathogen, the quantity of antibodies circulating in the blood stream may decrease in number to a quantity that is insufficient to combat a pathogen. Since antibodies have limited value in combating some of the more elusive viruses that hibernate in host cells, vaccines have limited value in destroying latent viruses.

[0011] The Human Immunodeficiency Virus demonstrates four factors which make this pathogen particularly elusive and a difficult infectious agent to eradicate from the body. First: the host for HIV is the T-Helper cell. The T-Helper cell is a key element in the immune system's response since it helps coordinate the body's defensive actions against pathogens seeking to invade the body's tissues. In cases of a bacterial infection versus a viral infection, T-Helper cells actively direct which immune cells will rev-up in response to the infectious agent and engage the particular pathogen. Since HIV infects and disrupts T-Helper cells, coordination of the immune response against the virus is disrupted, thus limiting the body's capacity to mount a proper response against the presence of the virus and produce a sufficient action to successfully eradicate the virus.

[0012] Second: again, latent viruses such as HIV, have a strategic advantage. When the immune system first recognizes a pathogen and begins to generate antibodies against a particular pathogen, the response is generally robust. Once time has passed and the immune system fails to detect an active threat, the production of antibodies against the particular pathogen diminishes. When HIV infects a T-Helper cell, the viral genome may lay dormant, sometimes for years before taking command of the T-Helper cell's biologic functions. HIV may, therefore, generate a very active initial immune response to its presence, but if the virus sits dormant inside T-Helper cells for months or years, the antibody response to the virus will diminish over time. There may not be an adequate quantity of circulating antibodies to actively engage the HIV virions as they migrate from the T-Helper cell that generated the copies to uninfected T-Helper cells that will serve as a new host to support further replication. If the immune system's response is insufficient during the period while the virus is exposed and vulnerable, it becomes extremely difficult for the body to eradicate the virus.

[0013] Third, when replicas of the Human Immunodeficiency Virus are released from their host cell, during the budding process the HIV virion coats itself with an exterior envelope comprised of a portion of the plasma membrane from the T-Helper cell that acted as the host for the virus. A T-Helper cell's plasma membrane is comprised of a lipid bilayer, a double layer of lipid molecules oriented with their polar ends at the outside of the membrane and the nonpolar ends in the membrane interior. The virus thus, in part, takes on an external appearance of a naturally occurring cell in the body. Since the exterior envelope of a HIV virion has the characteristics of a T-Helper cell it is more difficult for the immune system to recognize that it is a pathogen as it migrates through the body in search of another T-Helper cell to infect.

[0014]   Fourth, the Human Immunodeficiency Virus exhibits a very elusive mode of action which the virus readily utilizes to actively defeat the body's immune system.   HIV carries in its genome a segment of genetic material that directs an infected T-Helper cell to create and mount on the surface the plasma membrane a FasL cell-surface receptor.   Healthy T-Helper cells carry on the surface of their plasma membrane Fas cell-surface receptors.   The Fas cell-surface receptor when engaged by a FasL cell-surface receptor on another cell, initiates apoptosis in the cell carrying the Fas cell-surface receptor.   Apoptosis is a biologic process that causes a cell to terminate itself.   A T-Helper cell infected with the HIV virus carrying a FasL cell-surface receptor is therefore capable of killing noninfected T-Helper cells that the infected T-Helper cell encounters as it circulates the body.   The occurrence of AIDS is therefore propagated not only by the number of T-Helper cells that become incapacitated due to direct infection by HIV, but also by the number of noninfected T-Helper cells that are eliminated by coming in direct contact with infected T-Helper cells.

[0015]   Acquired Immune Deficiency Syndrome (AIDS) occurs as a result of the number of circulating T-Helper cells declining to a point where the immune system's capacity to mount a successful response against opportunistic infectious agents is significantly compromised.   The number of viable T-Helper cells declines either because they become infected with the HIV virus or because they have been killed by encountering a T-Helper cell infected with HIV.   When there is an insufficient population of non-HIV infected T-Helper cells to properly combat infectious agents such as Pneumocystis carinii or cytomegalo virus or other pathogens, the body becomes overwhelmed with the opportunistic infection and the patient becomes clinically ill. In cases where the combination of the patient's compromised immune system and medical assistance in terms of synthetic antibiotics intended to combat the opportunistic pathogens, fluids, intravenous nutrition and other treatments are not sufficient to sustain life, the body succumbs to the opportunistic infection and death ensues.

[0016]   The Human Immunodeficiency Virus locates its host by utilizing probes located on its envelope. The HIV virion has two types of glycoprotein probes attached to the outer surface of its exterior envelope. A glycoprotein is a structure comprised of a protein component and a lipid component. HIV utilizes a glycoprotein 120 (gp 120) probe to locate a CD4 cell-surface receptor on the plasma membrane of a T-Helper cell. The plasma membrane of the T-Helper cell is comprised of a lipid bilayer. Cell-surface receptors are anchored in the lipid bilayer. Once an HIV gp 120 probe has successfully engaged a CD4 cell-surface receptor on a T-Helper cell a conformational change occurs in the gp 120 probe and a glycoprotein 41 (gp 41) probe is exposed. The gp 41 probe's intent is to engage a CXCR4 or CCR5 cell-surface receptor on the plasma membrane of the same T-Helper cell. Once a gp 41 probe on the HIV virion engages a CXCR4 or CCR5 cell-surface receptor, the HIV virion opens an access portal through the T-Helper cell's plasma membrane.

[0017]   Once the virus has gained access to the T-Helper cell by opening a portal through the cell's outer membrane the virion inserts two positive strand RNA molecules approximately 9500 nucleotides in length. Inserted along with the RNA strands are the enzymes reverse transcriptase, protease and integrase. Once the virus's genome gains access to the interior of the T-Helper cell, in the cytoplasm the pair of RNA molecules are transformed to deoxyribonucleic acid by the reverse transcriptase enzyme. Following modification of the virus's genome to DNA, the virus's genetic information migrates to the host cell's nucleus. In the nucleus, with the assistance of the integrase protein, the virus's DNA becomes inserted into the

T-Helper cell's native DNA. When the timing is appropriate, the now integrated viral DNA, becomes read by the host cell's polymerase molecules and the virus's genetic information commands certain cell functions to carry out the replication process to construct copies of the human deficiency virus.

[0018] Present anti-viral therapy has been designed to target the enzymes that assist the HIV genome with the replication process. Anti-viral therapy is intended to interfere with the action of these replication enzymes. Part of the challenge of eradicating HIV is that once the virus inserts its genome into a T-Helper cell host, the viral genome may lay dormant until the proper circumstances evolve. The virus's genome may sit idle inside a T-Helper cell for years before becoming activated, causing drugs that interfere with HIV's life cycle to have limited effect on eliminating the virus from the body. Arresting the replication process does not insure that T-Helper cells infected with HIV do not continue to circulate the body killing noninfected T-Helper cells thus causing the patient to progress to a clinically apparent state of Acquired Immune Deficiency Syndrome and eventually succumbing to an opportunistic infection which eventually results in the death of the individual.

[0019] The outer layer of the HIV virion is comprised of a portion of the T-Helper cell's outer cell membrane. In the final stage of the replication process, as a copy of the HIV capsid, carrying the HIV genome, buds through the host cell's plasma membrane, the capsid acquires as its outermost shell a wrapping of lipid bilayer from the host cell's plasma membrane. Vaccines are generally comprised of pieces of a virus or bacterium, or copies of the entire virus or bacterium weakened to the point the pathogen is incapable of causing an infection. These pieces of a pathogen or copies of a nonvirulent pathogen prime the immune system such that a vaccine intent is to cause B-cells to produce antibodies that are programmed to seek out the surface characteristics of the pathogen comprising the vaccine. In the case of HIV, since the surface of the pathogen is an envelope comprised of lipid bilayer taken from the host T-Helper cell's plasma membrane, a vaccine comprised of portions of the exterior envelope of the HIV virions might not only target HIV virions, but might also have deleterious effects on the T-Helper cell population. Some antibodies produced to combat HIV infections may not be able to tell the difference between an HIV virion and a T-Helper cell, and such antibodies may act to coat and assist in the elimination of both targets. In such a scenario, since such a vaccine might cause a decline in the number of available T-Helper cells, it is conceivable that a vaccine comprised of portions of the external envelope of HIV virions might paradoxically induce clinically apparent AIDS in a patient that a vaccine has been administered.

[0020] It is clear that the traditional approach of utilizing antibiotics or providing vaccines to stimulate the immune system to produce endogenous antibodies, by themselves, is an ineffective strategy to manage a virus as elusive and deadly as HIV. Drugs that interfere with the replication process of HIV generally slow progression of the infection by the virus, but do not necessarily eliminate the virus from the body nor eliminate the threat of the clinical symptoms of AIDS. A new strategy is required in order to successfully combat the threat of HIV.

[0021] The Human Immunodeficiency Virus virion is much smaller in size than the red blood cells and white blood cells. The gp120 and gp 41 probes located on the surface of HIV are seeking to engage the CD4 and CXCR4 or CCR5 cell-surface receptors located on T-Helper cells. A filter mechanism could be fashioned to be comprised of a chamber that contains a filter medium constructed to engage HIV virions. Upon body fluids entering the chamber, such fluids would come in contact with the filter medium inside the chamber and HIV virions being carried in such fluid would come in contact with the surface features of the filter medium. As HIV's glycoprotein probes, gp120 and gp 41, engage the CD4 and CXCR4 or CCR5 cell-surface receptors mounted on the filter medium present in the chamber, the HIV virions carried in body fluids would adhere to the filter medium and either become stuck to the filter medium thus being retained inside the filter chamber as the body fluids exit the chamber, or by the action of the HIV probes engaging the filter medium cell-surface receptors HIV virions would eject their genome rendering the HIV virion incapable of infecting an endogenous T-Helper cell in the woman. Such a chamber could be fashioned to be comfortably placed in a woman's vagina. One version of the chamber would be fashioned such that the filter medium would be retained inside the chamber. Another version of the chamber would be fashioned such that the filter medium could be expressed from the chamber and the filter medium could mix freely with the body fluids present in the vagina.

[0022] The technology to make such filter mechanisms is readably available and could be quickly implemented for worldwide use to prevent infections by HIV virions.

[0023] A device, to accomplish the task of acting as a barrier and filtering out Human Immunodeficiency Virus virions, would be to construct a chamber, which inside the chamber would be present a filter medium, this filter medium constructed surface characteristics similar to the surface characteristics of a naturally occurring T-Helper cell, since, specifically, it is the cell-surface receptors affixed to the surface of a T-Helper cell that the HIV virion's probes are seeking. T-Helper cells are constructed with the outer membrane being comprised of a lipid bilayer. Cell-surface receptors are anchored into this lipid bilayer and the protein portion of the cell-surface receptor extends out and away from the surface of the T-Helper cell. Sheets of lipid bilayer constructed with a generous quantity of CD4, CXCR4 and CCR5 cell-surface receptors affixed to the surface, would attract and engage HIV virions as a surrogate target in place of endogenous T-Helper cells the HIV virions are seeking as a host.

[0024] A medical device could be constructed in a manner where a quantity of lipid bilayer fashioned in the shape of sheets or strips or spheres would be constructed with a generous quantity of CD4, CXCR4 and CCR5 cell-surface receptors affixed to the surface of the filter medium would be placed inside a chamber. The chamber would be fashioned to be inserted inside the vagina of a woman. Body fluids, a combination of vaginal secretions generated by the woman and pre-ejaculate and ejaculate generated by one or more a male partners, would pass through the filter chamber. As the body fluids pass across the surface of a sheet or strip or sphere of lipid bilayer, HIV virions would come in contact with CD4, CXCR4 and CXR5 cell-surface receptors present on the surface of the lipid bilayer and engage the cell-surface receptors. The HIV virions making contact with the lipid bilayer would either permanently adhere to the lipid bilayer or by engaging the cell-surface receptors on the lipid bilayer the HIV virions would be caused to eject their genome, which would neutralize the infectious threat of the HIV virions. The body fluids exiting the filter chamber would be cleared of HIV virions capable of infecting T-Helper cell endogenous to the woman's body.

[0025] A woman whom desired to become pregnant may be able to become pregnant from a sex partner with sperm and possibly not contract the Human Immunodeficiency Virus because the sperm would not accompanied by body fluids that carried HIV virions. A woman whom wished not to become pregnant might utilize a variation of the filter chamber device that in addition to containing the filter medium, also contained an agent that prevented sperm from being able to engage in zygosis and impregnate a viable egg present inside the woman. A woman whom wished not to become pregnant might use an alternative means of birth control, such as oral birth control pills, in place of a suppository device containing a spermicidal agent.

[0026] Since HIV virions are searching their environment for CD4, CXCR4 and CXR5 cell-surface receptors a filter material comprised of any hypoallergenic material suitable to attach CD4, CXCR4 and CXR5 cell-surface receptors or the protein portion of these receptors, to the surface of the material, could be placed inside the filter chamber and act as an effective filter medium. Body fluids, a combination of vaginal secretions generated by the woman, and pre-ejaculate and ejaculate generated by one or more a male partners, would pass through the filter chamber. As the body fluids pass across the surface of a sheet or strips or spheres of a hypoallergenic material with CD4, CXCR4 and CXR5 cell-surface receptors, HIV virions would come in contact with CD4, CXCR4 and CXR5 cell-surface receptors present on the surface of the hypoallergenic material and engage the cell-surface receptors. The HIV virions making contact with the cell-surface receptors affixed to the hypoallergenic material would either permanently adhere to the hypoallergenic material or by engaging the cell-surface receptors affixed to the surface of the hypoallergenic material the HIV virions would be caused to eject their genome, which would neutralize the infectious threat of the HIV virions. The body fluids exiting the filter chamber would be cleared of HIV virions capable of infecting T-Helper cell endogenous to the woman's body.

[0027] White blood cells are physically larger than red blood cells. Bacteria are generally much smaller than red blood cells. HIV virions are much smaller than bacteria. HIV is comprised of an outer envelope, an internal capsid and the viral genome. Because of its small size HIV can potentially maneuver into places in the body's tissues or crevasses between tissues where mobile cells are unable to go.

[0028] An approach to managing HIV would be to create a product that would be relatively the same size as HIV so that the product could penetrate into every location that HIV might migrate. HIV's probes are seeking the CD4 and CCR5 and

CXCR4 cell-surface receptors of a T-Helper cell, thus a product to challenge HIV could be equipped with the same cell-surface receptors as would be found on a naturally occurring T-Helper cell.

[0029]   Utilizing genetic machinery and a colony of T-Helper cells or a colony of hybrid T-Helper cells or a colony of specially designed host cells, a medically therapeutic modified virus or virus-like product approximately the size of a HIV virion could be manufactured in a similar manner as how HIV naturally replicates, except the product would carry the T-Helper cell cell-surface receptors CD4, CXCR4 and/or CCR5 instead of the glycoprotein probes associated with a naturally occurring HIV virion. The virus-like product would be constructed either with no genetic information present inside the capsid or genetic material to act as a filler, this genetic material being inert such that it could not carry out any useful function.

[0030]   Constructing a virus-like structure, that has affixed to its exterior cell-surface receptors intended to engage a virus, is referred to as a Scientifically Modulated And Reprogrammed Target (SMART) virus. Copies of such a SMART virus could be placed in a filter chamber. The diameter of the SMART virus could be increased to a size larger than the naturally occurring HIV virion to facilitate containing the SMART virus inside the filter chamber as the body fluids pass through the filter chamber. Body fluids could transit through the filter chamber containing a quantity of SMART virus. The SMART virus would be available within the walls of the chamber to engage HIV virions as the body fluids pass through the filter chamber.   As HIV virions make contact with SMART viruses the HIV virions would engage the SMART virus and become permanently attached and become trapped inside the chamber, or the HIV virions, upon engaging a SMART virus, would harmlessly eject the genetic material the HIV virion carries. Either trapping the HIV virion inside the filter chamber or causing the HIV virion to eject the genetic material that it carries, would neutralize the virulence of HIV and assist in managing the threat of AIDS. Copies of such a SMART virus could be fashioned such that they are expressed from the chamber through holes in the walls of the chamber to mix freely with the body fluids present in the vagina to engage HIV virions that may be present in the body fluids in the vagina.

[0031]   The most effective barrier in preventing a woman from contracting the Human Immunodeficiency Virus would be to construct the filter material in such a manner as to allow the filter medium to exit the filter chamber. A stimulus such as pressure applied to the exterior of a compressible filter chamber would cause the filter medium contained inside the filter chamber to be expressed from the filter chamber through the holes in the walls of the filter chamber.   Women are vulnerable to contracting the Human Immunodeficiency Virus by means of abrasions or lacerations incurred by the vaginal wall while engaging in sex or by the Human Immunodeficiency Virus virions gaining access to the inner portions of the woman's body by passing through the os of the cervix, then passing through the uterus, then passing through the fallopian tubes, finally ending up in the abdominal cavity. The filter chamber may assist in preventing HIV virions from penetrating the woman through the cervix, a filter medium that would be expressed into the vagina would coat the walls of the vagina, providing a secondary barrier in addition to the primary barrier created by the presence of the filter chamber to help prevent HIV virions from gaining access to the woman's internal tissues through abrasions or lacerations in the tissues of the vagina.

BRIEF SUMMARY OF THE INVENTION

[0032]   Initially the Human Immunodeficiency Virus is attracted to its host, the T-helper cell, by having its surface probes seek out a CD4 cell-surface receptor. Once HIV virion's gp 120 probe successfully engages a CD4 cell-surface receptor a conformation change occurs in the gp 120 probe and a gp 41 probe attempts to engage either a CXCR4 or a CCR5 cell-surface receptor located on the target T-Helper cell. Described here is a device that offers a surrogate target HIV virions are seeking. It is a device intended to remove the infectious threat of Human Immunodeficiency Virus virions from body fluids present in the vagina. Body fluids in the vagina enter a filter chamber that contains a filter medium that is placed in the vagina by the woman using the device when she wishes to use such the device to prevent an infection by the Human Immunodeficiency Virus. As the body fluids transit through the filter chamber the body fluids make contact with the filter medium present in the filter chamber. As the body fluids transit the filter chamber any HIV virions present in the body fluids have the opportunity to engage the three cell surface receptors the CD 4 receptor, the CCR5 receptor and the CXCR4 receptor which are well known to the medical and scientific community due to the fact they appear naturally on the surface of the Human T-Helper cell. A version of the medical device expresses the filter medium present inside the device's chamber, such that the filter medium is meant to be present inside of the vagina and engage HIV virions present in body fluids inside the vagina. Since the HIV virions engage cell-surface receptors located on the surface of the filter medium rather than located on the surface of endogenous T-Helper cells inside the body, the infectious nature of the HIV virions is neutralized by either the HIV virion becoming trapped by being attached the filter medium or the HIV virion is caused to harmlessly eject its genome. When HIV virions become trapped by the filter medium it is incapable of migrating further to successfully engaging endogenous T-Helper cells inside the body. When a HIV virion is caused to eject its genome, the HIV virion is incapable of infecting an endogenous T-Helper cell inside the body. Trapping the HIV virion or causing the HIV virion to harmlessly eject its genome leads to neutralizing the infectious threat of HIV, which leads to effectively averting AIDS. The residual chamber is removed from the vagina and appropriately discarded after the sexual encounter has been completed and the threat of infection by Human Immunodeficiency Virus virions is minimized.

DETAILED DESCRIPTION OF THE INVENTION

[0033]   The invention described herein is intended to neutralize the virulence of Human Immunodeficiency Virus virions carried in body fluids deposited in the vagina of a woman.

[0034]   Three cell receptors CD4, CCR5 and CXCR4 are well known to the medical and scientific community and appear naturally on the surface of the Human T-Helper cells. The HIV virion expresses gp 120 glycoprotein probes and glycoprotein 41 probes on its outer envelope. HIV utilizes the T-Helper cell as its host cell for the purposes of replication.

[0035]   In completing the virus's natural reproductive-cycle, HIV utilizes the gp 120 probe positioned on the exterior envelope of an HIV virion to locate and engage a T-Helper cell's CD4 exterior cell-surface receptor. Once the HIV's gp 120 has successfully engaged a CD 4 cell-surface receptor, the HIV virion's gp 41 probe engages either a CCR5 or CXCR4 exterior cell-surface receptor on the T-Helper cell. A filter medium present inside the inner chamber of a filter device, expressing CD4, CCR5 and CXCR4 cell-surface receptors offers a surrogate target expressing the cell-surface receptors HIV virions are seeking to engage.   When HIV virion's probes encounter a filter medium expressing CD4, CCR5 and CXCR4 cell-surface receptors, HIV's gp 120 probes would engage CD 4 exterior surface receptors, followed then by HIV's gp 41 probes engaging either CCR5 or CXCR4 exterior cell-surface receptors. Once the HIV gp 120 probes and gp 41 probes have engaged their respective cell-surface receptors affixed to the filter medium's exterior surface, the HIV is fixed to the surface of the filter medium and the HIV virion may eject RNA genome it carries. Since the HIV engaged a filter medium the HIV virion becomes affixed and trapped by the filter device and if the HIV virion ejects its RNA genome, the threat of the HIV virion being able to infect an endogenous T-Helper cell inside a body is effectively neutralized. The body fluids passing through such a filter becomes cleared of infectious HIV virions.

[0036] The medical device described herein, intended to neutralize infectious HIV virions in body fluids in the vagina of a woman, is comprised of a chamber, where body fluids enter into the chamber, the body fluids come into contact with a filter medium inside the chamber, the body fluids exit the chamber, the filter medium is retained inside the chamber. The filter medium inside the filter chamber may be comprised of several different materials and designs. The filter medium is intended to make available cell-surface receptors including CD 4, CCR5 and CXCR4 for HIV virions to engage. The filter medium may be comprised of a quantity of exogenous T-Helper cells. The filter medium may be comprised of a quantity of lipid bilayer sheets which are comprised of similar materials as found existing as the outer membrane of a T-Helper cell, and affixed to the said lipid bilayer sheets are glycoprotein cell-surface receptors including a quantity of CD4 cell-surface receptors, CXCR4 cell-surface receptors, CCR5 cell-surface receptors. The filter medium may be comprised of a quantity of modified viruses or virus-like structures with cell-surface receptors to include a quantity of CD4 cell-surface receptors, CXCR4 cell-surface receptors, CCR5 cell-surface receptors. The filter medium may be comprised of any appropriate hypoallergenic material, which can be affixed to the surface a quantity of CD4 cell-surface receptors, CXCR4 cell-surface receptors, CCR5 cell-surface receptors or simply the protein portion of the CD4 cell-surface receptors, CXCR4 cell-surface receptors, CCR5 cell-surface receptors.

[0037] The materials to be used to create the walls of such a filter chamber may any suitable hypoallergenic material include materials such as a flexible plastic, rigid plastic, cotton product, a paper product, latex, or a dissolvable material that dissolves and releases the filter medium contained inside the filter chamber once the filter chamber is placed in the vagina such that the filter medium is released into the vagina of the woman.

[0038] To carry out the process to manufacture a modified medically therapeutic virus, messenger RNA that would code for the general physical outer structures of the modified virus, such as instruction code to generate a modified HIV virion or a modified Hepatitis C virus virion or other virus virion or other virus-like structure, would be inserted into a host. The host may include devices such as a host cell or a hybrid host cell. The host may utilize DNA or RNA or a combination of genetic instructions in order to accomplish the construction of medically therapeutic modified virus virions. In some cases DNA or messenger RNA would be inserted into the host that would be coded to cause the production of surface probes that would be affixed to the surface of the virus virion that would target the glycoprotein probes affixed to the surface of an HIV virion. The copies of the medically therapeutic modified viruses or medically therapeutic virus-like structures, upon exiting the host, would be collected, stored and utilized as a medical treatment as necessary.

[0039] The medically therapeutic version of the modified virus and virus-like structures would be incapable of replication on its own due to the fact that the messenger RNA that would code for the replication process to produce copies of the virus or virus-like structure would not be present in the modified form of a virus or virus-like structure.

[0040] Lipid bilayer sheets can be manufactured and combinations of CD 4 cell-surface receptors, CXCR4 cell-surface receptors, CCR5 cell-surface receptors can be affixed to the surface, similar to the manner these cell-surface receptors are affixed to the surface of naturally occurring T-Helper cells, with the entire structure acting as a filter medium. Sheets of any appropriate hypoallergenic material can be manufactured and combinations of CD 4 cell-surface receptors, CXCR4 cell-surface receptors, CCR5 cell-surface receptors can be affixed to the surface with the entire structure acting as a filter medium. Sheets of any appropriate hypoallergenic material can be manufactured and combinations of the protein portion of the CD 4 cell-surface receptors, CXCR4 cell-surface receptors, CCR5 cell-surface receptors available to engage either glycoprotein probes on HIV or cell-surface receptors on a T-Helper cell, affixed to the surface of the hypoallergenic material with the entire structure acting as a filter medium.

[0041] The medical device described herein, intended to neutralize infectious HIV virions in body fluids in the vagina of a woman, is comprised of a chamber, where body fluids enter into the chamber, the body fluids come into contact with a filter medium, the body fluids exit the chamber, the filter medium is retained inside the chamber of the medical device. The chamber is to be fashioned to comfortably be placed in a woman's vagina. The filter medium inside the filter chamber may be comprised of several different materials and designs. The filter medium is intended to make available cell-surface receptors including CD 4, CCR5 and CXCR4, affixed to the surface of the filter medium similar to the manner these cell-surface receptors are affixed to the surface of naturally occurring T-Helper cells, for HIV virions to engage. The filter medium may be comprised of a quantity of exogenous T-Helper cells. The filter medium may be comprised of a quantity of lipid bilayer sheets which are comprised of similar materials as found existing as the outer membrane of a T-Helper cell, and affixed to the said lipid bilayer sheets are glycoprotein cell-surface receptors including a quantity of CD4 cell-surface receptors, CXCR4 cell-surface receptors, CCR5 cell-surface receptors. The filter medium may be comprised of a quantity of modified viruses or virus-like structures with cell-surface receptors to include a quantity of CD4 cell-surface receptors, CXCR4 cell-surface receptors, CCR5 cell-surface receptors. The filter medium may be comprised of any appropriate hypoallergenic material, which can be affixed to the surface a quantity of CD4 cell-surface receptors, CXCR4 cell-surface receptors, CCR5 cell-surface receptors or simply the protein portion of the CD4 cell-surface receptors, CXCR4 cell-surface receptors, CCR5 cell-surface receptors. The hypoallergenic material may be fashioned into the shape of a sheet, a strip or a sphere.

[0042] The medical device described herein, intended to neutralize infectious HIV virions in body fluids in the vagina of a woman, is comprised of a chamber, where body fluids enter into the chamber, the body fluids come into contact with a filter medium, the body fluids exit the chamber. Pressure applied to the outside of the chamber may cause the filter medium to be expressed from the chamber of the medical device into the vagina where the filter medium would mix with the body fluids present in the vagina. Once the chamber is placed inside the vagina, the walls of the chamber may dissolve causing the filter medium to be expressed from the chamber of the medical device into the vagina where the filter medium would mix with the body fluids present in the vagina. The chamber is to be fashioned to comfortably be placed in a woman's vagina. The filter medium present inside the filter chamber may be comprised of several different materials and designs. The filter medium is intended to make available cell-surface receptors including CD 4, CCR5 and CXCR4, affixed to the surface of the filter medium similar to the manner these cell-surface receptors are affixed to the surface of naturally occurring T-Helper cells, for HIV virions to engage. The filter medium may be comprised of a quantity of exogenous T-Helper cells. The filter medium may be comprised of a quantity of lipid bilayer sheets which are comprised of similar materials as found existing as the outer membrane of a T-Helper cell, and affixed to the said lipid bilayer sheets are glycoprotein cell-surface receptors including a quantity of CD4 cell-surface receptors, CXCR4 cell-surface receptors, CCR5 cell-surface receptors. The filter medium may be comprised of a quantity of modified viruses or virus-like structures with cell-surface receptors to include a quantity of CD4 cell-surface receptors, CXCR4 cell-surface receptors, CCR5 cell-surface receptors. The filter medium may be comprised of any appropriate hypoallergenic material, which can be affixed to the surface a quantity of CD4 cell-surface receptors, CXCR4 cell-surface receptors, CCR5 cell-surface receptors or simply the protein portion of the CD4 cell-surface receptors, CXCR4 cell-surface receptors, CCR5 cell-surface receptors. The hypoallergenic material may be fashioned into the shape of a sheet, a strip or a sphere. The filter medium may be suspended in a hypoallergenic fluid or cream.

[0043]   The filter chamber may be fashioned to allow sperm to enter and exit the chamber, thus allowing a woman to retain the possibility of becoming pregnant, but due to the presence of the filter medium, limit the chances of contracting the Human Immunodeficiency Virus.

[0044]   The filter medium may coexist with an agent that acts as a spermatocide to prevent sperm present in the vagina from being able to proceed from the vagina to fertilize an egg and cause the woman to become pregnant.

[0045]   The residual chamber is intended to be removed from the vagina and appropriately discarded after the sexual encounter has been completed and the threat of infection by Human Immunodeficiency Virus virions is minimized.

CLAIMS: Reserved.

A6: SCIENTIFICALLY MODULATED AND REPROGRAMMED TREATMENT (SMART) FAS/FASL VIRUS TECHNOLOGY INTENDED TO NEUTRALIZE T-HELPER CELLS INFECTED WITH THE HUMAN IMMUNODEFICIENCY VIRUS

INDIVIDUALS REQUESTING PATENT: Dr. Lane B. Scheiber, ScD and Dr. Lane B. Scheiber II, MD

CITIZENSHIP: Both United States Citizens

NUMBER OF CLAIMS: 15

ABSTRACT

Scientifically Modulated And Reprogrammed Treatment (SMART) Virus Fas/FasL technology is intended to terminate T-Helper cells infected with the Human Immunodeficiency Virus. The SMART-Fas/FasL Virus carrying Fas and FasL cell-surface receptors is capable of engaging a T-Helper cell infected by HIV that is expressing one or more FasL cell-surface receptors. When a T-Helper cell infected with HIV encounters a SMART-Fas/FasL Virus, the infected T-Helper cell's FasL cell-surface receptor will engage the SMART-Fas/FasL Virus's Fas receptor, then the SMART-Fas/FasL Virus's FasL will engage the infected T-Helper cell's Fas receptor, which will initiate apoptosis in the infected T-Helper cell. Given the HIV infected T-Helper cell will be triggered to die, HIV's safe haven inside the T-Helper cell will be eliminated and the threat of Acquired Immunodeficiency Syndrome caused by HIV is averted.

BACKGROUND OF THE INVENTION

Field of the Invention

This invention relates to any medical device intended to physically interact directly with T-Helper cells infected with the Human Immunodeficiency Virus (HIV) or infected with other virus, to neutralize the infectious threat of the virus.

Description of the Background Art

[0001] The Human Immunodeficiency Virus (HIV), which is responsible for Acquired Immunodeficiency Disease Syndrome (AIDS), threatens the lives of an estimated 170 millions of people worldwide. There are different strains of HIV that exist around the world. Most predominantly HIV-1 exists worldwide and HIV-2 is generally found in Western Africa, the western coastal regions of India and in Europe. Amongst HIV-1 and HIV-2 they can be further subdivided into different strains including an 'R5' strain which uses a CCR5 cell-surface receptor on a T-Helper cell to identify and access its host and an 'X4' strain which uses a CXCR4 cell-surface receptor located on a T-Helper cell to identify and access its host. The approach to controlling the disease caused by HIV has been the application of drugs directed at interfering with the replication process, in an attempt to slow down the rate of replication of the virus. Millions of people continue to die and the virus continues to pose an escalating worldwide threat despite current treatment strategies. The virus is generally communicated between individuals by contact with body fluids carrying intact HIV.

[0002] Though there are recognized differences between HIV-1 and HIV-2, for purposes of further discussion the term 'HIV' will refer to both HIV-1 and HIV-2, unless otherwise not-ed. HIV is a retrovirus with its genetic material in the form of two identical copies of a positive sense single stranded ribonucleic acid (RNA) molecule, each approximately 9500 nucleotides long. HIV is approximately 50 to 150 nm in diameter, about one seventieth the size of a white cell carrying the marker Cluster Designation 4 (CD4) exterior cell-surface receptor.

[0003] A eukaryote refers to a nucleated cell. Eukaryotes comprise nearly all plant and animal cells. Animal cells generally are comprised of a cell membrane, cytoplasm, a nucleus and organelles. The cell membrane consists of a lipid bilayer where two layers of lipid molecules oriented with their polar ends pointed outside of the membrane and their nonpolar ends points toward the inside of the membrane. Polarized ends of the lipid molecules are hydrophobic, therefore the lipid bilayer functions to control the movement of water, nutrients and hormones in and out of a cell. A variety of receptors affixed to the exterior of the lipid bilayer membrane assist in a cell communicating with its environment. The cytoplasm inside a cell, which forms the interior fluid matrix of the cell, is comprised of amino acids and nutrients. The nucleus is surrounded by a double membrane (often referred to as a nuclear membrane) and contains the majority of a cell's genetic material. Organelles are structures generally found in the cytoplasm that perform specialized functions of cells. Organelles found inside a cell may include the mitochondria, endoplasmic reticulum, Golgi complex, lysosomes, vacuoles.

[0004] Genetic material in a eukaryote is generally in the form of deoxyribonucleic acid (DNA) with the majority located in the nucleus of the cell, but DNA may also be found in the mitochondria of cells. By the process of transcription, a section of the DNA is read by a polymerase and a molecule of ribonucleic acid (RNA) is generated. DNA is comprised of sections of combinations of four nucleotides: adenine, cytosine, guanine, and thymine. When two strands of nucleotides are arranged together, such as in the double helix configuration of chromosomal DNA, adenine on one strand is always matched to thymine in the opposing strand, and cytosine on one strand is always matched to guanine in the opposing strand. RNAs generated by polymerases reading nuclear DNA are usually single stranded chains of nucleotides, constructed of similar adenine, cytosine and guanine nucleotides as DNA, but instead of 'thymine', RNAs are constructed with the nucleotide 'uracil'. RNAs are generally divided into three categories including messenger RNA (mRNA), ribosomal RNA (rRNA) and transfer RNA (tRNA). Messenger RNAs are considered positive sense and interact with ribosomes to generate protein molecules. Ribosomes read the code physically built into the messenger RNAs, and with the aid of rRNAs and tRNAs, generate protein molecules by bonding together amino acids in linear configurations as directed by the code on a messenger RNA.

[0005]   Blood cells are generally referred to as white blood cells and red blood cells. Thrombocytes, otherwise known as platelets, are flat disk-shaped cell fragments that circulate the blood to assist with clotting when required. White blood cells, also referred to as leukocytes, play an active role in the body's immune system. White blood cells are further divided into T-Cells and B-Cells. T-Helper cells, also known as CD4 T-lymphocytes or CD4 T-Cells, are a subset of white blood cells. T-Helper cells act to coordinate the body's immune response against infectious agents. A significant decline in the number of circulating T-Helper cells represents a state where the body is vulnerable to opportunistic infections such as pneumonia, fungal infections or other common ailments.

[0006]   Viruses are obligate intracellular parasites designed to infect cells often with great specificity to a particular cell type it uses as a host. Virion is a term that refers to a complete structure of a virus as it exists outside of a host cell. Viruses do not carry out any biologically active processes on their own when outside a host cell. A virus requires a host in order to reproduce itself. Viruses circulate the environment without the need for nutrition or energy production through respiration. Viruses are in essence a vehicle that carries the genetic programming instructions necessary to cause an appropriate host cell to generate identical copies of the same virus. Some viruses, such as HIV, do introduce to their host cells programming instructions that result in toxic effects to the body as a whole.

[0007] HIV is considered to be approximately spherical in shape and comprised of an outer lipid bilayer envelope, a matrix protein, a capsid, two strands of RNA, nucleocapsid protein and proteins to assist in the replication process. The virus's core or capsid is icosahedral in shape and acts as a protective shell to carry the genetic payload. The capsid is comprised of numerous copies of the capsid protein (p24), the number and arrangement of the capsid proteins determines the overall dimensions of the capsid shell; HIV uses approximately 2,000 capsid proteins (p24) to construct its capsid. The capsid carries the two single strands of RNA each containing a copy of the virus's nine genes, the nucleocapsid protein, reverse transcriptase, protease and integrase. The nucleocapsid protein causes the RNA to coil up so that it can fit inside the capsid. The protein matrix consisting of protein 17 (p17) covers the capsid. The HIV envelope is derived from the plasma membrane of the host cell as the virus buds or pushes through the host cell's plasma membrane as it exits and migrates from the host cell. Anchored in and projecting out from the HIV's lipid bilayer outer membrane, otherwise referred to as an envelope, are exterior probes well known to the medical and scientific community as glycoprotein 120 (gp 120) and glycoprotein 41 (gp 41). The term glycoprotein refers to a protein with a carbohydrate attached. The gp 41 probe is anchored to the outer envelope and is in close proximity to the gp 120 probe. The probes can be found arranged together into protein complexes, which may contain up to three gp 120 probes and three gp 41 probes. Protein complexes have been described as 'spikes'. It has been reported that an HIV outer envelope may project from ten to seventy-two said spikes.

[0008] A HIV virion transits the environment at large with its surface probes seeking to engage a human T-Helper cell. Human T-Helper cells express a number of cell-surface receptors on their outer plasma membrane including Cluster Designation 4 (CD4), Chemotactic Chemokine Receptor 5 (CCR5) and CX Chemokine Receptor 4 (CXCR4). HIV utilizes the human T-Helper cell, also known as a CD4 T-lymphocyte or CD4 T-Cell, as its host for the purpose of replicating copies of itself. To initiate its reproductive-cycle, the gp 120 probe on a HIV virion makes initial contact with a T-Helper cell's CD4 cell-surface receptor. Following the engagement of the gp 120 probe with the CD4 cell-surface receptor, the gp 120 probe alters its configuration to allow the HIV gp 41 probe to engage a second receptor on the surface of the T-Helper cell, either a CCR5 cell-surface receptor or a CXCR4 cell-surface receptor. Once the HIV virion's gp 120 probe has successfully engaged a T-Helper cell's CD4 cell-surface receptor and the HIV's gp 41 probe has successfully engaged the T-Helper cell's CCR5 or CXCR4 cell-surface receptor, then the HIV virion is able to transfer its capsid containing the two strands of ribonucleic acid (RNA) and the support proteins including reverse transcriptase, protease, and integrase into the T-Helper cell. Once the capsid has gained access to the interior of the T-Helper cell, utilizing the transferred HIV enzyme 'reverse transcriptase', the RNA molecules undergo reverse transcription to deoxyribonucleic acid (DNA). Protease helps modify HIV's genome. Aided by the integrase, the virus's RNA that has been transcribed into DNA migrates to the T-Helper cell's nucleus and is known to become inserted into the T-Helper cell's native DNA. The HIV genetic material then redirects the resources of the T-Helper cell to facilitate the manufacture of copies of HIV.

[0009] Most predominantly HIV-1 exists worldwide and HIV-2 is generally found in Western Africa, the western coastal regions of India and Europe. Amongst HIV-1 and HIV-2 that use CD4 as the initial cell-surface receptor to gain entry into a T-Helper cell, they can be further divided by an 'R5' strain which uses a CCR5 cell-surface receptor on a T-Helper cell to identify its host; an 'X4' strain which uses a CXCR4 cell-surface receptor located on a T-Helper cell to identify its host. It is also believed at least one strain of HIV-2 may infect a T-Helper cell without engaging a CD4 cell-surface receptor, but uses either a CCR5 or a CXCR4 cell-surface receptor on a T-Helper cell host. There has also been identified at least one strain of HIV-2 believed not utilize the CD4, CCR5 or the CXCR4 cell-surface receptors to engage a T-Helper cell host, the mode of entry utilized by this form or HIV virion is unknown at this time.

[0010] The Fas cell-surface receptor (also referred to as CD95 cell-surface receptor) appears naturally on the surface of T-Helper cells. The Fas cell-surface receptor, when triggered, will transmit into the cell a biologic signal to activate the process of apoptosis. Apoptosis is a natural process utilized to terminate a cell, resulting in cell death.

[0011] Naturally occurring T-Helper cells, not infected with HIV, help orchestrate the human body's immune response against infectious agents that threaten the health and integrity of the body. The HIV virus, by taking control and altering the function of the T-Helper cells in the body, creates a state of ill health. By redirecting the T-Helper cell's function to produce copies of the HIV virus rather than coordinate appropriate immune responses against potentially infectious agents leaves the body as a whole vulnerable to attack by other infectious agents that can do harm to the tissues of the body. In addition, the HIV genome carries a 'nef' gene. Once the HIV's DNA is inserted into the host cell's native DNA, the nef gene provides instructions for a Fas ligand (FasL) cell-surface marker to be manufactured and expressed on the surface of the infected T-Helper cell. Noninfected T-Helper cells (meaning not infected with HIV) express a Fas cell-surface marker. When a HIV infected T-Helper cell expressing the Fas ligand (FasL) cell-surface marker encounters a Fas cell-surface marker on a noninfected T-Helper cell, a lethal biologic signal is transmitted to the noninfected T-Helper cell. That is when the FasL cell-surface marker engages a Fas cell-surface marker, the process of apoptosis is triggered in the noninfected T-Helper cell. By triggering apoptosis in noninfected T-Helper cells, HIV infected T-Helper cells are capable of killing the noninfected T-Helper cells they encounter. The clinical ramifications of Acquired Immunodeficiency Syndrome (AIDS) occur when the number of noninfected T-Helper cells declines to the point the immune system is unable to defend the body as a whole from dangerous infectious agents that would attempt to invade the body's tissues.

[0012] T-Helper cells infected with HIV pose possibly the greatest threat to the integrity of a body's immune system by terminating noninfected T-Helper cells, which a critical number of noninfected T-Helper cells is needed to defend the body from infectious agents. Since the clinical characteristics of AIDS appears to coincide more with the decline of non-infected T-Helper cells below a critical number and not necessarily with the number of HIV infected T-Helper cells, controlling the population of HIV infected T-Helper cells or ridding the environment of HIV infected T-Helper cells would be a successful approach to managing AIDS.

BRIEF SUMMARY OF THE INVENTION

[0013] A Scientifically Modulated And Reprogrammed Treatment (SMART) Fas/FasL Virus is comprised of an inner capsid similar to the naturally occurring HIV icosahedral capsid. The SMART-Fas/FasL Virus capsid is encapsulated with a protein matrix similar to the protein matrix that encapsulates the HIV's capsid. A lipid bilayer envelope then encapsulates the matrix protein coat and capsid similar to the lipid bilayer that encapsulates the matrix protein of HIV. Two cell-surface receptors Fas and Fas ligand (FasL) would be fixed to the surface of the SMART-Fas/FasL Virus. The capsid of the medically therapeutic version of the SMART-Fas/FasL Virus would carry either no genetic payload or would carry RNA molecules that would not be capable of replicating the virus-like structure in the natural environment or causing any disease in any form of life. The amount of genetic payload or filler would relate to the intended size and stability of the SMART-Fas/FasL Virus. SMART-Fas/FasL Viruses are intended to engage T-Helper cells infected with HIV that are expressing the FasL cell-surface receptor. Once an infected T-Helper cell's FasL cell-surface receptor engages a Fas cell-surface receptor on the SMART-Fas/FasL Virus, the SMART-Fas/FasL Virus's FasL cell-surface receptor engages a Fas cell-surface receptor on the infected T-Helper cell. Once the infected T-Helper cell's Fas cell-surface receptor has been engaged, a biologic signal is triggered inside the infected T-Helper cell that initiates the process of apoptosis. The process of apoptosis terminates the infected T-Helper cell.

DETAILED DESCRIPTION

[0014]   Scientifically Modulated And Reprogrammed Treatment (SMART) Fas/FasL Virus technology is intended to neutralize T-Helper cells infected with the Human Immunodeficiency Virus. A Scientifically Modulated And Reprogrammed Treatment (SMART) Fas/FasL Virus is comprised of an inner capsid similar to the naturally occurring HIV icosahedral capsid. The SMART-Fas/FasL Virus capsid would be encapsulated with a protein matrix similar to the protein matrix that encapsulates the HIV's capsid. A lipid bilayer envelope then encapsulates the matrix protein coat and capsid similar to the lipid bilayer that encapsulates HIV's matrix protein and inner capsid. Two cell-surface receptors Fas (also known as CD98) and Fas ligand (FasL) would be fixed to the surface of the SMART-Fas/FasL Virus. The capsid of the therapeutic version of the SMART-Fas/FasL Virus would carry either no genetic payload or would carry RNA molecules that would not be capable of replicating the virus-like structure in the natural environment or causing any disease in any form of life. The amount of genetic payload or filler would relate to the intended stability of the SMART-Fas/FasL Virus. Within the SMART-Fas/FasL Virus's outer envelope are matrix protein and a capsid to act as the interior conformational structure to provide the appropriate size and shape to the outer envelope as needed for the intended use. The size of the SMART-Fas/FasL Virus ranges from 7 nanometer (nm) in thickness (the diameter of HIV is approximately 50 to 150 nm) to a diameter in the order of the size of a naturally occurring noninfected T-Helper cell, and up to a diameter of one meter. T-Helper cells are mobile structures and constantly alter their shape and size, but are approximately 3500 nm in diameter. The range in size of the SMART-Fas/FasL Virus is dependent upon the type of application for which the SMART-Fas/FasL Virus is intended to be utilized.

[0015] A SMART-Fas/FasL Virus is intended to engage a T-Helper cell infected with HIV that is expressing the FasL cell-surface receptor. Once an infected T-Helper cell's FasL cell-surface receptor engages a Fas cell-surface receptor on the said SMART-Fas/FasL Virus, the SMART-Fas/FasL Virus's FasL cell-surface receptor engages a Fas cell-surface receptor on the infected T-Helper cell. Once the infected T-Helper cell's Fas cell-surface receptor has been engaged, a biologic signal is triggered inside the infected T-Helper cell that initiates the process of apoptosis. Apoptosis is a naturally occurring biologic process present in cells that when initiated results in cell death. Activation of apoptosis terminates the infected T-Helper cell. In the event HIV is unable to successfully create additional copies of itself and unable to further threaten noninfected T-Helper cells, the threat of Acquired Immunodeficiency Disease Syndrome is successfully neutralized.

[0016] SMART-Fas/FasL Virus technology can be used as a cleaning device to neutralize and rid a surface or a fluid environment of HIV infected T-Helper cells. SMART-Fas/FasL Virus is intended to engage HIV infected T-Helper cells where ever it may exist.

[0017] HIV utilizes T-Helper cells as a natural factory for generating copies of HIV. HIV utilizes a fusion technique where the virion envelope fuses with the cellular membrane of the host cell and directly releases the capsid containing the RNA genome and replicating enzymes into the cytoplasm of the host cell. HIV utilizes enzymes created by its own genome and enzymes native to the T-Helper cell to generate the proteins it requires to construct copies of HIV. Once the appropriate copies of the RNA, nucleocapsid protein, integrase, protease, reverse transcriptase enzyme, capsid proteins, matrix protein and external probes have been manufactured and collected together, the capsid carrying the RNA genetic payload is enveloped by the matrix protein and pushes through the host cell's plasma membrane in a process called budding. The HIV copy becomes encapsulated in an envelope comprised of a lipid bilayer as it separates from the host cell and becomes an independent entity termed a virion. Probes stick out through the lipid bilayer envelope of the virion to seek the receptors located on an appropriate host cell.

[0018] To produce copies of the SMART-Fas/FasL Virus a T-Helper cell can be utilized, bacteria with a lipid bilayer membrane could be utilized, hybrid cells (combination of animal cell, plant cell or bacteria) could be utilized or other appropriate host cell could be utilized. The technology to manufacture viruses carrying a therapeutic DNA gene has already been worked out and implemented. The process to generate a medically therapeutic virus to target a particular type of cell is a matter of placing inside a host cell the appropriate genetic instructions and enzymes to facilitate the host cell to manufacture the intended 'medically therapeutic' virus.

[0019] In the case of the SMART-Fas/FasL Virus, the construction of the medically therapeutic copies of the SMART-FasL Virus include the appropriate instructions and biologic machinery necessary to generate the capsid proteins, matrix proteins, external cell-surface receptors Fas and FasL, any filling material to be placed inside the capsid and any cell instruction proteins necessary to stimulate and manage the budding process. The Fas cell-surface receptor is a naturally occurring cell-surface receptor on T-Helper cells. The genetic instruction code for manufacturing the FasL receptor and fixing it on the lipid bilayer as a receptor is available and carried in the HIV genome. The size of the capsid is dependent upon the quantity of capsid proteins used to construct the capsid. For descriptive purposes the use of the term 'capsid' is interchangeable with the term 'capsid shell'. Different naturally occurring viruses are constructed with a different size capsid depending upon the number and arrangement of capsid proteins utilized to construct a virus's capsid. The diameter of the SMART-Fas/FasL Virus is in part dependent upon the number and arrangement of capsid proteins used to construct the capsid. A genetic payload to act as a filler, incapable of stimulating a disease state in any form of life, may be required to fill the inside the capsid of some of the larger diameter SMART-Fas/FasL Viruses in order to support the successful construction of a particular size of SMART-Fas/FasL Virus and to facilitate the SMART-Fas/FasL Virus remaining sturdy enough and thus intact once released into the environment to enable it to successfully carry out its intended function.

[0020] The size of the SMART-Fas/FasL Virus is between 7 nm in thickness (the diameter of HIV is approximately 50 to 150 nm) to a diameter in the order of the size of a naturally occurring noninfected T-Helper cell, to a diameter of one meter. The size of the SMART-Fas/FasL Virus is variable due to the range of applications for which the SMART-Fas/FasL Virus is intended to be utilized. The SMART-Fas/FasL Virus may take on the shape of simply a relatively flat sheet of varying sizes which may be folded into various configurations, to spherical structures of varying sizes to irregularly shaped convoluted structures of varying sizes. The unique principle of intent is to engage infected T-Helper cells with Fas cell-surface receptors and FasL cell-surface receptors in whatever manner might terminate T-Helper cells infected with the Human Immunodeficiency Virus.

CLAIMS: Reserved.

A7: A VACCINE COMPRISED SPECIFICALLY OF PROTEIN SUBUNITS OF HUMAN IMMUNODEFICIENCY VIRUS'S GLYCOPROTEIN 120 PROBE TO PREVENT AND TREAT AN INFECTION CAUSED BY THE HUMAN IMMUNODEFICIENCY VIRUS

INDIVIDUALS REQUESTING PATENT: Dr. Lane B. Scheiber, ScD and Dr. Lane B. Scheiber II, MD

Claims: 1 independent claim, 6 dependent claims

ABSTRACT

The human immunodeficiency virus poses a significant threat to the health and well being of the world's population. Current strategies utilized to eradicate this deadly pathogen have not been effective. A vaccine comprised solely of protein subunits of the glycoprotein 120 probe as the active ingredient, can be effective in stimulating an individual's immune system to repel an HIV infection. The protein subunit of the glycoprotein 120 probe extends from the surface of HIV and is the unique identifier of an HIV virion. When protein subunits of HIV's glycoprotein probe are exclusively presented to the immune system, the antibodies generated will neutralize the glycoprotein 120 probes located on the surface of HIV virions, such that the virus's virions then are incapable of engaging a T-Helper cell and thus the infectious threat posed by HIV is averted.

BACKGROUND OF THE INVENTION

1. Field of the Invention

[0001]   This invention relates to any medical device introduced into the body, which is intended to cause an immune response against the human immunodeficiency virus to prevent or treat an infection caused by the human immunodeficiency virus.

2. Description of Background Art

[0002]   According to the Center for Disease control, in the United States it is estimated that as of December 2004 there have been 944,306 people infected with the Human Immunodeficiency Virus (HIV), and 56% of these individuals have died.   It is estimated there are at least 40,000 new cases of individuals infected with HIV in the United States per year with 25% of patients unaware they have contracted the virus. Further, it has been estimated by the World Health Organization that HIV infects 33 million people worldwide. After over twenty years of research and investigation, eradicating the ever-growing global humanitarian crisis posed by the HIV remains an elusive goal for the medical community.

[0003]   The Human Immunodeficiency Virus is ingeniously configured as well as a deadly virus. Viruses, in general, have been difficult to contain and eradicate due to their being obligate parasites and the fact they tend not to carry out biologic functions outside the cell the virus has targeted as its host. An intact, individual form of a virus, as it exists outside the boundaries of a host cell, is generally referred to as a 'virion'. The human body's immune system possesses innate mechanisms to repel viral infections once such a pathogen breaches the perimeter defenses and is recognized as an invader. If a cell is determined to be infected with a virus, neighboring cells may generate a defense response that causes neighboring cells to resist infection or if neighboring cells become infected, such cells shuts down biologic processes the virus might attempt to utilize for the purpose of replication. HIV virions possess several attributes that make them especially elusive, circumventing the immune system's routine defensive measures.

[0004] Bacteria generally have posed a much easier target for the medical community to eradicate compared to viral infections. Bacteria generally live and reproduce outside animal cells. When a white cell encounters a bacterium, the white cell engulfs the bacterium, encapsulates the pathogen, processes the identification of the pathogen and kills the pathogen utilizing acids and destructive enzymes. The white cell then alerts the B-cells of the immune system as to the identity of the intruding pathogen. A subpopulation of B-cells is created. This subpopulation of B-cells is dedicated to producing antibodies directed against the pathogen the circulating white cell encountered and identified. A variety of other cells, such as, dendritic cells, macrophages and circulating B-cells may also engage a pathogen and stimulate an immune response. Antibodies, generated by B-cells, traverse the blood and body tissues in search of the bacteria they were designed to repel. Antibodies attach to bacteria, coating the surface of bacteria, attempting to punch holes through a bacterium's cell wall and signal the cells comprising the immune system to the presence of the bacterium.

[0005] Viruses pose a much different challenge to the body's defense system than do bacteria. Since viruses generally do not carry out biologic processes outside their host cell, a virus virion can be destroyed, but there are no on-going internal biologic life-sustaining processes to terminate. A virus is simply comprised of one or more external shells, one or more segments of genetic material carried inside the core of the innermost shell, and many viruses contain one or more enzymes to assist in the replication of the virus. Antibodies can coat the exterior of a virus to make it easier for the white cells in the body to identify the pathogen, but the action of punching holes in the virus's external shell does not terminate any life functions. Many viruses only briefly circulate in the blood and tissues of the body, thus exist for only a limited time as an exposed and vulnerable entity.

[0006] Viruses utilize exterior probes to hunt down a cell in the body that will act as an appropriate host so that the virus can engage in the task of replicating of itself. Once the virus has found a proper host cell, the virus inserts its genome and any enzymes it carries into the host cell. The virus's genetic material takes command of cellular functions and the virus's genetic material diverts the host cell biologic machinery from normal cellular functions to engaging in constructing copies of the virus.

[0007] Once the virus has infected a host cell, the virus is in effect shielded from the body's immune system defense mechanisms by the cell membrane of the host cell. A virus which has infected a host cell, is generally only represented as 'genetic information' that often becomes intimately incorporated into the host cell's own DNA. Often, following the action of a virus's virion infecting a cell in the body, the presence of the virus can only be eradicated if the host cell is destroyed. Antibodies are generally designed to engage a bacteria or a virus and not to attack the naturally occurring tissues found in the body. Circulating white cells and the immune cells comprising lymph nodes and the immune cells comprising the spleen may or may not recognize that a cell, which has become a host for a virus, is carrying a virus's genetic material and is infected with a virus. If the immune system fails to identify a cell that has become infected with a virus, the virus's genetic material can proceed to force the infected cell to make copies of the virus. Since a virus is in essence simply a segment of genetic material, time is of no consequence regarding the life-cycle of the virus, and in some cases a virus's genome may exist for years without a need to activate until the pathogen's genetic programming senses the time is right to initiate the virus's replication process. The only opportunity the immune system may have to combat a latent virus is at the time when copies of the virus leave the host cell and circulate in the blood or tissues, in search of another perspective host cell.

[0008] The traditional medical approach to combating infectious agents such as bacteria have limited value in managing or eradicating aggressive viral infections, especially those that are latent viral infections. Synthetic antibiotics, generally used to augment the body's capacity to produce naturally occurring antibodies against bacterial infections, circulate the blood stream for limited periods of time and thus have little success in combating latent viruses that are protected by their host cell. Stimulating the body's immune system recognition by administering a vaccine may have limited value in combating latent viral infections. Vaccines generally are intended to introduce to the body's immune system an attenuated, noninfectious intact bacteria or virus, or pieces of a bacteria or virus so the immune system is able to recognize and process the infectious agent and generate antibodies directed to assist in killing the pathogen. Once the immune system has been primed to recognize an intruder, antibodies are generally produced by B-cells in generous quantities in an effort to repel an invader. Following the initial antibody response, the antibody production diminishes if the body fails to recognize evidence of a substantial ongoing active infection. Latent viruses may lie in wait inside the protective shelter of its host cell and not activate its reproductive cycle until a time where the innate antibody response by the body has declined to the point where it is in fact ineffective in intercepting the viral copies once the viral copies have been released into circulation.

[0009] The human immunodeficiency virus demonstrates three factors, which make this pathogen particularly challenging to seek out and eradicate. First: the host for HIV is the T-Helper cell. The T-Helper cell is a key element in the immune system's response since it helps coordinate the body's defensive actions against most pathogens seeking to invade the body's tissues. In cases of a bacterial infection versus a viral infection, T-Helper cells actively direct which immune cells will rev-up and engage the particular infection. Since HIV infects and disrupts T-Helper cells, coordination of the immune response against the virus is disrupted, thus limiting the body's capacity to mount an appropriate and effective response against the presence of HIV and eradicate the virus.

[0010] Second: again, latent viruses such as HIV have a strategic advantage. When the immune system first recognizes a pathogen's existence and begins to generate antibodies against a particular pathogen, the response is robust. Once time has passed and the immune system fails to detect an active threat, the production of antibodies against the particular pathogen diminishes. When HIV infects a T-Helper cell, the viral genome lays dormant, sometimes for years before taking command of the T-Helper cell's biologic functions. HIV may therefore generate a very active initial immune response to its presence, but if the virus sits dormant inside T-Helper cells for months or years, the antibody response to the virus will diminish over time. There may not be an adequate quantity of circulating antibodies to actively engage the HIV virions as they migrate from the T-Helper cell that generated the copies to uninfected T-Helper cells that will serve as a new host to support further replication. If the immune system's response is insufficient during the period while the virus is exposed and vulnerable, it becomes extremely difficult for the body to eradicate the virus. In addition, HIV has as its most outer surface an enveloped made from the T-Helper cell's own outer cell membrane; therefore much of the surface of an HIV virion would appear to the immune system to be naturally occurring tissue, not the surface characteristics generally recognizable as a pathogen.

[0011] The human immunodeficiency virus posses a third, very elusive mode of action, which the virus actively utilizes to defeat the body's immune system. HIV carries in its genome a segment of genetic material that directs an infected T-Helper cell to create and mount on its surface FasL receptors. T-Helper cells carry, on the surface of their outer cell membrane Fas receptors. A Fas receptor, when triggered, initiates apoptosis in the cell. Apoptosis is a biologic process that causes a cell to terminate itself. A T-Helper cell infected with the HIV virus is therefore capable of killing noninfected T-Helper cells that the infected T-Helper cell encounters as it traverses the body. The occurrence of AIDS is therefore enhanced not only by the number of T-Helper cells that become incapacitated due to direct infection by the HIV virus, but also by the number of noninfected T-Helper cells that are eliminated from circulation by coming in contact with infected T-Helper cells.

[0012] Acquired Immune Deficiency Syndrome (AIDS) occurs as a result of the number of circulating T-Helper cells declining to a point where the immune system's capacity to mount a successful response against opportunistic infectious agents is critically compromised. The number of viable T-Helper cells declines either because they become infected with the HIV virus or because they have been killed by encountering a T-Helper cell infected with HIV. When there is an insufficient population of non-HIV infected T-Helper cells to properly combat infectious agents such as Pneumocystis carinii or cytomegalovirus or other pathogens, the body becomes overwhelmed with the opportunistic infection and the patient becomes ill. In cases where the combination of the patient's compromised immune system and medical assistance in terms of synthetic antibiotics intended to combat the opportunistic pathogens, fluids, intravenous nutrition and other treatments are not sufficient to sustain life, the body succumbs to the opportunistic infection and death ensues.

[0013] The human immunodeficiency virus's outermost shell is referred to as its envelope. HIV locates its host by utilizing probes affixed to the outer surface of the envelope. The HIV virus has at least two types of glycoprotein probes attached to the outer surface of its envelope. HIV utilizes a glycoprotein probe 120 (gp 120) to locate a CD4 cell-surface receptor on a T-Helper cell. Once an HIV gp 120 probe has successfully engaged a CD4 cell surface-receptor on a T-Helper cell a conformational change occurs in the probe and a glycoprotein 41 (gp 41) probe is exposed on HIV's surface. The gp 41 probe's intent is to engage a CXCR4 or CCR5 cell-surface receptor on the same T-Helper cell. Once a gp 41 probe on the HIV virion engages a CXCR4 or CCR5 cell-surface receptor, HIV opens an access port through the T-Helper cell's outer membrane.

[0014] Once the virus procures an access port into the T-Helper cell, the HIV virion inserts into the T-Helper cell two positive strand RNA molecules approximately 9500 nucleotides in length. Inserted along with the RNA strands are the enzymes: reverse transcriptase, protease and integrase. Once the virus's genome gains access to the interior of the T-Helper cell, in the cytoplasm, the pair of RNA molecules are transformed to deoxyribonucleic acid by the reverse transcriptase enzyme. Following modification of the virus's genome to DNA, the virus's genetic information migrates to the host cell's nucleus. In the nucleus, with the assistance of the integrase protein, the virus's DNA becomes inserted into the T-Helper cell's native DNA. When the timing is appropriate, the now integrated viral DNA becomes read by a host cell's polymerase molecule and the virus's genetic information commands certain cell functions to carry out the replication process to construct copies of the human deficiency virus.

[0015] The outer layer of the HIV virion is comprised of a portion of the T-Helper cell's outer cell membrane. In the final stage of the replication process, as a copy of the HIV internal shell referred to as a capsid, which carries the HIV genome, buds through the host cell's outer membrane, the capsid acquires as its outermost shell, a wrapping of lipid bilayer, which it harvests from the host cell's outer membrane. Vaccines are generally comprised of copies of a particular virus or a bacterium, weakened to the point the pathogen is incapable of causing an infection, or a vaccine is often comprised of pieces of a virus or bacteria. In the case of HIV, since the surface of this pathogen is an envelope comprised of lipid bilayer taken from the host T-Helper cell's outer membrane, a vaccine might not only target HIV virions, but might also have deleterious effects on the T-Helper cell population. Antibodies produced to combat HIV infections may not be able to differentiate between the surface of an infectious HIV virion and a noninfected T-Helper cell, and such antibodies may act to coat and assist in the elimination of both targets. In such a scenario, since the vaccine might cause a decline in the number of available T-Helper cells, it is conceivable that such a vaccine might paradoxically induce clinically apparent AIDS in a non-HIV infected patient whom received such a vaccine.

[0016] It is clear that the traditional approach of utilizing antibiotics or providing vaccines to stimulate the immune system to produce endogenous antibodies, by themselves, is an ineffective strategy to manage a virus as elusive and deadly as HIV. Drugs that interfere with the replication process of HIV generally slow progression of the infection by the virus, but do not eliminate the virus from the body nor the threat of the clinical symptoms of AIDS. A new strategy is desperately needed in order to successfully combat HIV and prevent the occurrence of AIDS.

[0017] In effect, it has been reported that recent vaccines designed to prevent HIV infections have had limited effect. HIV has been regarded as a pathogen that possess the capacity to create a high rate of genetic mutation and thus copies of the virus can readily adapt features that help it circumvent the effects of the antiviral drugs currently in use to combat the virus. It has been reported that given the length of time HIV infects an individual, new, more resistant strains of the virus will appear in the same patient as a result of the introduction of anti-viral therapies, to the point that single drug therapy intended to slow down the virus's replication process is well recognized 'not' to be an effective treatment strategy.

[0018] A recent approach to creating a vaccine against HIV has been to take a subset of genetic material from an HIV virion and place this inside an alternative virus, in at least one case the virus 'adenovirus' has been used.   A weakened form of adenovirus was to be introduced into the body and engaged by the immune system.   Once white cells had engulfed the weakened adenovirus, the immune system was to become alerted to the presence of HIV by recognizing the existence of the HIV genetic material carried by the adenovirus. The intent was to stimulate cytotoxic white cells to recognize and kill HIV virions and cell infected by HIV. This innovative approach to managing HIV infections has yet to be proven to be successful. HIV's genetic material is generally never exposed to the surveillance apparatuses of the immune system; though as a result of the function of HIV's genetic material it is conceivable that a cell infected with HIV may demonstrate on its outer surface one or more cell-surface markers that could indicate the cell is infected with the virus. This approach has yet to be found to be practical or effective.

[0019] It is understood that the B-cells of the immune system, when activated, are capable of generating antibodies not only directed against viruses, bacteria, cellular parasites, but also 'foreign proteins'. If an insect or reptile venom, which generally consists of one or more proteins, is injected into a body, and if sufficient time is allowed and the victim does not have a fatal reaction to the venom, the victim's B-cells will generate antibodies against the foreign proteins comprising the venom. Injectable medications that consist of one or more proteins may stimulate the B-cells of the immune system to generate antibodies against the medication. Often protein-based medications, such as insulin, are therefore designed and constructed to appear to the immune system as identical as possible to the naturally occurring human protein it is supplementing. The closer a protein intended to provide a medical treatment, appears to the body like the endogenous protein it is supplementing, in theory, the less likely the medical treatment protein will generate an immune response against the medication.

[0020] The unique surface feature of the human immune deficiency virus are, in fact, its surface probes. The remainder of the surface envelope of an HIV virion is comprised of, and appears as, the outer cell membrane of a T-Helper cell. Affixed to the exterior surface of an HIV virion are a quantity of gp 120 probes and gp 41 probes, which represent the distinguishing features of the pathogen.

[0021] Since the introduction of a protein alone into the body can create an immune response and cause antibodies to be formed, taking simply the glycoprotein probes, which are unique to HIV might act as the basis of an effective vaccine. The two HIV probes gp 120 and gp 41 are constructed of a combination of protein and lipid structures. Inserting into the body a quantity of intact or partially intact gp 120 and gp 41 probes, like one would insert a traditional vaccine, might produce an immune response by the B-cells directed solely against the presence of these probes. Since the probes only occur on the surface of HIV virions, antibodies created by the B-cells of the immune system specifically against such probes would target HIV virions and not T-Helper cells.

[0022] In addition, despite the genetic variation that the HIV virus might undergo, since the T-Helper cell's CD4, CXCR4, and CCR5 cell-surface receptors do not appreciably change their construct over time, it stands to reason the construct of HIV's gp 120 probes and gp 41 probes cannot undergo substantial physical change. HIV's probes need to remain relatively standard in their construct if HIV intends to maintain its capability to successfully access T-Helper cells. Where medications directed at slowing down the virus's replication process may see a decline in their effectiveness due to a defensive genetic variation by the virus, a vaccine made solely of the protein subunit of HIV's gp 120 probes should not diminish in its effectiveness despite HIV's attempt to mutate. The design of HIV's probes is dependent upon the construct of the T-Helper cells' cell-surface receptors. If the T-Helper cells' cell-surface receptors do not change in their physical construct, the construct of the protein subunit of HIV's gp 120 probe cannot be substantially altered otherwise HIV risks becoming incapable of propagating itself.

[0023]   A eukaryote refers to a nucleated cell.   Eukaryotes comprise nearly all animal and plant cells. A human eukaryote or nucleated cell is comprised of an exterior lipid bilayer plasma membrane, cytoplasm, a nucleus, and organelles. The exterior plasma membrane defines the perimeter of the cell, regulates the flow of nutrients, water and regulating molecules in and out of the cell, and has embedded into its structure receptors that the cell uses to detect properties of the environment surrounding the cell membrane. The cytoplasm acts as a filling medium inside the boundaries of the plasma cell membrane and is comprised mainly of water and nutrients such as amino acids, oxygen, and glucose. The nucleus, organelles, and ribosomes are suspended in the cytoplasm. The nucleus contains the majority of the cell's genetic information in the form of double stranded deoxyribonucleic acid (DNA). Organelles generally carry out specialized functions for the cell and include such structures as the mitochondria, the endoplasmic reticulum, storage vacuoles, lysosomes and Golgi complex. Floating in the cytoplasm, but also located in the endoplasmic reticulum and mitochondria are ribosomes. Ribosomes are protein structures comprised of several strands of proteins that combine and couple to a messenger ribonucleic acid (mRNA) molecule. More than one ribosome may be attached to a single mRNA at a time. Ribosomes decode genetic information in a mRNA molecule and manufacture proteins to the specifications of the instruction code physically present in the mRNA molecule.

[0024] The majority of the deoxyribonucleic acid (DNA) comprises the chromosomes, double stranded helical structures located in the nucleus of the cell. DNA in a circular form, can also be found in the mitochondria, the powerhouse of the cell, an organelle that assists in converting glucose into usable energy molecules. DNA represents the genetic information a cell needs to manufacture the materials it requires to sustain life and to replicate. Genetic information is stored in the DNA by arrangements of four nucleotides referred to as: adenine, thymine, guanine and cytosine. DNA represents instruction coding, that in the process known as transcription, the DNA's genetic information is decoded by transcription protein complexes referred to as polymerases, to produce ribonucleic acid (RNA). RNA is a single strand of genetic information comprised of coded arrangements of four nucleotides: adenine, uracil, guanine and cytosine. Some types of RNAs are classified as messenger RNAs (mRNA), transport RNAs (tRNA) and ribosomal RNAs (rRNA).

[0025] Proteins are comprised of a series of amino acids bonded together in a linear strand, sometimes referred to as a chain; a protein may be further modified to be a structure comprised of one or more similar or differing strands of amino acids bonded together. Insulin is a protein structure comprised of two strands of amino acids, one strand comprised of 21 amino acids long and the second strand comprised of 30 amino acids, the two strands attached by two disulfide bridges. There are an estimated 30,000 different proteins the cells of the human body may manufacture. The human body is comprised of a wide variety of cells, many with specialized functions requiring unique combinations of proteins and protein structures such as glycoproteins (a protein combined with a carbohydrate) to accomplish the required task or tasks a specialized cell is designed to perform. Certain forms of glycoproteins are known to be utilized as cell-surface receptors. Messenger RNAs (mRNA) are created by transcription of DNA; they exit the nucleus of the cell, and are utilized as protein manufacturing templates by ribosomes. A ribosome is a protein complex that manufactures proteins by deciphering the instruction code located in a mRNA molecule. When a specific protein is needed, pieces of the ribosome complex bind around the strand of a mRNA that carries the specific instruction code that will generate the required protein. The ribosome traverses the mRNA strand and deciphers the genetic information coded into the sequence of nucleotides that comprise the mRNA molecule.

[0026] Transport RNAs (tRNA) are constructed in the nucleus or in the mitochondria, and are coded for one of the 20 amino acids the cells of the human body use to construct proteins. Once a tRNA is created by transcription of the DNA, the tRNA seeks out the type of amino acid it has been coded for and attaches to that specific amino acid. The tRNA then delivers the amino acid it carries to a ribosome that is waiting for that specific amino acid. Proteins are manufactured by the ribosomes binding together sequences of amino acids. The order by which the amino acids are bonded together is dictated by the way the mRNA is constructed and how the ribosome interprets the information encoded in the string of nucleotides present in the mRNA strand.

[0027] A sequence of three nucleotides present in a mRNA molecule represents a unit of information referred to as a codon. Codons code for all of the 20 amino acids used to construct protein molecules and also for START and STOP commands. In the process known as translation, the ribosome decodes the codons present in the mRNA, initiating the protein manufacturing process at a START codon, then interfacing with tRNAs carrying the amino acids that match the sequence of codons in the mRNA as the ribosome traverses the length of the mRNA molecule. The ribosome functions as a protein factory by taking amino acids delivered by tRNAs and binding the amino acids together in the order dictated by the sequence of codon instructions coded into the mRNA template as directed by the manner of the nucleic acid arrangement in the mRNA molecule. Protein synthesis ceases when a ribosome encounters a STOP code. The protein molecule is released by the ribosome.

[0028]   It is well known to the medical scientific community the method of generating proteins for medical treatment purposes. Insulin is a common protein generated for medical treatment purposes. Bacteria, animal cells or hybrid cells comprised of a bacteria-animal cell combination can be utilized as factories to build large quantities of specific proteins. DNA specific for the desired protein can be introduced into the intended factory cell. The factory cell will then decipher the DNA using innate biologic mechanisms and from the DNA, generate mRNA. The mRNA, specific for the desired protein, then acts as a template for the construction of the desired protein. The mRNA is read by ribosomes and the protein molecule is created. The protein subunit of the glycoprotein 120 probe can be generated in large volumes in a similar manner.

[0029]   HIV's RNA genome consists of two identical positive sense single stranded RNA approximately 9500 nucleotides in length. The core genes comprising the RNA genome consist of the genes known as Gag, Pro, Pol and Env. The Gag gene translates into molecules of capsid proteins. The Pro gene translates into protease molecules. The Pol gene translates into molecules of reverse transcriptase. The Env gene translates into the envelope proteins. The Env gene carries the instruction coding for the amino acid sequence and physical construct characteristics, in RNA format, for the molecular structure of the protein subunit of the glycoprotein 120 probe.

Brief Summary of the Invention

[0030] A medical treatment device comprised of a quantity of protein subunits of the glycoprotein 120 probe, these protein subunits of the glycoprotein 120 probes similar in construct to the protein subunit of the glycoprotein 120 probes found on the surface of a naturally occurring human immunodeficiency virus virion generally known to the medical scientific community as the glycoprotein 120 probe. These protein subunits of the glycoprotein 120 probe are to be held in suspension in a hypoallergenic medium formulated to keep intact the protein subunits of the glycoprotein 120 probe, intended to be introduced into the body, whereby the introduction of the protein subunits of the glycoprotein 120 probe is intended to stimulate the production of antibodies against the protein subunit of glycoprotein 120 probes with the intention to generate a defensive immune response by the body in the form of antibodies directed against the presence of the human immunodeficiency virus. The objective of the vaccine to cause the body to generate antibodies intended to engage the protein subunit of the glycoprotein 120 probe and only the protein subunit of the glycoprotein 120 probe, as it is affixed to the surface of a HIV virion, rendering the HIV virion unable to attach to a host cell by blocking the protein subunit of the glycoprotein 120 probes. By generating an antibody to engage and block the protein subunit of the glycoprotein 120 probes as they exist on the surface of a HIV virion, this would cause the HIV virions to be unable to engage CD4 T-Helper cells, thus incapable of further infecting cells in the body. By generating an antibody to engage and only engage the protein portion of the glycoprotein 120 probe will produce a safe, practical, and effective vaccine to prevent and treat those at risk for developing AIDS.

Detailed Description of the Invention

[0031] Vaccines created to combat infectious medical diseases are generally comprised of a liquid medium that carries in suspension intact virus or bacteria of a particular strain that has been weakened to the point it is unable to generate an infection, or a vaccine is comprised of pieces of a virus or bacteria of a particular strain. The weakened, but intact virus or bacteria or the pieces of a virus or bacteria are meant to activate the immune system of the individual receiving the vaccine, such that the individual's immune system will generate antibodies against the intact virus or bacteria or the portions of the virus or bacteria the immune system is exposed to by way of the vaccine.

[0032] Due to the fact that the exterior surface of a human immunodeficiency virus is comprised of essentially the same material as the outer membrane of a T-Helper cell, introducing to the immune system weakened HIV virions or portions of HIV's exterior envelope may lead to a vaccine that has deleterious effects on the individual's T-Helper cell population. Antibodies generated by the immune system directed against the surface characteristics of a T-Helper cell may lead to antibodies seeking out and engaging endogenous T-Helper cells, rendering these endogenous T-Helper cells ineffective. If the antibodies generated by such a vaccine were robust enough in their action, the vaccine could lead to generating an AIDS-like clinical picture due to a reduction in the number of effective circulating T-Helper cells.

[0033] A vaccine that introduced portions of the internal structures of the HIV virion would generally be ineffective since the internal structures of HIV are never exposed to the immune system as HIV virions traverse the body in search of a host cell.

[0034] Vaccines are generally only effective if they are targeted against a structure that is specific to the pathogen and a structure that is readily exposed to the immune system and vulnerable to the immune system's defense mechanisms. The unique identifiers of the human immunodeficiency virus are the two known glycoprotein probes that exist on the surface of HIV's virion. The glycoprotein 120 probe and the glycoprotein 41 probe are unique to HIV, and are the structures on the surface of HIV's virion that the virus utilizes to seek out and engage a perspective T-Helper cell host. The glycoprotein 41 probe is usually hidden by the glycoprotein 120 probe until the glycoprotein 120 probe has engaged a CD4 cell-surface receptor. Once the glycoprotein 120 probe engages a CD4 cell-surface receptor on a T-Helper cell, a conformational change occurs in the 120 probe and the underlying glycoprotein 41 probe is exposed. The exposed glycoprotein 41 probe is then capable of engaging a CXCR4 or CCR5 cell-surface receptor present on the T-Helper cell.

[0035]   Glycoproteins are generally comprised of two subunits, a lipid molecular subunit and a protein molecular subunit. The lipid portion of the glycoprotein acts as an anchor to hold the glycoprotein structure fixed into the bilayer lipid envelope that comprises the surface the of the HIV virion. The protein subunit of the glycoprotein probe extends out from the bilayer lipid envelope and acts to engage a cell-surface receptor on the surface of a prospective host cell. The protein portion of the glycoprotein is generally what would be exposed on the surface of an HIV virion and would be the unique identifier of an HIV virion.

[0036]   Antibodies are generated by the immune system in response to the presence of a virus, bacteria, or foreign substance identified in the fluids or tissues within the outer boundaries of the body. Antibodies are intended to act to compromise the outer surface of a pathogen, or antibodies are to coat the exterior of a virus, bacteria or foreign substance to make the pathogen or foreign substance easier for the immune system to identify and clear from the body. Antibodies may differ in construction and function depending upon the virus, bacteria or foreign substance identified by the immune system. Further, antibodies may differ in construction and function depending upon the portion of the virus, portion of the bacteria or portion of the foreign substance presented to and identified by the immune system.

[0037] A vaccine comprised of intact glycoprotein 120 probes or intact glycoprotein 41 probes may be ineffective in stimulating the necessary immune response due the antibodies may not be constructed properly to engage the working portion of the glycoprotein probes, specifically the protein subunit of the glycoprotein 120 probe due to the fact this is the unique identifier of HIV and the protein portion of the glycoprotein 120 probe is the only portion of the HIV probes that is generally exposed. A vaccine comprised of only the protein subunit of the glycoprotein 120 probe is necessary to act as an effective stimulant of the immune system. Such a vaccine can be effective only if not accompanied by any other portion of the HIV virion. It is critical to the effectiveness and success of the described vaccine that no portion of the outer envelope of the HIV virion other than the protein portion of the glycoprotein 120 probe accompany the protein subunits of the glycoprotein 120 probe when introduced into the body as a vaccine. In addition, no portion of the glycoprotein 120 probe other than the protein subunit accompany the protein subunits of the glycoprotein 120 probe when introduced into the body as a vaccine.

[0038] A vaccine to prevent and treat HIV infections would be comprised of a quantity of protein subunits of the glycoprotein 120 probe, these protein subunits of the glycoprotein 120 probe being similar in construct to the protein subunit of the glycoprotein 120 probes found on the surface of a naturally occurring human immunodeficiency virus virion. These protein subunits of the glycoprotein 120 probe being utilized as a vaccine, would be held in suspension in a hypoallergenic medium intended to be introduced into the body, whereby the introduction of the protein subunits of the glycoprotein 120 probe is intended stimulate the production of antibodies against the protein subunit of the glycoprotein 120 probes to generate a defensive immune response by a body against the presence of the human immunodeficiency virus while not generating an immune response to the hypoallergenic medium.

[0039] The mechanism to produce protein molecules of a particular design is well known to the medical community. Bacteria or animal cells or hybrid cells can be readily fashioned to act as biologic factories to produce large quantities of proteins of a particular construct. Inside a cell utilized to act as a factory, messenger RNA designed to construct the protein subunit of the glycoprotein 120 probe can interact with ribosomes to produce quantities of the protein. The instruction coding for the messenger RNAs to be used is readily available in the HIV RNA genome in the location of the Env gene. HIV's Env gene carries the instruction coding for the amino acid sequence and physical construct characteristics of the molecular structure of the protein subunit of the glycoprotein 120 probe. Once such protein subunits of the glycoprotein 120 probe is produced in quantity by bacteria, animal cells, or hybrid cells, an appropriate quantity would be placed in a hypoallergenic suspension medium to be used as a vehicle to deliver the quantity of these protein subunits of the glycoprotein 120 probe into the body.

[0040] The hypoallergenic suspension is meant to act as a medium to facilitate delivery of the protein subunits of the glycoprotein 120 probe into the body. The hypoallergenic suspension is meant specifically not to generate an immune response so that the immune system will direct its sole response against the protein subunits of the glycoprotein 120 probe suspended in the medium. The hypoallergenic suspension medium is meant to act to preserve the structure of the protein subunits of the glycoprotein 120 probe prior to and during delivery of the hypoallergenic suspension into the body. The hypoallergenic suspension medium containing the quantity of protein subunits of the glycoprotein 120 probe may be injected into the body, or may be administered by an oral route or administered by a rectal route or administered by a vaginal route in women or aerosolized and inhaled.

CLAIMS: Reserved.

A8: MEDICAL TREATMENT DEVICE FOR TREATING AIDS BY UTILIZING MODIFIED HUMAN IMMUNODEFICIENCY VIRUS VIRIONS TO INSERT ANTI-VIRAL MEDICATIONS INTO T-HELPER CELLS

INDIVIDUALS REQUESTING PATENT: Dr. Lane B. Scheiber, ScD and Dr. Lane B. Scheiber II, MD

NUMBER OF CLAIMS: 3 independent claims, 17 dependent claims

ABSTRACT

The medical device by which a modified Human Immunodeficiency Virus or virus-like structure is used as a transport medium to carry a payload of a quantity of anti-viral drug molecules to T-Helper cells in the body. The modified Human Immunodeficiency Virus or virus-like structure makes contact with a T-Helper cell by means of the modified virus's exterior probes or virus-like structure's exterior probes. Once the exterior probes engage the T-Helper cell's receptors, the modified virus or virus-like structure inserts into the T-Helper cell the quantity of medically therapeutic anti-viral drug molecules it is carrying. The anti-viral drug molecules exhibit an anti-viral effect when present inside the T-Helper cells thus assisting in repelling an infection by the Human Immunodeficiency Virus and the use of such a device significantly lowers the occurrence of unwanted deleterious side effects.

BACKGROUND OF THE INVENTION

1. Field of the Invention

This invention relates to any medical treatment device intended to treat a medical condition in the body by utilizing a modified virus to insert a drug into cells of the body.

Description of Background Art

[0001]   The approach to treating the AIDS epidemic has been to administer to patients anti-viral drugs to combat infection of T-Helper cells by the Human Immunodeficiency virus. This approach has produced limited success. Side effects of these anti-viral drugs has in some cases posed a deterrent to the success of such therapy.

[0002] Many drugs used to treat medical diseases have limited success and incomplete compliance by patients due to the fact that drugs often cause unwanted side effects when healthy cells suffer delirious effects of the drug. A drug introduced into the body by means of an oral route, inhaled route, rectal suppository or an injectable manner may affect every cell it comes in contact with rather than limiting its effects to the specific tissues or specific cells that the drug is intended to exert an effect on to generate a medically therapeutic outcome. Adverse side effects generated by systemic effects of drugs may be minimized by limiting the delivery of a drug to specific target cells or specific tissues in the body.

[0003]   A eukaryote refers to a nucleated cell. Eukaryotes comprise nearly all animal and plant cells. A human eukaryote or nucleated cell is comprised of an exterior lipid bilayer plasma membrane, cytoplasm, a nucleus, and organelles.   The exterior plasma membrane defines the perimeter of the cell, regulates the flow of nutrients, water and regulating molecules in and out of the cell, and has embedded into its structure cell-surface receptors that the cell uses to detect properties of the environment surrounding the cell membrane. Cytoplasm refers to the entire contents inside the cell except for the nucleus and acts as a filling medium inside the boundaries of the plasma cell membrane. Cytosol refers to the semifluid portion of the cytoplasm minus the mitochondria and the endoplasmic reticulum. The nucleus, organelles, and ribosomes are suspended in the cytosol. Nutrients such as amino acids, oxygen and glucose are present in the cytosol. The nucleus contains the majority of the cell's genetic information in the form of double stranded deoxyribonucleic acid (DNA). Organelles generally carry out specialized functions for the cell and include such structures as the mitochondria, the endoplasmic reticulum, storage vacuoles, lysosomes and Golgi complex. Floating in the cytoplasm, but also located in the endoplasmic reticulum and mitochondria are ribosomes. Ribosomes are protein structures comprised of several strands of proteins that combine and couple to a messenger ribonucleic acid (mRNA) molecule. More than one ribosome may be attached to a single mRNA at a time. Ribosomes decode genetic information coded in a mRNA molecule and manufacture proteins to the specifications of the instruction code physically present in the mRNA molecule.

[0004] The majority of the deoxyribonucleic acid (DNA) in a cell is present in the form of chromosomes, the double stranded helical structures located in the nucleus of the cell. DNA in a circular form, can also be found in the mitochondria, the powerhouse of the cell, an organelle that assists in converting glucose into usable energy molecules. DNA represents the genetic information a cell needs to manufacture the materials it requires to develop to its mature form, sustain life and to replicate. Genetic information is stored in the DNA by arrangements of four nucleotides referred to as: adenine, thymine, guanine and cytosine. DNA represents instruction coding, that in the process known as transcription, the DNA's genetic information is decoded by transcription protein complexes referred to as polymerases, to produce ribonucleic acid (RNA). RNA is a single strand of genetic information comprised of coded arrangements of four nucleotides: adenine, uracil, guanine and cytosine. The physical difference in the construction of a DNA molecule versus a RNA molecule is that DNA utilizes the nucleotide 'thymine', while RNA molecules utilize the nucleotide 'uracil'. RNAs are generally classified as messenger RNAs (mRNA), transport RNAs (tRNA) and ribosomal RNAs (rRNA).

[0005] Proteins are comprised of a series of amino acids bonded together in a linear strand, sometimes referred to as a chain; a protein may be further modified to be a structure comprised of one or more similar or differing strands of amino acids bonded together. A protein comprised of one or more strands of amino acids (referred to as subunits) may be referred to as a protein complex. Insulin is a protein structure comprised of two strands of amino acids, one strand comprised of 21 amino acids long and the second strand comprised of 30 amino acids; the two strands attached by two disulfide bridges. There are an estimated 30,000 different proteins the cells of the human body may manufacture. The human body is comprised of a wide variety of cells, many with specialized functions requiring unique combinations of proteins and protein structures such as glycoproteins (a protein combined with a carbohydrate) to accomplish the required task or tasks a specialized cell is designed to perform. Forms of glycoproteins are known to be utilized as cell-surface receptors.

[0006] Viruses are obligate parasites. Viruses simply represent a carrier of genetic material and by themselves viruses are unable to replicate or carry on any form of biologic function outside their host cell. Viruses are generally comprised of one or more shells constructed of one or more layers of protein or lipid material, and inside the outer shell or shells, a virus carries a genetic payload that represents the instruction code necessary to replicate the virus, and protein enzymes to help facilitate the genetic payload in the function of replicating copies of the virus once the genetic payload has been delivered to a host cell. Located on the outer shell or envelope of a virus are probes. The function of a virus's probes is to locate and engage a host cell's receptors. The virus's surface probes are designed to detect, make contact with and functionally engage one or more receptors located on the exterior of a cell type that will offer the virus the proper environment in which to construct copies of itself. A host cell is a cell that provides the virus the proper biochemical machinery for the virus to successfully replicate itself.

[0007] Protected by the outer coat generally comprised of an envelope or capsid or envelope and capsid, viruses carry a genetic payload in the form of deoxyribonucleic acid (DNA) or ribonucleic acid (RNA). Once a virus's exterior probes locate and functionally engage the surface receptor or receptors on a host cell, the virus inserts its genetic payload into the interior of the host cell. In the event a virus is carrying a DNA payload, the virus's DNA travels to the host cell's nucleus and is known to become inserted into the host cell's own native DNA. In the case where a virus is carrying its genetic payload as RNA, the virus inserts the RNA payload into the host cell and may also insert one or more enzymes to facilitate the RNA being utilized properly to replicate copies of the virus. Once inside the host cell, some species of virus facilitate their RNA being converted to DNA. Once the viral RNA has been converted to DNA, the virus's DNA travels to the host cell's nucleus and is known to become inserted into the host cell's native DNA. Once a virus's genetic material has been inserted into the host cell's native DNA, the virus's genetic material takes command of certain cell functions and redirects the resources of the host cell to generate copies of the virus. Other forms of RNA viruses bypass the need to use the host cell's nuclear DNA and simply utilize portions of its innate viral genome to act as messenger RNA (mRNA). RNA viruses that bypass the host cell's DNA, cause the cell, in general, to generate copies of the necessary parts of the virus directly from the virus's RNA genome. When a virus's genome directly acts as a template, then similar to the cell's messenger RNA, the virus's RNA is read by the cell's ribosomes and proteins necessary to complete the virus's replication process are generated.

[0008] Current state of gene therapy generally refers to efforts directed toward inserting an exogenous subunit of DNA into a vehicle such as a naturally occurring virus. The vehicle is intended to insert the exogenous subunit of DNA into a target cell. The exogenous DNA subunit then migrates to the target cell's nucleus. The exogenous DNA subunit then inserts into the native DNA of the cell. This represents a permanent alteration of the cell's nuclear DNA. At some point, the nuclear transcription proteins read the exogenous DNA subunit's nucleotide coding to produce the intended cellular response. The approach described within the scope of this text involves a medically therapeutic drug as a payload versus DNA or RNA as a payload. DNA is comprised of the nucleotides adenine, thymine, guanine and cytosine. RNA is composed of the nucleotides adenine, uracil, guanine and cytosine. DNA codes acts as a template to code for the manufacture of RNA molecules. RNA acts as a template coding for the manufacture of proteins, which are composed of amino acids. A drug acts to function as a participant in a chemical reaction, as either a catalyst of the reaction or with another substance to produce one or more additional substances, these additional substances often having different properties. A safer, more effective treatment of many diseases may be approached by utilizing modified viruses as vehicles to transport a medically therapeutic drug molecules to specific cells in the body with the intent to have the drug exert an effect only on those cells to which the modified virus virions deliver the drug.

[0009] The Human Immunodeficiency Virus (HIV) is an ingeniously configured, deadly virus. Viruses, in general, have been difficult to contain and eradicate due to their being obligate parasites and the fact they tend not to carry out biologic functions outside the cell the virus has targeted as its host. An intact, individual form of a virus, as it exists outside the boundaries of a host cell, is generally referred to as a 'virion'. The human body's immune system possesses innate mechanisms to repel viral infections once such a pathogen breaches the perimeter defenses and is recognized as an invader. If a cell is determined to be infected with a virus, neighboring cells may generate a defense response that causes neighboring cells to resist infection or if neighboring cells become infected, such cells shuts down biologic processes the virus might attempt to utilize for the purpose of replication. HIV virions possess several attributes that make them especially elusive, circumventing the immune system's routine defensive measures.

[0010]   Acquired Immune Deficiency Syndrome (AIDS) occurs as a result of the number of circulating T-Helper cells declining to a point where the immune system's capacity to mount a successful response against opportunistic infectious agents is critically compromised. The number of viable T-Helper cells declines either because they become infected with the HIV virus or because they have been killed by encountering a T-Helper cell infected with HIV. When there is an insufficient population of non-HIV infected T-Helper cells to properly combat infectious agents such as Pneumocystis carinii or cytomegalovirus or other pathogens, the body becomes overwhelmed with the opportunistic infection and the patient becomes ill. In cases where the combination of the patient's compromised immune system and medical assistance in terms of synthetic antibiotics intended to combat the opportunistic pathogens, fluids, intravenous nutrition and other treatments are not sufficient to sustain life, the body succumbs to the opportunistic infection and death ensues.

[0011]   The human immunodeficiency virus's outermost shell is referred to as its envelope. HIV locates its host by utilizing probes affixed to the outer surface of the envelope. The HIV virus has at least two types of glycoprotein probes attached to the outer surface of its envelope. HIV utilizes a glycoprotein probe 120 (gp 120) to locate a CD4 cell-surface receptor on a T-Helper cell. Once an HIV gp 120 probe has successfully engaged a CD4 cell surface-receptor on a T-Helper cell a conformational change occurs in the probe and a glycoprotein 41 (gp 41) probe is exposed on HIV's surface. The gp 41 probe's intent is to engage a CXCR4 or CCR5 cell-surface receptor on the same T-Helper cell. Once a gp 41 probe on the HIV virion engages a CXCR4 or CCR5 cell-surface receptor, HIV opens an access port through the T-Helper cell's outer membrane.

[0012]   Once the virus procures an access port into the T-Helper cell, the HIV virion inserts into the T-Helper cell two positive strand RNA molecules approximately 9500 nucleotides in length. Inserted along with the RNA strands are the enzymes: reverse transcriptase, protease and integrase. Once the virus's genome gains access to the interior of the T-Helper cell, in the cytoplasm, the pair of RNA molecules are transformed to deoxyribonucleic acid by the reverse transcriptase enzyme. Following modification of the virus's genome to DNA, the virus's genetic information migrates to the host cell's nucleus. In the nucleus, with the assistance of the integrase protein, the virus's DNA becomes inserted into the T-Helper cell's native DNA. When the timing is appropriate, the now integrated viral DNA becomes read by a host cell's polymerase molecule and the virus's genetic information commands certain cell functions to carry out the replication process to construct copies of the human deficiency virus.

[0013]   The outer layer of the HIV virion is comprised of a portion of the T-Helper cell's outer cell membrane. In the final stage of the replication process, as a copy of the HIV internal shell referred to as a capsid, which carries the HIV genome, buds through the host cell's outer membrane, the capsid acquires as its outermost shell or envelope, a wrapping of lipid bilayer, which it harvests from the host cell's outer membrane.

[0014]   There is currently no vaccine or cure for AIDS. Current therapies are in the form of antiretroviral therapy. Combination therapy is often used to interfere with HIV replication inside an infected T-Helper cell.   Anti-viral therapy includes nucleoside analogue reverse transcriptase inhibitors (NARTI), protease inhibitors and non-nucleoside reverse transcriptase inhibitor (NNRTI).

[0015]   A means of treating AIDS could be to take the naturally occurring Human Immunodeficiency Virus (HIV) which is an RNA virus and replace HIV's innate genome with a quantity of anti-viral drug molecules. HIV already posses the means to locate and infect T-Helper cells, which act as the natural host for HIV replication. Modified HIV virions could be utilized to carry anti-viral drugs directly to infected as well as non-infected T-Helper cells. Utilizing modified HIV virions to directly insert antiviral drugs directly in a patient's T-Helper cells would prevent HIV from being able to infect a patient's T-Helper cell population and thus stop AIDS from occurring or progressing in a patient.   HIV may affect other cell lines that possess CD4 cell-surface markers, so utilizing modified HIV virions that have their exterior glycoprotein probes altered to engage specific target cells in the body to directly insert antiviral drugs directly into any cell with CD4 cell-surface receptors, other than limited to just T-Helper cells, may also prevent HIV from being able to infect a patient and thus stop AIDS from occurring or progressing in a patient.

BRIEF SUMMARY OF THE INVENTION

[0016]   The medical treatment device comprised of a modified virus or virus-like structure is used as a transport medium to carry a payload consisting of a quantity of anti-viral drug molecules to T-Helper cells in the body. The modified virus or virus-like structure makes contact with a T-Helper cell by means of the virus's exterior probes or virus-like structure's exterior probes. Once the exterior probes engage the target cell's receptors, the modified virus or virus-like structure inserts into the T-Helper cell the quantity of medically therapeutic anti-viral drug molecules it is carrying.

DETAILED DESCRIPTION

[0017] Viruses or virus-like structures can be fashioned to act as transport vehicles to carry and deliver medically therapeutic drug molecules directly to specific cells. The medically therapeutic drug carried by therapeutic modified viruses or virus-like structures would supply the cells of the body with the drug without interfering or harming other cells in the body.

[0018] Naturally occurring viruses can be altered by replacing the genetic material the virus would carry, with medically therapeutic drug molecules that would have a medically beneficial therapeutic effect on cells. The naturally occurring virus would then carry and deliver to its natural target cell the payload of medically therapeutic drug molecules.

[0019] Naturally occurring viruses can be further modified to have their naturally occurring glycoprotein surface probes replaced by glycoprotein surface probes that target specific cells in the body. Viruses modified to carry and deliver medically therapeutic drug molecules as the payload, further modified to have their glycoprotein surface probes, that cause the modified virus to engage specific cells in the body, provides a device whereby specific cells in the body can be targeted and this device embodies a means of providing to a specific type of cell in the body a drug to participate in chemical reactions with the intent to accomplish a medically therapeutic outcome.

[0020] Virus-like structures can be constructed with similar physical characteristics to naturally occurring viruses and be fashioned to carry medically therapeutic drug molecules as the payload and have located on the surface glycoprotein probes that engage specific cells in the body. Viruses-like structures carrying medically therapeutic drug molecules as the payload, constructed to have their glycoprotein surface probes engage specific cells in the body, and deliver to those specific cells the drug the virus-like structures carry provides a device whereby specific cells in the body can be targeted and this device embodies a means of providing to a specific type of cell in the body a drug to participate in chemical reactions with the intent to accomplish a medically therapeutic outcome. The advantage of a virus-like structure is that the physical dimensions of the virus-like structure can be adjusted to accommodate variations in the physical size of the payload of medically therapeutic drug molecules, yet maintain a means of engaging targeted cells in the body and delivering to those targeted cells the drug molecules required to accomplish the desired medical therapeutic outcome. A second advantage of utilizing virus-like structures is to be able to change the surface characteristics of the transport vehicle to prevent the body's immune system from reacting to the presence of the therapeutic modified virus and destroying the modified virus before it is able to deliver the payload it carries to the cells it has been designed to target. HIV utilizes an exterior envelope comprised of the surface membrane of its host, the T-Helper cell, which acts as a disguise to fool the body's immune system detection resources. Virus-like structures could be fashioned, similar to HIV, to have as an exterior envelope a surface that resembles a cell's outer membrane in order to avoid detection by the body's immune system to improve survivability and functionality of the virus-like structure.

[0021] Replicating viruses and constructing viruses to carry DNA payloads is a form of manufacturing technology that has already been well established and is in use facilitating the concept of gene therapy. Replicating viruses and designing these viruses to carry drug as the genetic payload would incorporate similar techniques as already proven useful in current DNA gene therapy technologies.

[0022] To carry out the process to manufacture a modified medically therapeutic Human Immunodeficiency Virus virions, DNA or RNA that would code for the general physical structures of the Human Immunodeficiency Virus virion would be inserted into a host. The host may include devices such as a host cell or a hybrid host cell. The host may utilize DNA or RNA or a combination of genetic instructions in order to accomplish the construction of medically therapeutic virus virions. The DNA or messenger RNA molecules to create the medically therapeutic virus virions would direct the cells to generate copies of the medically therapeutic Human Immunodeficiency Virus virions carrying a medically therapeutic drug payload. In some cases DNA or messenger RNA would be inserted into the host that would be coded to cause the production of surface probes that would be affixed to the surface of the Human Immunodeficiency Virus virions that would target the surface receptors on specific cells in the body other than the T-Helper cells the Human Immunodeficiency Virus virions naturally targets. DNA or messenger RNA would direct the host to generate copies of the medically therapeutic drug molecules that would provide a therapeutic action, or alternatively the medically therapeutic drug molecules would be artificially introduced into the host; these medically therapeutic drug molecules would take the place of the Human Immunodeficiency Virus's innate genome as its payload. The medical treatment form of the Human Immunodeficiency Virus carrying medically therapeutic drug molecules would be produced, assembled and released from a host. Virus-like structures would be generated in similar fashion using a host such as host-cells or hybrid host cells. The copies of the medically therapeutic Human Immunodeficiency Virus virions or virus-like structures, upon exiting the host, would be collected, stored and utilized as a medical treatment as necessary.

[0023]   A means of treating AIDS could be to take the naturally occurring Human Immunodeficiency Virus (HIV) which is an RNA virus and replace HIV's innate genome with a quantity of anti-viral drug molecules.   Anti-viral therapies include nucleoside analogue reverse transcriptase inhibitors (NARTI), protease inhibitors or non-nucleoside reverse transcriptase inhibitor (NNRTI).   HIV already posses the means to locate and infect T-Helper cells, which act as the natural host for HIV replication.   Modified HIV virions could be utilized to carry antiviral drugs directly to infected as well as non-infected T-Helper cells.   Utilizing modified HIV virions to directly insert antiviral drugs directly in a patient's T-Helper cells would prevent HIV from being able to infect a patient's T-Helper cell population and thus stop AIDS from occurring or progressing in a patient. HIV may affect other cell lines that possess CD4 cell-surface markers, so utilizing modified HIV virions that have their exterior glycoprotein probes altered to engage specific target cells in the body to directly insert antiviral drugs directly into any cell with CD4 cell-surface receptors, other than limited to T-Helper cells, may also prevent HIV from being able to infect a patient and thus stop AIDS from occurring or progressing in a patient.

[0024]   The modified Human Immunodeficiency Virus virions and virus-like structures would be incapable of replication on their own due to the fact that the messenger RNA that would code for the replication process to produce copies of the virus or virus-like structure would not be present in the modified form of the   Human Immunodeficiency   Virus virions or virus-like structure.

[0025]   In review, the medical device described in this text includes taking a naturally occurring Human Immunodeficiency Virus virion and altering its payload so that it transports medically therapeutic drug molecules to a T-Helper cell it is naturally designed to infect, but instead of delivering its own genetic payload, it delivers the medically therapeutic drug molecules it is carrying, <u>and</u> the medical device described in this text includes taking a naturally occurring Human Immunodeficiency Virus virion and altering its payload so that it carries medically therapeutic drug molecules to cells and alter the virus's glycoprotein probes so that it is capable of infecting specific targeted cells, but instead of delivering its own genetic payload, it delivers the medically therapeutic drug molecules it is carrying to a specific target cell, and the medical device described in this text includes taking a virus-like structure, which carries medically therapeutic drug molecules to cells, affixed to the surface glycoprotein probes so that it is capable of delivering medically therapeutic drug molecules it is carrying to specific target cells.

[0026] The described medical device includes a quantity of modified Human Immunodeficiency Virus virions or virus-like structures would be introduced into a patient's blood stream or tissues so that the modified virus could deliver the medially therapeutic anti-viral drug payload that it carries to T-Helper cells in the body.

[0027] The described medical device includes a quantity of modified Human Immunodeficiency Virus virions or virus-like structures introduced into a patient's blood stream or tissues so that the modified virus or virus-like structure could deliver the medially therapeutic anti-viral drug payload that it carries to the specific target cells in the body that the modified Human Immunodeficiency Virus's or virus-like structure's exterior glycoprotein probes are constructed to engage.

[0028] By utilizing the described method to provide the T-Helper cells of the body with therapeutic anti-viral drug molecules in an effort to enhancing the capacity of T-Helper cells to prevent infection by HIV and in cells already infected with HIV to combat HIV to prevent the virus from using the T-Helper cell as a host to manufacture copies of the virus, which will result the betterment of medical management for patients infected with HIV who may progress to AIDS or already have AIDS

CLAIMS: Reserved.

A9: METHOD FOR CURING AND PREVENTING AC-QUIRED IMMUNE DEFICIENCY SYNDROME BY ALTERING CELL-SURFACE RECEPTORS IN PRECURSOR T-HELPER CELLS AND MATURE T-HELPER CELLS TO PREVENT HU-MAN IMMUNODEFICIENCY VIRUS VIRIONS ACCESS TO MATURE T-HELPER CELLS

INDIVIDUALS REQUESTING PATENT: Dr. Lane B. Scheiber, ScD and Dr. Lane B. Scheiber II, MD

NUMBER OF CLAIMS: 3 independent claims, 26 dependent claims

ABSTRACT

The medical method by which a modified Human Immuno-deficiency Virus or virus-like structure is used as a transport medium to carry a medically therapeutic ribonucleic acid to precursor T-Helper cells and mature T-Helper cells to prevent AIDS. The modified Human Immunodeficiency Virus or virus-like structures make contact with precursor T-Helper cells or mature T-Helper cells by means exterior probes. Once the exterior probes engage the precursor T-Helper cells' or mature T-Helper cells' cell-surface receptors, the modified virus or virus-like structures inserts into the cells the medically therapeutic ribonucleic acid they are carrying. The medically therapeutic ribonucleic acid causes T-Helper cells to express an altered cell-surface receptor on their surface thus thwarting HIV virions from being able to gain access to such cells, thus preventing AIDS.

BACKGROUND OF THE INVENTION

1. Field of the Invention

[0001] This invention relates to any medical device that is intended to alter the cell-surface receptors on precursor T-Helper cells or mature T-Helper cells in order to make an individual immune to an infection by the Human Immunodeficiency Virus.

2. Description of Background Art

[0002] It has been estimated by the Center for Disease Control that in the United States 55,000 to 60,000 new cases of Human Immunodeficiency Virus (HIV) are occurring each year. It is thought that there are 900,000 people currently infected with HIV in the United States, with many victims not aware that they have contracted the virus. Further, it has been estimated that the Human Immunodeficiency Virus (HIV), the pathogen that causes Acquired Immune Deficiency Syndrome (AIDS), has infected as many as 30-60 million people around the globe.

[0003] The presence of HIV was first came to the attention of those in the United States in 1981, when there appeared an outbreak of Kaposi's Sarcoma and Pneumocystis carinii pneumonia in gay men in New York and California. After over twenty-five years of research and investigation, eradicating the ever growing global humanitarian crisis posed by the HIV remains an elusive goal for the medical community. It is estimated the virus has already killed 25 million citizens of this planet.

[0004] The Human Immunodeficiency Virus has been previously referred to as human T-Lymphotrophic virus III (HTLV-III), lymphadenopathy-associated virus (LAV), and AIDS-associated retrovirus (ARV). Infection with HIV may occur by the virus being transferred by blood, semen, vaginal fluid, or breast milk. Four major means of transmission of HIV include unprotected sexual intercourse, contaminated needles, breast milk, and transmission from an infected mother to her baby at birth.

[0005] HIV is an ingeniously constructed very deadly virus, which represents the most challenging pathogen the worldwide medical community faces to date. A pathogen may be a bacterium, virus, or other organism that may cause disease. Viruses in general, have been difficult to contain and eradicate due to the fact they are obligate parasites and tend not to carry out any biologic functions outside the cell the virus has targeted as its host. A virus when it exists outside the boundaries of a cell is generally referred to as a virion. HIV virions posses several attributes that make them very elusive and difficult to destroy.

[0006] For purposes of this text, the term 'body' refers to the material part of a man or a woman, generally including the head, neck, trunk, extremities and all usual internal structures. The terms 'body' and 'human body' are interchangeable.

[0007] Bacterial infections have posed an easier target for the medical community to eradicate from the body. Bacteria generally live and reproduce outside animal cells. Bacteria, like animal cells, carryout biologic functions. A large multi-celled organism such as the human body combats bacterial infections with a combined force of white cells, antibodies, complements and its lymphatic system. White cells circulate the body in search of bacteria. When a white cell encounters a bacterium, the white cell engulfs the bacterium, encapsulates the pathogen, processes the identification of the pathogen and kills the pathogen utilizing acids and destructive enzymes. The white cell then alerts the B-cells of the immune system as to the identity of the intruding bacterium. A subpopulation of B-cells is generated, dedicated to producing antibodies directed against the particular pathogen the circulating white cell encountered and identified. Antibodies, generated by B-cells, traverse the blood and body tissues in search of the bacteria they were designed to repel. Once an antibody encounters a bacterium it is targeted to attack, the antibody attaches to the bacterium's outer wall. The effect antibodies have in coating the outside of a bacterium is to assist the white cells and the other components of the immune system in recognizing the bacterium, so that appropriate defensive action can be taken against the pathogen. Some antibodies, in addition to coating the bacterium, will act to punch holes through the bacterium's outer wall. If the integrity of the bacterium's cell wall is breached, this action generally leads to the death of the bacterium. Complements are primitive protein structures that circulate the blood stream in search of anything that appears consistent with a bacteria cell wall. Complements are indiscriminant. Once the complement proteins locate any form of bacterial cell wall, the complement proteins organize, and much like antibodies, act in concert to punch one or more holes though a bacterium's cell wall to compromise the viability of the bacterium. The lymphatic system is a diffuse network of thin walled vessels that drain excess water from extracellular fluids and join to form the thoracic duct and right lymph duct, which empty into the venous system near the heart. Lymph nodes are present at different locations in the body and screen the fluid transiting the lymphatic system, called lymph, to remove pathogens. Cells in the spleen screen the blood in search of bacteria. When a bacterial pathogen is identified, such as by antibodies coating the surface, the bacterium is taken out of circulation and terminated.

[0008] Viruses pose a much different infectious vector to the body's defense system than either bacteria or cellular parasites. Since viruses do not carry out biologic processes outside their host cell, a virus can be destroyed, but they cannot be killed. A virus is simply comprised of one or more external shells and a portion of genetic material. The virus's genetic information is carried in the core of the virus. Antibodies can coat the exterior of a virus to make it easier for the white cells in the body to identify the viral pathogen, but the action of punching holes in the virus's external shell by antibodies or complement proteins does not necessarily kill the virus. Viruses also only briefly circulate in the blood and tissues of the body as an exposed entity. Using exterior probes, a virus hunts down a cell in the body that will act as an appropriate host so that the virus can replicate. Once the virus has found a proper host cell, the virus inserts its genome into the host cell. To complete its life-cycle, the virus's genetic material takes command of cellular functions and directs the host cell to make replicas of the virus.

[0009] Once the virus's genome has entered a host cell, the virus is in effect shielded from the body's immune system defense mechanisms. Inside a host cell, the presence of the virus is generally only represented as genetic information incorporated into the host cell's DNA. Once a virus has infected a cell in the body, the presence of the virus can only be eradicated if the host cell is destroyed. Antibodies and complements are generally designed not to attack the autologous tissues of the body. Circulating white cells and the immune cells which comprise lymph nodes and the spleen may or may not recognize that a cell, which has become a host for a virus, is infected with a virus's genome. If the immune system fails to identify a cell that has become infected with a virus, the virus's genetic material can proceed to force the infected cell to make copies of the virus. Since a virus is in essence simply a segment of genetic material, time is of no consequence to the life-cycle of the virus and a virus's genome may be carried for years by the host without a need to activate; such viruses are often termed latent viruses. A virus's genetic material may sit idle in a host cell for an extended period of time until the pathogen's programming senses the time is right to initiate the virus's replication process or an action of the host cell triggers the virus to replicate. The only opportunity for the immune system to destroy a latent virus is when copies of the virus leave the host cell and circulate in the blood or tissues in search of another perspective host cell.

[0010] The traditional medical approach to combating infectious agents such as bacteria and cellular parasites, therefore has limited value in managing or eradicating elusive or latent viral infections. Synthetic antibiotics, generally used to augment the body's capacity to produce naturally occurring antibodies against bacterial infections, have little success in combating latent viral infections. Stimulating the body's immune system's recognition of a virus by administering a vaccine also has had limited success in combating elusive viral infections. Vaccines generally are intended to introduce to the body pieces of a bacteria or virus, or an attenuated, noninfectious intact bacteria or virus so that the immune system is able to recognize and process the infectious agent and generate antibodies directed to assist in killing the pathogen. Once the immune system has been primed to recognize an intruder, antibodies will be produced by the immune system in great quantities in an effort to repel an invader. Over time, as the immune system down-regulates its antibody production in response to a lack of detecting the presence of the intruding pathogen, the quantity of antibodies circulating in the blood stream may decrease in number to a quantity that is insufficient to combat a pathogen. Since antibodies have limited value in combating some of the more elusive viruses that hibernate in host cells, vaccines have limited value in destroying latent viruses.

[0011] The Human Immunodeficiency Virus demonstrates four factors which make this pathogen particularly elusive and a difficult infectious agent to eradicate from the body. First: the host for HIV is the T-Helper cell. The T-Helper cell is a key element in the immune system's response since it helps coordinate the body's defensive actions against pathogens seeking to invade the body's tissues. In cases of a bacterial infection versus a viral infection, T-Helper cells actively direct which immune cells will rev-up in response to the infectious agent and engage the particular pathogen. Since HIV infects and disrupts T-Helper cells, coordination of the immune response against the virus is disrupted, thus limiting the body's capacity to mount a proper response against the presence of the virus and produce a sufficient action to successfully eradicate the virus.

[0012]   Second: again, latent viruses such as HIV, have a strategic advantage. When the immune system first recognizes a pathogen and begins to generate antibodies against a particular pathogen, the response is generally robust. Once time has passed and the immune system fails to detect an active threat, the production of antibodies against the particular pathogen diminishes. When HIV infects a T-Helper cell, the viral genome may lay dormant, sometimes for years before taking command of the T-Helper cell's biologic functions. HIV may, therefore, generate a very active initial immune response to its presence, but if the virus sits dormant inside T-Helper cells for months or years, the antibody response to the virus will diminish over time. There may not be an adequate quantity of circulating antibodies to actively engage the HIV virions as they migrate from the T-Helper cell that generated the copies to uninfected T-Helper cells that will serve as a new host to support further replication. If the immune system's response is insufficient during the period while the virus is exposed and vulnerable, it becomes extremely difficult for the body to eradicate the virus.

[0013]   Third, when replicas of the Human Immunodeficiency Virus are released from their host cell, during the budding process the HIV virion coats itself with an exterior envelope comprised of a portion of the plasma membrane from the T-Helper cell that acted as the host for the virus. A T-Helper cell's plasma membrane is comprised of a lipid bilayer, a double layer of lipid molecules oriented with their polar ends at the outside of the membrane and the nonpolar ends in the membrane interior. The virus thus, in part, takes on an external appearance of a naturally occurring cell in the body. Since the exterior envelope of a HIV virion has the characteristics of a T-Helper cell it is more difficult for the immune system to recognize that it is a pathogen as it migrates through the body in search of another T-Helper cell to infect.

[0014] Fourth, the Human Immunodeficiency Virus exhibits a very elusive mode of action which the virus readily utilizes to actively defeat the body's immune system. HIV carries in its genome a segment of genetic material that directs an infected T-Helper cell to create and mount on the surface the plasma membrane a FasL cell-surface receptor. Healthy T-Helper cells carry on the surface of their plasma membrane Fas cell-surface receptors. The Fas cell-surface receptor when engaged by a FasL cell-surface receptor on another cell, initiates apoptosis in the cell carrying the Fas cell-surface receptor. Apoptosis is a biologic process that causes a cell to terminate itself. A T-Helper cell infected with the HIV virus carrying a FasL cell-surface receptor is therefore capable of killing noninfected T-Helper cells that the infected T-Helper cell encounters as it circulates the body. The occurrence of AIDS is therefore propagated not only by the number of T-Helper cells that become incapacitated due to direct infection by HIV, but also by the number of noninfected T-Helper cells that are eliminated by coming in direct contact with infected T-Helper cells.

[0015] Acquired Immune Deficiency Syndrome (AIDS) occurs as a result of the number of circulating T-Helper cells declining to a point where the immune system's capacity to mount a successful response against opportunistic infectious agents is significantly compromised. The number of viable T-Helper cells declines either because they become infected with the HIV virus or because they have been killed by encountering a T-Helper cell infected with HIV. When there is an insufficient population of non-HIV infected T-Helper cells to properly combat infectious agents such as Pneumocystis carinii or cytomegalo virus or other pathogens, the body becomes overwhelmed with the opportunistic infection and the patient becomes clinically ill. In cases where the combination of the patient's compromised immune system and medical assistance in terms of synthetic antibiotics intended to combat the opportunistic pathogens, fluids, intravenous nutrition and other treatments are not sufficient to sustain life, the body succumbs to the opportunistic infection and death ensues.

[0016] The Human Immunodeficiency Virus locates its host by utilizing probes located on its envelope. The HIV virion has two types of glycoprotein (gp) probes attached to the outer surface of its exterior envelope. A glycoprotein is a structure comprised of a protein component and a lipid component. HIV utilizes a glycoprotein 120 (gp 120) probe to locate a Cluster Designation (CD) 4 cell-surface receptor on the plasma membrane of a T-Helper cell. The plasma membrane of the T-Helper cell is comprised of a lipid bilayer. Cell-surface receptors are anchored in the lipid bilayer. Once an HIV gp 120 probe has successfully engaged a CD4 cell-surface receptor on a T-Helper cell a conformational change occurs in the gp 120 probe and a glycoprotein 41 (gp 41) probe is exposed. The gp 41 probe's intent is to engage a CXCR4 or CCR5 cell-surface receptor on the plasma membrane of the same T-Helper cell. Once a gp 41 probe on the HIV virion engages a CXCR4 or CCR5 cell-surface receptor, the HIV virion opens an access portal through the T-Helper cell's plasma membrane.

[0017] Once the virus has gained access to the T-Helper cell by opening a portal through the cell's outer membrane the virion inserts two positive strand RNA molecules approximately 9500 nucleotides in length. Inserted along with the RNA strands are the enzymes reverse transcriptase, protease and integrase. Once the virus's genome gains access to the interior of the

T-Helper cell, in the cytoplasm the pair of RNA molecules are transformed to deoxyribonucleic acid by the reverse transcriptase enzyme. Following modification of the virus's genome to DNA, the virus's genetic information migrates to the host cell's nucleus. In the nucleus, with the assistance of the integrase protein, the virus's DNA becomes inserted into the T-Helper cell's native DNA. When the timing is appropriate, the now integrated viral DNA, becomes read by the host cell's polymerase molecules and the virus's genetic information commands certain cell functions to carry out the replication process to construct copies of the human deficiency virus.

[0018] Present anti-viral therapy has been designed to target the enzymes that assist the HIV genome with the replication process. Anti-viral therapy is intended to interfere with the action of these replication enzymes. Part of the challenge of eradicating HIV is that once the virus inserts its genome into a T-Helper cell host, the viral genome may lay dormant until the proper circumstances evolve. The virus's genome may sit idle inside a T-Helper cell for years before becoming activated, causing drugs that interfere with HIV's life cycle to have limited effect on eliminating the virus from the body. Arresting the replication process does not insure that T-Helper cells infected with HIV do not continue to circulate the body killing noninfected T-Helper cells thus causing the patient to progress to a clinically apparent state of Acquired Immune Deficiency Syndrome and eventually succumbing to an opportunistic infection which eventually results in the death of the individual.

[0019] The outer layer of the HIV virion is comprised of a portion of the T-Helper cell's outer cell membrane. In the final stage of the replication process, as a copy of the HIV capsid, carrying the HIV genome, buds through the host cell's plasma membrane, the capsid acquires as its outermost shell a wrapping of lipid bilayer from the host cell's plasma membrane. Vaccines are generally comprised of pieces of a virus or bacterium, or copies of the entire virus or bacterium weakened to the point the pathogen is incapable of causing an infection. These pieces of a pathogen or copies of a nonvirulent pathogen prime the immune system such that a vaccine intent is to cause B-cells to produce antibodies that are programmed to seek out the surface characteristics of the pathogen comprising the vaccine. In the case of HIV, since the surface of the pathogen is an envelope comprised of lipid bilayer taken from the host T-Helper cell's plasma membrane, a vaccine comprised of portions of the exterior envelope of the HIV virions might not only target HIV virions, but might also have deleterious effects on the T-Helper cell population. Some antibodies produced to combat HIV infections may not be able to tell the difference between an HIV virion and a T-Helper cell, and such antibodies may act to coat and assist in the elimination of both targets. In such a scenario, since such a vaccine might cause a decline in the number of available T-Helper cells, it is conceivable that a vaccine comprised of portions of the external envelope of HIV virions might paradoxically induce clinically apparent AIDS in a patient that a vaccine has been administered.

[0020] It is clear that the traditional approach of utilizing antibiotics or providing vaccines to stimulate the immune system to produce endogenous antibodies, by themselves, is an ineffective strategy to manage a virus as elusive and deadly as HIV. Drugs that interfere with the replication process of HIV generally slow progression of the infection by the virus, but do not necessarily eliminate the virus from the body nor eliminate the threat of the clinical symptoms of AIDS. A new strategy is required in order to successfully combat the threat of HIV.

[0021] A eukaryote refers to a nucleated cell. Eukaryotes comprise nearly all animal and plant cells. A human eukaryote or nucleated cell is comprised of an exterior lipid bilayer plasma membrane, cytoplasm, a nucleus, and organelles. The exterior plasma membrane defines the perimeter of the cell, regulates the flow of nutrients, water and regulating molecules in and out of the cell, and has embedded into its structure cell-surface receptors that the cell uses to detect properties of the environment surrounding the cell membrane. Cytoplasm refers to the entire contents inside the cell except for the nucleus and acts as a filling medium inside the boundaries of the plasma cell membrane. Cytosol refers to the semifluid portion of the cytoplasm minus the mitochondria and the endoplasmic reticulum. The nucleus, organelles, and ribosomes are suspended in the cytosol. Nutrients such as amino acids, oxygen and glucose are present in the cytosol. The nucleus contains the majority of the cell's genetic information in the form of double stranded deoxyribonucleic acid (DNA). Organelles generally carry out specialized functions for the cell and include such structures as the mitochondria, the endoplasmic reticulum, storage vacuoles, lysosomes and Golgi complex. Floating in the cytoplasm, but also located in the endoplasmic reticulum and mitochondria are ribosomes. Ribosomes are protein structures comprised of several strands of proteins that combine and couple to a messenger ribonucleic acid (mRNA) molecule. More than one ribosome may be attached to a single mRNA at a time. Ribosomes decode genetic information coded in a mRNA molecule and manufacture proteins to the specifications of the instruction code physically present in the mRNA molecule.

[0022] The majority of the deoxyribonucleic acid (DNA) in a cell is present in the form of chromosomes, the double stranded helical structures located in the nucleus of the cell. DNA in a circular form, can also be found in the mitochondria, the powerhouse of the cell, an organelle that assists in converting glucose into usable energy molecules. DNA represents the genetic information a cell needs to manufacture the materials it requires to develop to its mature form, sustain life and to replicate. Genetic information is stored in the DNA by arrangements of four nucleotides referred to as: adenine, thymine, guanine and cytosine. DNA represents instruction coding, that in the process known as transcription, the DNA's genetic information is decoded by transcription protein complexes referred to as polymerases, to produce ribonucleic acid (RNA). RNA is a single strand of genetic information comprised of coded arrangements of four nucleotides: adenine, uracil, guanine and cytosine. The physical difference in the construction of a DNA molecule versus a RNA molecule is that DNA utilizes the nucleotide 'thymine', while RNA molecules utilize the nucleotide 'uracil'. RNAs are generally classified as messenger RNAs (mRNA), transport RNAs (tRNA) and ribosomal RNAs (rRNA).

[0023] The nucleic acids comprising the DNA are arranged in a biologic code format. Adenine is 'A'; Thymine is 'T'; Cytosine is 'C'; Guanine is 'G'. It is believed that the DNA is divided into segments of three nucleic acids. A segment of three nucleic acids is referred to as a codon. Given there are four different nucleic acids and three nucleic acids are used to comprise a codon, there are 64 possible combinations. Most of the combinations are thought to code for amino acids, the building blocks of proteins. There are 20 amino acids. As an example, the three nucleic acid codon 'TCA' codes for the amino acid Serine. As another example, the three nucleic acid codon 'GCA' codes for the amino acid Alanine. Three of the codons are considered STOP codes. STOP codons are biologic signals to terminate events, such as reading and deciphering of the genetic code. The three STOP codes are represented in the DNA by the codons: 'TAA', 'TAG', and 'TGA'. Since RNA is comprised of coded arrangements of the four nucleotides: adenine, uracil, guanine and cytosine, the three STOP codes are represented in the messenger RNA as the three codons: 'UAA', 'UAG' and 'UAG'.

[0024] Proteins are generated when ribosomes decipher the genetic code present on a strand of messenger RNA. Each codon represents an amino acid. Some of the twenty amino acids have more than one codon that codes for the same amino acid. Ribosomes build proteins by stringing together amino acids as dictated by the codons present on messenger

RNA. When a protein is being generated by ribosomes, the ribosomes cease reading the messenger RNA when they encounter any of the three STOP codons; the presence of a STOP code terminates production of the polypeptide chain by the ribosomes. The polypeptide chain is then released from the ribosome and represents an individual protein.

[0025] Proteins are comprised of a series of amino acids bonded together in a linear strand, sometimes referred to as a chain; a protein may be further modified to be a structure comprised of one or more similar or differing strands of amino acids bonded together. A protein comprised of one or more strands of amino acids (referred to as subunits) may be referred to as a protein complex. Insulin is a protein structure comprised of two strands of amino acids, one strand comprised of 21 amino acids long and the second strand comprised of 30 amino acids; the two strands attached by two disulfide bridges. There are an estimated 30,000 different proteins the cells of the human body may manufacture. The human body is comprised of a wide variety of cells, many with specialized functions requiring unique combinations of proteins and protein structures such as glycoproteins (a protein combined with a carbohydrate) to accomplish the required task or tasks a specialized cell is designed to perform. Forms of glycoproteins are known to be utilized as cell-surface receptors.

[0026] Viruses are obligate parasites. Viruses simply represent a carrier of genetic material and by themselves viruses are unable to replicate or carry on any form of biologic function outside their host cell. Viruses are generally comprised of one or more shells constructed of one or more layers of protein or lipid material, and inside the outer shell or shells, a virus carries a genetic payload that represents the instruction code necessary to replicate the virus, and protein enzymes to help facilitate the genetic payload in the function of replicating copies of the virus once the genetic payload has been delivered to a host cell. Located on the outer shell or envelope of a virus are probes. The function of a virus's probes is to locate and engage a host cell's receptors. The virus's surface probes are designed to detect, make contact with and functionally engage one or more receptors located on the exterior of a cell type that will offer the virus the proper environment in which to construct copies of itself. A host cell is a cell that provides the virus the proper biochemical machinery for the virus to successfully replicate itself.

[0027] Protected by the outer coat generally comprised of an envelope or capsid or envelope and capsid, viruses carry a genetic payload in the form of deoxyribonucleic acid (DNA) or ribonucleic acid (RNA). Once a virus's exterior probes locate and functionally engage the surface receptor or receptors on a host cell, the virus inserts its genetic payload into the interior of the host cell. In the event a virus is carrying a DNA payload, the virus's DNA travels to the host cell's nucleus and is known to become inserted into the host cell's own native DNA. In the case where a virus is carrying its genetic payload as RNA, the virus inserts the RNA payload into the host cell and may also insert one or more enzymes to facilitate the RNA being utilized properly to replicate copies of the virus. Once inside the host cell, some species of virus facilitate their RNA being converted to DNA. Once the viral RNA has been converted to DNA, the virus's DNA travels to the host cell's nucleus and is known to become inserted into the host cell's native DNA. Once a virus's genetic material has been inserted into the host cell's native DNA, the virus's genetic material takes command of certain cell functions and redirects the resources of the host cell to generate copies of the virus. Other forms of RNA viruses bypass the need to use the host cell's nuclear DNA and simply utilize portions of its innate viral genome to act as messenger RNA (mRNA). RNA viruses that bypass the host cell's DNA, cause the cell, in general, to generate copies of the necessary parts of the virus directly from the virus's RNA genome. When a virus's genome directly acts as a template, then similar to the cell's messenger RNA, the virus's RNA is read by the cell's ribosomes and proteins necessary to complete the virus's replication process are generated.

[0028]   The Plague or Black Death ravaged Europe between 1347 to 1350 and claimed nearly a quarter of all who lived in Europe at the time. The bubonic plague was caused by Yersinia pestis, a bacterium that lived inside rats and could be spread to humans by the bite of a flea. Yersinia binds to white blood cells and injects a toxin into the white blood cell to stun the immune system, allowing Yersinia to flourish without being attacked by the immune system. The belief is that Yersinia uses the CCR5 cell-surface receptor on white blood cells to target white blood cell and bind to them. Those who were born without the gene for CCR5 or carried a mutant gene for the CCR5 cell-surface receptor were protected from the Black Death. Today, some of the descendants of the survivors of the Black Plaque are resistant to becoming infected by HIV.

[0029]   Once the 120 gp probe on an HIV virion engages a CD4 cell-surface receptor on a T-Helper cell, to gain access and infect the T-Helper cell the HIV virion's gp 41 probe must successfully engage a CXCR4 or CCR5 cell-surface receptor on the T-Helper cell. If a HIV virion's gp 41 probe is unable to properly engage a CXCR4 or CCR5 cell-surface receptor an access portal will not open up on the surface of the T-Helper cell and the cell membrane will remain impenetrable. At least one mutant CCR5 gene has been identified in the population. The mutation to the CCR5 gene is in the form of a missing 32-base section of the gene. Those who carry two copies of the mutant CCR5 gene have no CCR5 receptors on the surface of their cells and have a significantly lower rate of infection with HIV than those that carry normal CCR5 genes. Those who carry one mutant CCR5 gene have fewer CCR5 cell-surface receptors on the surface of their cells and though they may become infected with HIV, the mutation retards the onset of clinically apparent AIDS.

[0030]   T-Helper cells undergo a complex maturation process to become a mature T-Helper cell.   Precursor T-Helper cells are originally derived from stem cells located in the bone marrow.   As precursor T-Helper cells progress through the maturation process to become a mature T-Helper cell cell-surface receptors (sometimes referred to as markers) change. Precursor T-Helper cells lack certain cell-surface receptors found on mature T-Helper cells. Stem cells present in the bone marrow may express CD 7 and CD34 cell-surface markers that are not present on mature T-Helper cells. Precursor T-Helper cells released from the bone marrow are generally do not carry CD4 or CD8 cell-surface receptors and are often termed 'double negative' cells, meaning they do not express either one of these cell surface receptors on their surface.   Precursor T-Helper cells sometimes referred to as precursor T-Lymphocytes migrate from the bone marrow to thymus to undergo further maturation. The thymus is a gland in the neck which cultivates immature T-Helper cells through various stages of development until a mature form of T-Helper cell is reached and released into circulation. As a result of the stages of the maturation process precursor T-Helper cells continue to change some of the cell-surface receptors expressed on their surface.   At one point in the maturation process, precursor T-Helper cells will express both CD4 and CD8 cell-surface receptors and be termed as double positive cells. As the precursor T-Helper cell continues to mature it will lose the expression of either the CD8 cell-surface receptors. Mature T-Helper cells express CD4 cell-surface receptors on their surface, but do not express CD 8 cell-surface receptors. Other cell-surface receptors that are expressed include CD25, CD38 and CD44.

[0031]   Current state of gene therapy generally refers to efforts directed toward inserting an exogenous subunit of DNA, that are 'known genes' as they occur in nature, into a vehicle such as a naturally occurring virus. The vehicle is intended to insert the exogenous subunit of DNA into a target cell. The exogenous DNA subunit then migrates to the target cell's nucleus. The exogenous DNA subunit then inserts into the native DNA of the cell. This represents a permanent alteration of the cell's nuclear DNA. At some point, the nuclear transcription proteins read the exogenous DNA subunit's nucleotide coding to produce the intended cellular response.

[0032] An approach to defeating HIV from infecting healthy mature T-Helper cells would be to insert into precursor T-Helper cells a means to alter the genes that code for the CXCR4 cell-surface receptor or the CCR5 cell-surface receptor, thus producing mature T-Helper cells that do not express these cell-surface receptors or express altered, biologically nonfunctional forms of these cell-surface receptors. By generating T-Helper cells that do not express CXCR4 or CCR5 cell-surface receptors, or by generating T-Helper cells that do not express biologically functional CXCR4 or CCR5 cell-surface receptors makes these T-Helper cells impervious to infection by Human Immunodeficiency Virus virions. The natural selection process caused by the Yersinia pestis demonstrates that a substantial number of people possess mutant genes which cause T-Helper cells not express CCR5 cell-surface receptors and apparently such individuals live normal lives; thus such an alteration to cell-surface receptors does not produce a readily apparent harmful effect.

[0033] Since during the maturation process a precursor T-Helper cell expresses a CD8 cell-surface receptor and then removes this CD8 cell-surface receptor from its surface; there exits biologic instruction code and a mechanism inside the cell to remove a cell-surface receptor from the surface of a T-Helper cell or alter the cell-surface receptor such that it becomes biologically nonfunctional. Utilizing this natural process of removing or altering cell-surface receptors already present in cells, leads to removing or altering cell-surface receptors present on existing cell to make such cell impervious to infection. Removal of CXCR4 cell-surface receptors and CCR5 cell-surface receptors from the surface of mature T-Helper cells or making CXCR4 cell-surface receptors and CCR5 cell-surface receptors nonfunctional would make mature T-Helper cells impervious to infection by either Human Immunodeficiency Virus virions and Yersinia pestis and possibly other infectious pathogens.

[0034] Utilizing the natural process that a cell possesses to remove or alter cell-surface markers that exist on the surface of the cell, could lead to causing T-Helper cells infected with the Human Immunodeficiency Virus genome that are expressing FasL cell-surface receptors that terminate healthy T-Helper cells to remove their FasL receptor or alter the FasL receptor such that the FasL receptor becomes biologically nonfunctional. Removing the threat of infected T-Helper cells utilizing their FasL cell-surface receptors from terminating healthy T-Helper cells would help avert a person infected with HIV from progressing to AIDS.

[0035] The method described within the scope of this text involves utilizing modified virus virions to deliver to specific target cells such as stem cells, precursor T-Helper cells and mature T-Helper cells a medically therapeutic RNA genome as a payload. As with HIV, the RNA genome would be converted to DNA by enzymes and then inserted into the native DNA of the target cell to produce a biologic response. The biologic response would include causing a cell-surface receptor not to be expressed on the surface of the cell, or causing an altered form of a cell-surface receptor to be expressed on the surface of the cell, or causing removal of a cell-surface receptor from the surface of the cell, or causing alteration to an existing cell-surface receptor being expressed on the surface of the cell to produce a medically therapeutic outcome.

[0036] A means of treating AIDS could be to take the naturally occurring Human Immunodeficiency Virus (HIV) which is an RNA virus and replace HIV's innate genome with a genome that codes for either prevention of the CXCR4 or CCR5 cell-surface receptors from being expressed, or expression of nonfunctional CXCR4 or CCR5 cell-surface receptors or removal of existing CXCR4 or CCR5 cell-surface receptors. HIV already posses the means to locate and infect T-Helper cells, which act as the natural host for HIV replication. Modified HIV virions could be utilized to carry their modified genome to either precursor T-Helper cells or mature T-Helper cells. Utilizing modified HIV virions to insert modified genome in a patient's T-Helper cells would prevent HIV by altering the cell-surface receptors of the patient's T-Helper cell population, preventing HIV from being able to access T-Helper cells and thus stop AIDS from occurring or progressing in a patient.

BRIEF SUMMARY OF THE INVENTION

[0037] The medical treatment device comprised of a modified virus or virus-like structure is used as a transport medium to carry a payload consisting of a modified genome that alters the CXCR4 or CCR5 cell-surface receptors present on the surface of the T-Helper cells in the body. The modified virus or virus-like structure makes contact with a precursor T-Helper cell or mature T-Helper cell by means of the virus's exterior probes or virus-like structure's exterior probes. Once the exterior probes engage the precursor target cells' or mature T-Helper cells' cell-surface receptors, the modified virus or virus-like structure inserts into the precursor T-Helper cells or mature T-Helper cells the modified genome it is carrying. As the precursor T-Helper cell matures it will either not express CXCR4 or CCR5 cell-surface receptors or it will express biologically nonfunctional CXCR4 or CCR5 cell surface receptors. Mature T-Helper cells with either remove their CXCR4 or CCR5 cell-surface receptors from the outer membrane or the existing CXCR4 or CCR5 cell-surface receptors will be made nonfunctional. By removing functional CXCR4 and CCR5 cell-surface receptors from the surface of mature T-Helper cells prevents HIV virions from being able to gain access to mature T-Helper cells and thus prevents AIDS.

DETAILED DESCRIPTION

[0038] The medical treatment method described herein is a means of making the immune system impervious to infection by pathogens that utilize cell-surface receptors located on cells comprising the immune system to gain access to the cells that constitute the immune system. To make cells impervious to infection is a simple function of preventing such cells from ever expressing the cell-surface receptors that make them vulnerable to infection or alter the cell-surface receptors in a manner that prevents the cell-surface receptor from being used by a pathogen to gain access to the cell. It is known that the Human Immunodeficiency Virus utilizes its gp120 probe to engage the CD4 cell-surface receptor on its host the T-Helper cell. Once the gp120 probe has successfully engaged a CD4 cell-surface receptor, the HIV virion utilizes its gp41 probe to engage either a CXCR4 or CCR5 cell-surface receptor affixed to the surface of the T-Helper cell. Following successful engagement of a CXCR4 or CCR5 cell-surface receptor, the HIV virion is able to open a portal through the outer membrane of the T-Helper cell and insert into the T-Helper cell the HIV RNA genome and the enzymes needed to activate HIV's RNA genome. It is known that individuals that lack the gene to express a CCR5 cell-surface receptor on the surface of their T-Helper cells are immune to infection by the Human Immunodeficiency Virus.

[0039] T-Helper cells undergo a complex maturation process before they are released into circulation as mature T-Helper cells. Stem cells in the bone marrow produce precursor T-lymphocytes that leave the bone marrow and travel to the thymus gland. In the thymus gland these precursor T-lymphocytes or precursor T-Helper cells undergo various stages of development. As a precursor T-Helper cell develops into a mature T-Helper cell various cell-surface receptors are expressed on the surface of the precursor T-Helper cell. Some of the cell-surface receptors are expressed on the surface of the precursor T-Helper cell for a short time and then removed from the surface of the cell.

[0040]   The medical treatment method described herein takes the concept that if a T-Helper cell does not express a cell-surface receptor that makes it vulnerable to infection by a pathogen then the cell is impervious to that pathogen and develops this concept into a practical treatment strategy to prevent infection by pathogens. Altering the genes that control the expression of the cell-surface receptors that make a cell vulnerable to infection prevents the infection. In the case of infection by the Human Immunodeficiency Virus altering the genes that control the expression of the CXCR4 and CCR5 cell-surface receptors prevents T-Helper cells from becoming infected by the Human Immunodeficiency Virus or other pathogens such as Yersinia pestis. The medical treatment method targets a precursor form of T-Helper cell as it develops but before it expresses either the CXCR4 or CCR5 cell-surface receptors on its outer membrane. Altering the genes that control the expression of the CXCR4 and CCR5 cell-surface receptors in a manner that prevents expression of these genes before the cell-surface receptors are generated dictates that the mature form of the T-Helper cell will not express either the CXCR4 cell-surface receptor or the CCR5 cell-surface receptor on its surface.

[0041]   Viruses such as the Human Immunodeficiency Virus insert their genome into a cell, this genome gets transported from the cytoplasm to the nucleus of the cell, and then this genome gets inserted into the nuclear DNA of the cell. The Human Immunodeficiency Virus is designed to target T-Helper cells, and insert genetic material into T-Helper cells. The medical treatment method described herein is to take a modified form of a virus and use this modified virus to insert medically beneficial genetic material into specific cells to produce a medically beneficial response. In the case of preventing AIDS, the method is comprised of utilizing a modified virus to seek out and engage precursor T-Helper cells, whether this be stem cells or precursor T-Helper cells located in the bone marrow, in transit to the thymus gland or present in the thymus gland and insert into the precursor T-Helper cells genetic instruction code that alters the genes responsible for the CXCR4 and CCR5 cell-surface receptors. The modified virus would be generated with glycoprotein probes that would engage cell-surface receptors located on either stem cells or precursor T-Helper cells, that are unique to these cells, and offer the proper means for the modified virus to gain access to the precursor T-Helper cells so that the modified virus can deliver the medially therapeutic genome it carries to the precursor T-Helper cells. Cell-surface receptors such as CD7, CD 34, CD38, CD44 may designate precursor T-Helper cells. The presence of both the CD4 and CD8 cell-surface receptors designates a precursor form of T-Helper cell. Modified virus virions could use glycoprotein probes that seek out these cell-surface receptors in order to find and engage the proper precursor T-Helper cells.

[0042] STOP codes are biologic instructions that tell the polymerase molecules, that read and decipher the nuclear DNA, when to stop deciphering the code. Several forms of STOP codes have been defined. Utilizing the Universal Code the codons, comprised of three nucleic acids, designated TAA, TAG, and TGA represent STOP codes. Therefore, if a polymerase molecule which is reading a segment of nuclear DNA encounters a section that is comprised of three nucleic acids arranged as TAA, TAG, or TGA, the polymerase recognizes this particular instruction code as an instruction to cause the polymerase molecule to cease reading any further instruction code at that location in the nuclear DNA. Other biologic coding may interfere with the reading of the nuclear DNA and terminate deciphering of the nuclear DNA.

[0043] It is known that individuals that lack a 32-base segment in both CCR5 genes that they possess will not express a CCR5 cell-surface receptor on the surface of their mature T-Helper cells and such individuals are resistant to infection by the Human

Immunodeficiency Virus. The medically therapeutic method described herein creates an alteration to CCR5 cell-surface receptor genes by inserting into the CCR5 cell-surface receptor genes a STOP code. This STOP code may occur anywhere in the gene to prevent the gene from being deciphered properly by a polymerase molecule. Mimicking Mother Nature, the STOP code could be inserted into the gene at the point along the gene's nucleic acid sequence that prevents the 32-base segment from being read in the gene similar to the naturally occurring gene mutation that results in individuals being resistant to the Yersinia pestis pathogen. STOP codes as seen in DNA are represented by any of the three codons: 'TAA', 'TAG', and 'TGA'. STOP codes as seen in messenger RNA are represented by any of the three codons: 'UAA', 'UAG', and 'UGA'.

[0044] The medical treatment method described herein is comprised of a virus that is modified in such a fashion that it seeks out precursor T-Helper cells, the virus further modified to carry medically therapeutic genetic instruction code and insert this medically therapeutic instruction code into the precursor T-Helper cell, with the intention that this medically therapeutic instruction code will alter the CXCR4 or CCR5 cell-surface gene in such a manner that the mature T-Helper cell will not express either a CXCR4 cell-surface receptor or a CCR5 cell-surface receptor on the surface of its outer membrane.

[0045] It is known that as cells develop toward maturation, immature precursor cells may express certain cell-surface receptors for a period of time and then either cause the cell-surface receptor to become nonfunctional or remove the cell-surface receptor from the surface of the cell. As precursor T-Helper cells proceed through a very complex maturation process to become mature T-Helper cells, certain cell-surface receptors are expressed on the surface of the precursor T-Helper cell and then later altered to be nonfunctional or removed from the surface of the precursor T-Helper cell.

Given that there is a natural process already in existence to cause an existing cell-surface receptor affixed to the outside membrane of a cell to be altered to become nonfunctional or to be physically removed from the surface of the cell, this feature can be utilized to remove unwanted cell-surface receptors from existing cells to produce a beneficial medically therapeutic outcome. In a patient infected with Human Immunodeficiency Virus, the patient's healthy, noninfected T-Helper cells are vulnerable to infection by the Human Immunodeficiency Virus by the fact the noninfected cells express CXCR4 or CCR5 cell-surface receptors on their surface. Modifying the Human Immunodeficiency Virus to carry a biologic instruction code to cause a healthy noninfected T-Helper cell to make the CXCR4 and CCR5 cell-surface receptors it expresses on its surface to either become nonfunctional or remove these cell-surface receptors from the surface of its outer membrane will result in noninfected T-Helper cells being impervious to infection by the Human Immunodeficiency Virus. Further, modifying the Human Immunodeficiency Virus to carry a biologic instruction code to cause infected T-Helper cells to make the FasL cell-surface receptors it carries to become nonfunctional or cause the FasL cell-surface receptors to be removed from the surface will prevent infected T-Helper cells from triggering apoptosis in noninfected T-Helper cells, which will prevent AIDS from occurring.

[0046] Viruses or virus-like structures can be fashioned to act as transport vehicles to carry and deliver medically therapeutic genetic material, representing a quantity of either RNA segments or DNA segments, directly to specific precursor T-Helper cells or mature T-Helper cells.

[0047] Naturally occurring viruses can be altered by replacing the genetic material the virus would carry, with medically therapeutic RNA genome molecules that would have a medically beneficial therapeutic effect on precursor T-Helper cells and on mature T-Helper cells.

[0048] Naturally occurring viruses can be further modified to have their naturally occurring glycoprotein surface probes replaced by glycoprotein surface probes that target specific cells in the body. Viruses modified to carry and deliver medically therapeutic RNA genome molecules as the payload, further modified to have their glycoprotein surface probes, that cause the modified virus to engage specific precursor T-Helper cells or mature T-Helper cells in the body, provides a method whereby specific cells in the body can be targeted and cell-surface receptors that appear or would appear on the surface of mature T-Helper cells are altered to produce a medically therapeutic result.

[0049] Virus-like structures can be constructed with similar physical characteristics to naturally occurring viruses and be fashioned to carry medically therapeutic RNA molecules as their payload and have located on the surface glycoprotein probes that engage precursor T-Helper cells or mature T-Helper cells in the body. Viruses-like structures carrying medically therapeutic drug molecules as their payload, constructed to have their glycoprotein surface probes engage specific cells in the body, and deliver to those specific cells the drug the virus-like structures carry provides a device whereby specific cells in the body can be targeted and this device embodies a means of providing to a specific type of cell in the body a drug to participate in chemical reactions with the intent to accomplish a medically therapeutic outcome. The advantage of a virus-like structure is that the physical dimensions of the virus-like structure can be adjusted to accommodate variations in the physical size of the payload, yet maintain a means of engaging targeted cells in the body and delivering to those targeted cells the medically therapeutic RNA genome molecules required to accomplish the desired medical therapeutic outcome. A second advantage of utilizing virus-like structures is to be able to change the surface characteristics of the transport vehicle to prevent the body's immune system from reacting to the presence of the therapeutic modified virus and destroying the modified virus before it is able to deliver the payload it carries to the cells it has been designed to target. HIV utilizes an exterior envelope comprised of the surface membrane of its host, the T-Helper cell, which acts as a disguise to fool the body's immune system detection resources. Virus-like structures could be fashioned, similar to HIV, to have as an exterior envelope a surface that resembles a cell's outer membrane in order to avoid detection by the body's immune system to improve survivability and functionality of the virus-like structure.

[0050] Replicating viruses and constructing viruses to carry DNA payloads is a form of manufacturing technology that has already been well established and is in use facilitating the concept of gene therapy. Replicating viruses and designing these viruses to carry drug as the genetic payload would incorporate similar techniques as already proven useful in current DNA gene therapy technologies.

[0051] To carry out the process to manufacture a modified medically therapeutic Human Immunodeficiency Virus virions, DNA or RNA that would code for the general physical structures of the Human Immunodeficiency Virus virion would be inserted into a host. The host may include devices such as a host cell or a hybrid host cell. The host may utilize DNA or RNA or a combination of genetic instructions in order to accomplish the construction of medically therapeutic virus virions. The DNA or messenger RNA molecules to create the medically therapeutic virus virions would direct the cells to generate copies of the medically therapeutic Human Immunodeficiency Virus virions carrying a medically therapeutic drug payload. In some cases DNA or messenger RNA would be inserted into the host that would be coded to cause the production of surface probes that would be affixed to the surface of the Human Immunodeficiency Virus virions that would target the surface receptors on specific cells in the body other than the T-Helper cells the Human Immunodeficiency Virus virions naturally targets. DNA or messenger RNA would direct the host to generate copies of the medically therapeutic RNA genome molecules that would provide a therapeutic action; these medically therapeutic RNA genome molecules would take the place of the Human Immunodeficiency Virus's innate genome as its payload. The medical treatment form of the Human Immunodeficiency Virus carrying medically therapeutic RNA genome molecules would be produced, assembled and released from a host. Virus-like structures would be generated in similar fashion using a host such as host-cells or hybrid host cells. The copies of the medically therapeutic Human Immunodeficiency Virus virions or virus-like structures, upon exiting the host, would be collected, stored and utilized as a medical treatment as necessary.

[0052] A method of preventing and treating AIDS could be to take the naturally occurring Human Immunodeficiency Virus (HIV) which is an RNA virus and replace HIV's innate genome with a quantity of medially therapeutic RNA molecules. Utilizing modified virus virions to insert medically therapeutic RNA genome molecules into precursor T-Helper cells or mature T-Helper cells, the instruction code carried in the RNA genome that will alter cell-surface genes in the precursor T-Helper cells or cause existing cell-surface receptors to become nonfunctional in mature T-Helper cells would prevent HIV from being able to infect a patient's T-Helper cell population and thus stop AIDS from occurring or progressing in a patient.

[0053] The modified Human Immunodeficiency Virus virions and virus-like structures would be incapable of replication on their own due to the fact that the messenger RNA that would code for the replication process to produce copies of the virus or virus-like structure would not be present in the modified form of the Human Immunodeficiency Virus virions or virus-like structure.

[0054] The described medical method includes a quantity of modified Human Immunodeficiency Virus virions or modified viruses or virus-like structures introduced into a patient's blood stream or tissues so that the modified virus or virus-like structure could deliver the medially therapeutic RNA genome payload that it carries to precursor T-Helper cells or mature T-Helper cells in the body. By utilizing the described method to provide the precursor T-Helper cells of the body with a modified genome to create an altered CXCR4 and CCR5 cell-surface receptors to be expressed on mature T-Helper cells prevents infection by HIV and prevents progression to AIDS.

CLAIMS: Reserved.

APPENDIX B:
Patent Applications to Cure Diabetes, Eliminate Obesity and Fatigue, and Halt Aging

B1: ADAPTABLE MESSENGER RIBONUCLEIC ACID MEDICAL TREATMENT DEVICE TO MANAGE DIABETES MELLITUS

INDIVIDUALS REQUESTING PATENT: Dr. Lane B. Scheiber, ScD and Dr. Lane B. Scheiber II, MD

NUMBER OF CLAIMS: 20

ABSTRACT

Diabetes mellitus is a disease of elevated blood glucose, often directly related to a deficiency in insulin production or insulin receptor production. The innovative strategy of treatment described here utilizes modified viruses to act as a transport vehicle to deliver to target cells in the body, messenger RNA molecules. Delivering to the beta cells in the body the messenger RNA molecules needed to construct insulin or insulin receptors will lead to enhanced production of biologically active insulin or insulin receptors by beta cells as necessary, which will lead to correcting deficiencies in insulin or insulin receptors the result of which will help properly regulate blood glucose levels throughout the body utilizing innate regulatory mechanisms.

BACKGROUND OF THE INVENTION

Field of the Invention

This invention relates to any medical device intended to correct a protein deficiency in the body by increasing the intracellular production of the deficient protein by utilizing a modified virus to insert one or more messenger ribonucleic acid molecules into one or more cells of the body.

DESCRIPTION OF BACKGROUND ART

[0001]   Diabetes mellitus represents an important health issue that affects a significant portion of the world population. In the United States, about 16 million people suffer from diabetes mellitus. Every year, about 650,000 additional people are diagnosed with the disease. Diabetes mellitus is the seventh leading cause of all deaths.

[0002]   Diabetes mellitus represents a state of hyperglycemia, a serum blood sugar that is higher than what is considered the normal range for humans. Glucose, a six-carbon molecule, is a form of sugar. Glucose is absorbed by the cells of the body and converted to energy by the processes of glycolysis, the Krebs cycle and phosphorylation. Insulin, a protein, facilitates the absorption of glucose into cells. Normal range for blood sugar in humans is generally defined as a fasting blood plasma glucose level of between 70 to 110 mg/dl. For descriptive purposes, the term 'plasma' refers to the fluid portion of blood. Diabetes mellitus is classified as Type One and Type Two. Type One diabetes mellitus is insulin dependent, which refers to the condition where there is a lack of sufficient insulin circulating in the blood stream and insulin must be provided to the body in order to properly regulate the blood glucose level. When insulin is required to regulate blood glucose level in the body, this condition is often referred to as insulin dependent diabetes mellitus (IDDM). Type Two diabetes mellitus is noninsulin dependent, often referred to as noninsulin dependent diabetes mellitus (NIDDM), meaning the blood glucose level can be managed without insulin, but by means of diet, exercise or intervention with oral medications. Type Two diabetes mellitus is considered a progressive disease, the underlying pathogenic mechanisms including pancreatic beta cell (also often designated as β-Cell) dysfunction and insulin resistance.

[0003] The pancreas serves as an endocrine gland and an exocrine gland. Functioning as an endocrine gland the pancreas produces and secretes hormones including insulin and glucagon. Insulin acts to reduce levels of glucose circulating in the blood. Beta cells secrete insulin into the blood when a higher than normal level of glucose is detected in the serum. For purposes of this description the terms 'blood', 'blood stream' and 'serum' refer to the same substance. Glucagon acts to stimulate an increase in glucose circulating in the blood. Beta cells in the pancreas secrete glucagon when a low level of glucose is detected in the serum.

[0004] Glucose enters the body and then the blood stream as a result of the digestion of food. The beta cells of the Islets of Langerhans continuously sense the level of glucose in the blood and respond to elevated levels of blood glucose by secreting insulin into the blood. Beta cells produce the protein 'insulin' in the endoplasmic reticulum and store the insulin in vacuoles until it is needed. When beta cells detect an increase in the glucose level in the blood, beta cells release insulin into the blood from the said storage vacuoles.

[0005] Insulin is a protein. An insulin protein consists of two chains of amino acids, an alpha chain and a beta chain, linked by two disulfide (S-S) bridges. The alpha chain consists of 21 amino acids. The beta chain consists of 30 amino acids.

[0006] Insulin interacts with the cells of the body by means of a cell-surface receptor termed the 'insulin receptor' located on the exterior of a cell's 'outer membrane', otherwise known as the 'plasma membrane'. Insulin interacts with muscle and liver cells by means of the insulin receptor to rapidly remove excess blood sugar when the glucose level in the blood is higher than the upper limit of the normal physiologic range. Recognized functions of insulin include stimulating cells to take up glucose from the blood and convert it to glycogen to facilitate the cells in the body to utilize glucose to generate biochemically usable energy, and to stimulate fat cells to take up glucose and synthesize fat.

[0007] Diabetes Mellitus may be the result of one or more factors. Causes of diabetes mellitus may include: (1) mutation of the insulin gene itself causing miscoding, which results in the production of ineffective insulin molecules; (2) mutations to genes that code for the 'transcription factors' needed for transcription of the insulin gene in the DNA to create messenger RNAs which facilitates the manufacture of the insulin molecule; (3) mutations of the gene encoding for the insulin receptor, which produces inactive or an insufficient number of insulin receptors; (4) mutation to the gene encoding for glucokinase, the enzyme that phosphorylates glucose in the first step of glycolysis; (5) mutations to the genes encoding portions of the potassium channels in the plasma membrane of the beta cells, preventing proper closure of the channel, thus blocking insulin release; (6) mutations to mitochondrial genes that as a result, decreases the energy available to be used facilitate the release of insulin, therefore reducing insulin secretion; (7) failure of glucose transporters to properly permit the facilitated diffusion of glucose from plasma into the cells of the body.

[0008] A eukaryote refers to a nucleated cell. Eukaryotes comprise nearly all animal and plant cells. A human eukaryote or nucleated cell is comprised of an exterior lipid bilayer plasma membrane, cytoplasm, a nucleus, and organelles. The exterior plasma membrane defines the perimeter of the cell, regulates the flow of nutrients, water and regulating molecules in and out of the cell, and has embedded into its structure receptors that the cell uses to detect properties of the environment surrounding the cell membrane. The cytoplasm acts as a filling medium inside the boundaries of the plasma cell membrane and is comprised mainly of water and nutrients such as amino acids, oxygen, and glucose. The nucleus, organelles, and ribosomes are suspended in the cytoplasm. The nucleus contains the majority of the cell's genetic information in the form of double stranded deoxyribonucleic acid (DNA). Organelles generally carry out specialized functions for the cell and include such structures as the mitochondria, the endoplasmic reticulum, storage vacuoles, lysosomes and Golgi complex. Floating in the cytoplasm, but also located in the endoplasmic reticulum and mitochondria are ribosomes. Ribosomes are protein structures comprised of several strands of proteins that combine and couple to a messenger ribonucleic acid (mRNA) molecule. More than one ribosome may be attached to a single mRNA at a time. Ribosomes decode genetic information in a mRNA molecule and manufacture proteins to the specifications of the instruction code physically present in the mRNA molecule.

[0009] The majority of the deoxyribonucleic acid (DNA) comprises the chromosomes, double stranded helical structures located in the nucleus of the cell. DNA in a circular form, can also be found in the mitochondria, the powerhouse of the cell, an organelle that assists in converting glucose into usable energy molecules. DNA represents the genetic information a cell needs to manufacture the materials it requires to sustain life and to replicate. Genetic information is stored in the DNA by arrangements of four nucleotides referred to as: adenine, thymine, guanine and cytosine. DNA represents instruction coding, that in the process known as transcription, the DNA's genetic information is decoded by transcription protein complexes referred to as polymerases, to produce ribonucleic acid (RNA). RNA is a single strand of genetic information comprised of coded arrangements of four nucleotides: adenine, uracil, guanine and cytosine. Some types of RNAs are classified as messenger RNAs (mRNA), transport RNAs (tRNA) and ribosomal RNAs (rRNA).

[0010] Proteins are comprised of a series of amino acids bonded together in a linear strand, sometimes referred to as a chain; a protein may be further modified to be a structure comprised of one or more similar or differing strands of amino acids bonded together. Insulin is a protein structure comprised of two strands of amino acids, one strand comprised of 21 amino acids long and the second strand comprised of 30 amino acids, the two strands attached by two disulfide bridges. There are an estimated 30,000 different proteins the cells of the human body may manufacture. The human body is comprised of a wide variety of cells, many with specialized functions requiring unique combinations of proteins and protein structures such as glycoproteins (a protein combined with a carbohydrate) to accomplish the required task or tasks a specialized cell is designed to perform. Forms of glycoproteins are known to be utilized as cell-surface receptors. Messenger RNAs (mRNA) are created by transcription of DNA, they exit the nucleus of the cell, and are utilized as protein manufacturing templates by ribosomes. A ribosome is a protein complex that manufactures proteins by deciphering the instruction code located in a mRNA molecule. When a specific protein is needed, pieces of the ribosome complex bind around the strand of a mRNA that carries the specific instruction code that will generate the required protein. The ribosome traverses the mRNA strand and deciphers the genetic information coded into the sequence of nucleotides that comprise the mRNA molecule.

[0011] Transport RNAs (tRNA) are constructed in the nucleus or in the mitochondria, and are coded for one of the 20 amino acids the cells of the human body use to construct proteins. Once a tRNA is created by transcription of the DNA, the tRNA seeks out the type of amino acid it has been coded for and attaches to that specific amino acid. The tRNA then delivers the amino acid it carries to a ribosome that is waiting for that specific amino acid. Proteins are manufactured by the ribosomes binding together sequences of amino acids. The order by which the amino acids are bonded together is dictated by the way the mRNA is constructed and how the ribosome interprets the information encoded in the string of nucleotides present in the mRNA strand.

[0012] A sequence of three nucleotides present in a mRNA molecule represents a unit of information referred to as a codon. Codons code for all of the 20 amino acids used to construct protein molecules and also for START and STOP commands. In the process known as translation, the ribosome decodes the codons present in the mRNA, initiating the protein manufacturing process at a START codon, then interfacing with tRNAs carrying the amino acids that match the sequence of codons in the mRNA as the ribosome traverses the length of the mRNA molecule. The ribosome functions as a protein factory by taking amino acids delivered by tRNAs and binding the amino acids together in the order dictated by the sequence of codon instructions coded into the mRNA template as directed by the manner of the nucleic acid arrangement in the mRNA molecule. Protein synthesis ceases when a ribosome encounters a STOP code. The protein molecule is released by the ribosome.

[0013] The insulin molecule is a protein produced by beta cells located in the pancreas. The 'insulin messenger RNA' is created in a cell by transcribing the insulin gene from nuclear DNA in the nucleus of the cell. The native messenger RNA (mRNA) for insulin then travels to the endoplasmic reticulum, where numerous ribosomes engage these mRNA molecules. Many ribosomes may be attached to a single strand of mRNA simultaneously, each generating an identical copy of the protein as dictated by the information encoded in the mRNA. Insulin is produced by ribosomes translating the information in a mRNA molecule coded for the insulin protein, which produce strands of amino acids that are coded for an immature form of the biologically active insulin molecule referred to as 'pro-insulin'. Once the pro-insulin molecule is generated it then undergoes modification by several enzymes including prohormone convertase one (PC1), prohormone convertase two (PC2) and carboxypeptidase E, which results in the production of a biologically active insulin molecule. Once the biologically active insulin protein is generated it is stored in a vacuole in the beta cell to await being released into the blood stream.

[0014] The insulin receptor, prohormone convertase one (PC1), prohormone convertase two (PC2) and carboxypeptidase E are produced in a similar fashion as to how pro-insulin and insulin are produced in a beta cell. A messenger RNA is transcribed from DNA, specific for either the insulin receptor, prohormone convertase one (PC1), prohormone convertase two (PC2) or carboxypeptidase E. When a messenger RNA coded for an insulin receptor is present and available, ribosomes will attach to the mRNA and generate insulin receptor proteins. When a messenger RNA coded for either prohormone convertase one (PC1), prohormone convertase two (PC2) or carboxypeptidase E is present and available, ribosomes will attach to the mRNA, decode the instructions in the mRNA molecule and generate the protein.

[0015] Insulin receptors, which appear on the surface of cells, offer binding sites for insulin circulating in the blood. When insulin binds to an insulin receptor, the biologic response inside the cell causes glucose to undergo processing in the cytoplasm. Processed glucose molecules then enter the mitochondria. The mitochondria further process the modified glucose molecules to produce usable energy in the form of adenosine triphosphate molecules (ATP). Thirty-eight ATP molecules may be generated from one molecule of glucose during the process of aerobic respiration. ATP molecules are utilized as an energy source by biologic processes throughout the cell.

[0016] The current medical therapeutic approach to the management of diabetes mellitus has produced limited results. Patients with diabetes generally struggle with an inadequate production of insulin, or an ineffective release of biologically active insulin molecules, or a release of an insufficient number of biologically active insulin molecules, or an insufficient production of cell-surface receptors, or a production of ineffective cell-surface receptors, or a production of ineffective insulin molecules that are unable to interact properly with insulin receptors to produce the required biologic effect. Type One diabetes requires administration of exogenous insulin. The traditional approach to Type Two diabetes has generally first been to adjust the diet to limit the caloric intake the individual consumes. Exercise is used as an initial approach to both Type One and Type Two diabetes as a means of up-regulating the utilization of fats and sugar so as to reduce the amount of circulating plasma glucose. When diet and exercise are inadequate in properly managing Type Two diabetes, oral medications are often introduced. The action of sulfonylureas, a commonly prescribed class of oral medication, is to stimulate the beta cells to produce additional insulin receptors and enhance the insulin receptors' response to insulin. Biguanides, another form of oral treatment, inhibit gluconeogenesis, the production of glucose in the liver, thereby attempting to reduce plasma glucose levels. Thiazolidinediones (TZDs) lower blood sugar levels by activating peroxisome proliferator-activated receptor gamma (PPAR-γ), a transcription factor, which when activated regulates the activity of various target genes, particularly ones involved in glucose and lipid metabolism. If diet, exercise and oral medications do not produce a satisfactory control of the level of blood glucose in a diabetic patient, exogenous insulin is injected into the body in an effort to normalize the amount of glucose present in the serum. Insulin, a protein, has not successfully been made available as an oral medication to date due to the fact that proteins in general become degraded when they encounter the acid environment present in the stomach.

[0017] Despite strict monitoring of blood glucose and potentially multiple doses of insulin injected throughout the day, many patients with diabetes mellitus still experience devastating adverse effects from elevated blood glucose levels. Microvascular damage and elevated tissue sugar levels contribute to such complications as renal failure, retinopathy involving the eyes, neuropathy, and accelerated heart disease despite aggressive efforts to maintain the blood sugar within the physiologic normal range using exogenous insulin by itself or a combination of exogenous insulin and one or more oral medications. Diabetes remains the number one cause of renal failure in this country. Especially in diabetic patients that are dependent upon administering exogenous insulin into their body, though dosing of the insulin may be four or more times a day and even though this may produce adequate control of the blood glucose level to prevent the clinical symptoms of hyperglycemia; this does not unerringly supplement the body's natural capacity to monitor the blood sugar level minute to minute, twenty-four hours a day, and deliver an immediate response to a rise in blood glucose by the release of insulin from beta cells as required. The deleterious effects of diabetes may still evolve despite strict and persistent control of the glucose level in the blood stream.

[0018] The current treatment of diabetes may be augmented by the unique approach to utilizing modified viruses as vehicles to transport biologically active messenger ribonucleic acids (mRNA) coded to facilitate the manufacture of pro-insulin and insulin and the enzymes utilized to modify proinsulin to the biologically active insulin molecule and messenger ribonucleic acids (mRNA) coded to manufacture insulin receptors.

[0019] Viruses are obligate parasites. Viruses simply represent a carrier of genetic material and by themselves viruses are unable to replicate or carry on any form of biologic function outside their host cell. Viruses are generally comprised of one or more shells constructed of one or more layers of protein or lipid material, a genetic payload that represents the instruction code necessary to replicate the virus, and protein enzymes to help facilitate the genetic payload in the function of replicating copies of the virus once the genetic payload has been delivered to a host cell. Located on the outer shell or envelope of a virus are probes. The function of a virus's probes is to locate and engage a host cell's receptors. The virus's surface probes are designed to detect, make contact with and functionally engage one or more receptors located on the exterior of a cell type that will offer the virus the proper environment in which to construct copies of itself. A host cell provides the virus the proper biochemical machinery for the virus to successfully replicate itself.

[0020] Protected by the outer coat or envelope, viruses carry a genetic payload in the form of deoxyribonucleic acid (DNA) or ribonucleic acid (RNA). Once a virus's exterior probes locate and functionally engage the surface receptor or receptors on a host cell, the virus inserts its genetic payload into the interior of the host cell. In the event a virus is carrying a DNA payload, the virus's DNA travels to the host cell's nucleus and is known to become inserted into the host cell's own native DNA. In the case where a virus is carrying its genetic payload as RNA, the virus inserts the RNA payload into the host cell and may also insert one or more enzymes to facilitate the RNA being utilized properly to replicate copies of the virus. Once inside the host cell, some species of virus facilitate their RNA being converted to DNA. Once the viral RNA has been converted to DNA, the virus's DNA travels to the host cell's nucleus and is known to become inserted into the host cell's native DNA. Once a virus's genetic material has been inserted into the host cell's native DNA, the virus's genetic material takes command of certain cell functions and redirects the resources of the host cell to generate copies of the virus. Other forms of RNA viruses bypass the need to use the nuclear DNA and simply utilize portions of the viral genome to act as mRNA. RNA viruses that bypass the host cell's DNA, cause the cell to in general generate copies of the necessary parts of the virus directly from the virus's RNA genome.

[0021] The Hepatitis C virus (HCV) is a positive sense RNA virus, meaning a type of RNA that is capable of bypassing the need for involving the host cell's nucleus by having its RNA genome function as messenger RNA. Hepatitis C infects liver cells. The Hepatitis C genome becomes divided once it gains access to the interior of a liver host cell. Portions of the subdivisions of the Hepatitis C genome directly interact with ribosomes to produce proteins necessary to construct copies of the virus.

[0022] HCV belongs to the Flaviviridae family and is the only member of the Hepacivirus genus. There are considered to be at least 100 different strains of Hepatitis C virus based on genome sequencing variability.

[0023] HCV is comprised of an outer lipoprotein envelope and an internal nucleocapsid. The genetic payload is carried within the nucleocapsid. In its natural state, present on the surface of the outer envelope of the Hepatitis C virus are probes that detect receptors present on the surface of liver cells. The glycoprotein E1 probe and the glycoprotein E2 probe have been identified to be affixed to the surface of HCV. The E2 probe binds with high affinity to the large external loop of a CD81 cell-surface receptor. CD81 is found on the surface of many cell types including liver cells. Once the E2 probe has engaged the CD81 cell-surface receptor, cofactors on the surface of HCV's exterior envelope engage either or both the low density lipoprotein receptor (LDLR) or the scavenger receptor class B type I (SR-BI) present on the liver cell in order to effect the mechanism to facilitate HCV breaching the cell membrane and inserting its RNA genome payload through the plasma cell membrane of the liver cell into the liver cell. Upon successful engagement of the HCV surface probes with a liver cell's cell-surface receptors, HCV inserts the single strand of RNA and other payload elements it carries into the liver cell targeted to be a host cell. The HCV RNA genome then interacts with enzymes and ribosomes inside the liver cell in a translational process to produce the proteins required to construct copies of the protein components of HCV. The HCV genome undergoes a method of transcription to replicate copies of the virus's RNA genome. Inside the host, pieces of the HCV virus are assembled together and ultimately loaded with a copy of the HCV genome. Replicas of the original HCV then escape the host cell and migrate the environment in search of additional host liver cells to infect and continue the replication process.

[0024] The HCV's naturally occurring genetic payload consists of a single molecule of linear positive sense, single stranded RNA approximately 9600 nucleotides in length. By means of a translational process a polyprotein of approximately 3000 amino acids is generated. This polyprotein is cleaved post translation by host and viral proteases into individual viral proteins which include: the structural proteins of C, E1, E2, the nonstructural proteins NS1, NS2, NS3, NS4A, NS4B, NS5A, NS5B, p7 and ARFP/F protein. Hepatitis C virus's proteins direct the host liver cell to construction copies of the Hepatitis C virus. A membrane associated replicase complex consisting of the virus's nonstructural proteins NS3 and NS5B facilitate the replication of the viral genome. The membrane of the endoplasmic reticulum appears to be the site of protein maturation and viral assembly. Once copies of the Hepatitis C Virus are generated, they exit the host cell and each copy of

HCV migrates in search of another appropriate liver cell that will act as a host to continue the replication process.

[0025] Hepatitis C virus offers a naturally occurring vehicle mechanism to transport and insert medically therapeutic messenger ribonucleic acid (mRNA) molecules into specific targeted cells of the human body. The surface probes present on the Hepatitis C virus's outer protein coat can be modified to seek out specific receptors on specific target cells. Once the modified Hepatitis C virus's probes properly engage the cell-surface receptors on a target cell, the modified Hepatitis C virus would insert into the target cell one or more medically therapeutic mRNAs for the purpose of having the target cell generate proteins to achieve a medical therapeutic response.

[0026] Current state of gene therapy generally refers to efforts directed toward inserting an exogenous subunit of DNA into a vehicle such as a virus. The vehicle is intended to insert the exogenous subunit of DNA into a target cell. The exogenous DNA subunit then migrates to the target cell's nucleus. The exogenous DNA subunit then inserts into the native DNA of the cell. This represents a permanent alteration of the cell's nuclear DNA. The nuclear transcription proteins then read the exogenous DNA subunit's nucleotide coding to produce the intended cellular response. The approach described hereunder involves RNA versus DNA. DNA is comprised of the nucleotides adenine, thymine, guanine and cytosine. RNA is composed of the nucleotides adenine, uracil, guanine and cytosine. DNA codes for the manufacture of RNAs, which are composed of nucleotides. RNA codes for the manufacture of proteins, which are composed of amino acids. The virus chosen as the transport vehicle, Hepatitis C virus, is a RNA virus versus a virus that naturally carries a DNA genome.

[0027] Beta cells located in the Islets of Langerhans in the pancreas are thought to have at least one unique identifying surface receptor. The exterior receptor GPR40 appears specific to beta cells located in the Islets of Langerhans in the pancreas. A virus equipped with a surface probe designed to engage the GPR40 beta cell receptor, could travel the blood stream of the body until it locates a GPR40 receptor on a beta cell, engage the receptor with its surface probe, and then insert the genetic payload it carries into the beta cell. A genetic payload such as one or more messenger RNAs could be used to enhance proper protein production by cells deficient in a particular protein. Hormones are proteins that circulate the body and stimulate biologic activity specific to the hormone's role. In the case of a deficiency of a hormone, production of a deficient hormone could be enhanced by inserting one or more messenger RNAs into specific target cells in the body to stimulate production of the required hormone. In the case of diabetes mellitus, utilizing a modified Hepatitis C virus as a vehicle, messenger RNA molecules could be inserted into beta cells, coded for any protein the individual's beta cells are deficient in producing, with the intention of generating an adequate insulin production and adequate release of insulin into the blood to meet the body's needs.

[0028] The utilization of positive sense messenger RNA, does not permanently alter the cell's DNA. Messenger RNAs degrade and become unusable after a time. Use of RNA as a therapeutic modality offers a therapeutic opportunity that could have a reversible or an attenuatable effect when required. Messenger RNA also bypasses the action of decoding the DNA and errors or deficiencies that might occur during transcription. By employing a medically therapeutic virus to carry messenger RNA to cells, deficiencies of any of the approximately 30,000 proteins that comprise the tissues that exist in the body and on the surface of the body can be successfully treated or averted.

BRIEF SUMMARY OF THE INVENTION

[0029] A modified virus is used as a transport medium to carry a payload of one or more messenger ribonucleic acid (RNA) molecules. The modified virus makes contact with a target beta cell located in the Islets of Langerhans in the pancreas by means of the modified virus's exterior probes including one or more probes meant to engage GPR40 exterior cell-surface receptors on a beta cell. Once the virus's exterior probes engage the target cell's receptors, the modified virus inserts into the target cell one or more messenger ribonucleic acid (mRNA) molecules it is carrying. Messenger RNA molecules inserted into the cell act as native messenger RNA molecules and either interact with the cell's ribosomes in the process of protein synthesis or interact with the cell's native enzymes and undergo further modification until the delivered messenger RNA molecule is capable of interacting with the cell's ribosomes in the process of protein synthesis. Medical disease states such as diabetes mellitus that are the result of a deficiency of one or more proteins can be successfully treated by utilizing viruses to insert the proper messenger RNA molecules, into specific cells to enhance the production of proteins that are identified as being deficient, thus correcting the deficiency. The deficiency of insulin production is a prime example of a medical condition that is capable of being corrected by modifying a virus to transport messenger RNA molecules coded for the pro-insulin molecule, the insulin molecule, the insulin receptor molecule, prohormone convertase one (PC1), prohormone convertase two (PC2), and/or carboxypeptidase E, delivering such messenger RNAs to beta cells for the purpose of enhancing the beta cells' production of the insulin molecule and/or the insulin receptor.

DETAILED DESCRIPTION

[0030] Diabetes mellitus is a medical condition often recognized when an individual's fasting blood glucose level is persistently higher than the generally accepted normal range

314

of 60-110 mg/dl. An elevated blood glucose level may occur as the result of a lack of sufficient insulin; a lack of sufficient biologically effective insulin; a deficiency of the number of insulin receptors available to interact with insulin; a deficiency in the number of biologically active insulin receptors available to properly interact with insulin; insufficient release of insulin into the blood stream.

[0031] Insulin, a protein, is generated in beta cells located in the Islets of Langerhans in the pancreas. Insulin is produced by decoding DNA through a process called transcription. Initially, transcription of the DNA produces a messenger ribonucleic acid (mRNA) molecule coded for the pro-insulin molecule. This mRNA coded for the 'pro-insulin' molecule, is then decoded by one or more ribosomes through a process called translation to produce a chain of amino acids that is referred to as the 'pro-insulin' molecule. The 'pro-insulin' molecule is modified by enzymes to produce the biologically active 'insulin' protein. Insulin molecules are stored in vacuoles in the beta cells of the pancreas. Insulin is released from storage vacuoles in response to a rise in the level of glucose in the blood. Other proteins are manufactured in a similar fashion as pro-insulin and insulin.

[0032] Errors in the DNA or errors that occur in the process that generates the messenger RNA or a deficiency in the number of messenger RNA or a deficiency in the number of biologically active messenger RNA results in a deficiency of, or errors in the 'pro-insulin' molecule. Deficiencies in the biologically active enzymes intended to modify the 'pro-insulin' molecule to produce the biologically active insulin protein may result in deficiencies in adequate insulin production.

[0033] Correcting deficiencies or errors associated with the production of the protein insulin would correct diabetes mellitus, when diabetes mellitus is related to an insufficient quantity of biologically active insulin.

[0034] The Hepatitis C virus (HCV) is comprised of an outer lipoprotein envelope and an internal nucleocapsid. The virus's genetic payload is carried within the nucleocapsid. The HCV's naturally occurring genetic payload consists of a single molecule of linear positive sense, single stranded RNA approximately 9600 nucleotides in length, which includes: the structural proteins of C, E1, E2, the nonstructural proteins NS1, NS2, NS3, NS4A, NS4B, NS5A, NS5B, p7 and ARFP/F protein. Present on the surface of the outer envelope of the Hepatitis C virus are probes that detect receptors present on the surface of liver cells. The glycoproteins E1 and E2 have been identified to be affixed to the surface of HCV. Portions of the Hepatitis C virus genome, when separated into individual pieces, behave like messenger RNA. Naturally occurring HCV is constructed with surface probes fashioned to recognize a receptor on the surface of a liver cell. Once the naturally occurring HCV's surface probe E2 engages a liver cell's CD81 receptor, and cofactors on the surface of HCV's exterior envelope engage the low density lipoprotein receptor (LDLR) or the scavenger receptor class B type I (SR-BI) on the liver cell, HCV then has the opportunity to insert its RNA genetic payload into the engaged target liver cell.

[0035] Replicating viruses and constructing viruses to carry DNA payloads is a form of manufacturing technology that has already been well established and is in use facilitating gene therapy. Replicating viruses and designing these viruses to carry messenger ribonucleic acid as the genetic payload would incorporate similar techniques as already proven useful in current gene therapy technologies.

[0036] To carry out the process to manufacture a modified medically therapeutic Hepatitis C virus, messenger RNA would be inserted into the host that would code for the general physical outer structures of the Hepatitis C virus. Messenger RNA would be inserted into the host that would generate surface probes that would target the surface receptors on beta cells.

Messenger RNA would be inserted into the host that would generate copies of the messenger RNA that would provide a therapeutic action that would take the place of the Hepatitis C virus's innate genome. Therapeutic messenger RNA that would act as the modified HCV's genome would encode for proteins that would include the pro-insulin molecule, the insulin molecule, the insulin receptor, the enzyme prohormone convertase one, the enzyme prohormone convertase two, the enzyme carboxypeptidase E. Similar to how copies of a naturally occurring Hepatitis C virus is produced, assembled and released from a host cell, copies of the modified medically therapeutic Hepatitis C virus would be produced, assembled and released from a host cell.

[0037] To treat the various different forms of diabetes mellitus various combinations of messenger RNA would be inserted into the host, and the host would produce copies of modified Hepatitis C virus that target beta cells and carry a genetic payload consisting of messenger RNA molecules that would consist of one or more copies of a messenger RNA that codes for the insulin molecule, the insulin receptor, the enzyme prohormone convertase one, the enzyme prohormone convertase two, the enzyme carboxypeptidase E. Depending upon the physical size of the messenger RNAs and the available space inside the modified Hepatitis C virus more than one type of messenger RNA may be packaged into a single modified Hepatitis C virus, which would produce more than one therapeutic action in a cell.

[0038] The modified Hepatitis C virus would be incapable of replication on its own due to the fact that the messenger RNA that a naturally occurring Hepatitis C virus would normally carry would not be present in the modified form of the Hepatitis C virus.

[0039] To treat diabetes, a quantity of modified Hepatitis C virus would be introduced into a patient's blood stream or tissues so that the modified virus could deliver the therapeutic genetic payload that it carries to beta cells in the pancreas. When the probes on the surface of the modified Hepatitis C virus engage a cell-surface receptor or receptors on a beta cell, the modified Hepatitis C virus will insert its therapeutic payload of messenger RNA into the beta cell to enhance the beta cell's biologic function of producing insulin and/or insulin receptors.

[0040] By providing beta cells with the above-mentioned messenger RNAs, the capacity of beta cells to carrying out the biologic processes of producing insulin and recognizing and responding to blood glucose levels is enhanced, which results in an efficient means to control the glucose levels in the blood stream on a constant and persistent basis utilizing innate regulatory mechanisms and thus diabetes mellitus can be effectively treated and the harmful effects of this disease can be averted.

CLAIMS: Reserved.

B2: METHOD FOR TREATING DIABETES MELLITUS, OBE-
SITY, CHRONIC FATIGUE, AGING, AND OTHER MEDICAL
CONDITIONS BY UTILIZING MODIFIED VIRUS VIRIONS TO
INSERT MESSENGER RIBONUCLEIC ACID MOLECULES
INTO CELLS

INDIVIDUALS REQUESTING PATENT: Dr. Lane B. Scheiber,
ScD and Dr. Lane B. Scheiber II, MD

NUMBER OF CLAIMS: 3 independent claims, 17 dependent
claims

ABSTRACT

The common link between diabetes mellitus, obesity, chronic
fatigue and even aging may be related to deficiencies involving
a body's metabolism of glucose and the ability to optimally
conduct the necessary biologic processes of aerobic respiration.
Utilizing a modified form of virus to deliver to cells in the body
the messenger RNA molecules needed to construct insulin
receptors and generate the enzymes that participate in the
processes of glycolysis, the tricarboxylic acid cycle, oxidative
phosphorylation and anaerobic respiration will lead to greater
utilization of blood glucose and a more efficient and sustained
production of the energy molecules that fuel the metabolic
processes of the cell. Greater utilization of blood glucose will
correct problems associated with diabetes, obesity, chronic
fatigue, and aging.

BACKGROUND OF THE INVENTION

Field of the Invention

This invention relates to any medical method intended to correct a protein deficiency in the body by increasing the intracellular production of the deficient protein by utilizing a modified virus to insert messenger ribonucleic acid molecules into cells of the body.

Description of Background Art

[0001] Diabetes and obesity represent two very widespread and extremely important health issues across the United States. Both conditions affect a significant portion of the population and result in significant morbidity and mortality. In the United States, about 16 million people suffer from diabetes mellitus. Every year, about 650,000 additional people are diagnosed with the disease. Diabetes mellitus is the seventh leading cause of all deaths. According to the National Institutes of Health, in the United States, 97 million adults are overweight or obese. About 22.5 percent of the population is obese, up from 13 percent in 1960. Obesity and diabetes mellitus are linked disorders in many patients. Studies show that individuals who are 20 percent or more overweight run a greater risk of developing diabetes mellitus, hypertension, coronary heart disease, stroke, arthritis, and some forms of cancer.

[0002] Chronic fatigue syndrome (CFS) is characterized by extreme fatigue that has persisted in excess of six months. CFS occurs most commonly in people in their 40s and 50s. CFS is estimated to affect one million people in the United States, with estimated tens of millions with similar symptoms of fatigue that do not meet the strict criteria to make a formal diagnosis. CFS results in significant loss of productivity by the individuals affected by this condition, thus having a negative impact on the work-force in general.

[0003] Aging affects the entire scope of the population. The characteristics of aging may be related to a lack of sufficient sustained energy production and therefore a progressive decline in an individual's cellular capacity to sufficiently fuel biologic processes requiring energy. The mitochondria are the powerhouses of the cells, converting sugars such as glucose to energy molecules such as adenosine triphosphate (ATP). A liver cell may contain as many as 2500 mitochondria. If the mitochondria lack a sufficient amount of any of the required enzymes to complete the process of metabolizing glucose to energy molecules such as ATP, necessary biologic functions may not be available to engage in cellular functions as needed. It has been estimated that in a person's lifetime, between the ages of 35 to 50 years old, there occurs a fifty percent decline in the mitochondria's capacity to produce energy. As an individual ages, there is a further decline in mitochondrial output capacity.

[0004] Diabetes mellitus, obesity, chronic fatigue, and aging may all be linked to the vital process of glucose metabolism. Providing the body with the means of maintaining an optimum level of glucose metabolism and aerobic respiration may provide the means to effectively manage the above-mentioned four major health conditions.

[0005] Diabetes mellitus represents a state of hyperglycemia, which is generally defined as a serum blood sugar that is higher than what is considered the normal range for humans. Glucose, a six-carbon molecule, represents a form of sugar. Glucose is absorbed by the cells of the body through passive diffusion and is converted to energy by the biologic processes of glycolysis, the tricarboxylic acid (TCA) cycle and oxidative phosphorylation. Insulin, a protein, facilitates the absorption of glucose into cells. Normal range for blood glucose in humans is generally defined as a fasting blood plasma glucose level of between 70 to 110 mg/dl. An alternative means of measuring the blood glucose level is by measuring the glucose level stored inside red blood cells in the blood, which provides information regarding the average blood glucose spanning several weeks, rather than a real-time blood glucose level represented in a blood plasma glucose level. Measurement of glycated hemoglobin (Hgb A1C) provides an estimate of diabetic control over the preceding three months, with a normal value for nondiabetic patients being approximately 6% and values for a poorly controlled diabetic being 7-12%. For purposes of this description the terms "plasma' and 'serum' refer to the same substance, which is the fluid (noncellular) portion of blood.

[0006] Diabetes mellitus is generally classified as Type One and Type Two. Type One diabetes mellitus is insulin dependent, and refers to the condition where there is an insufficient quantity of insulin molecules circulating in the blood stream compared to the quantity required to maintain the blood glucose level within the recognized normal range. In Type One diabetes mellitus insulin must be provided to the body in order to properly regulate the blood plasma glucose level. When insulin is required to regulate the blood glucose level in the body, this condition is often referred to as insulin dependent diabetes mellitus (IDDM). Type Two diabetes mellitus is not dependent upon insulin and is often referred to as noninsulin dependent diabetes mellitus (NIDDM), meaning the blood glucose level can be managed without treatment with exogenous insulin, and is generally managed by means of diet, exercise or intervention with oral medications. Type Two diabetes mellitus is considered a progressive disease, with the underlying pathogenic mechanisms including pancreatic beta cell (often designated as β-Cell) dysfunction and insulin resistance.

[0007] The pancreas serves as an endocrine gland and an exocrine gland. Functioning as an endocrine gland, the pancreas produces and secretes hormones including the hormones insulin and glucagon. Insulin acts to reduce levels of glucose circulating in the blood. Beta cells secrete insulin into the blood when a higher than normal level of glucose is detected in the serum. Glucagon is an antagonistic hormone to insulin, which acts to stimulate an increase in glucose circulating in the blood. Alpha cells in the pancreas secrete glucagon into the blood when a low level of glucose is detected in the blood.

[0008]   Glucose generally enters the body and then the blood stream as a result of the digestion of food. For purposes of this description, 'blood' and 'blood stream' refer to the same substance, which is generally considered to be blood as a whole including plasma and blood cells. The beta cells of the Islets of Langerhans continuously sense the level of glucose in the blood and respond to elevated levels of blood glucose by secreting insulin into the blood. Beta cells produce the protein 'insulin' in the endoplasmic reticulum and store the insulin in vacuoles until the insulin is needed. When beta cells detect an increase in the glucose level in the blood, the beta cells release insulin into the blood plasma from said storage vacuoles.

[0009]   Insulin is a protein. An insulin molecule consists of two chains of amino acids, an alpha chain and a beta chain, linked by two disulfide (S-S) bridges. The alpha chain consists of 21 amino acids. The beta chain consists of 30 amino acids.

[0010]   Insulin interacts with the cells of the body by means of a cell-surface receptor termed the 'insulin receptor' located on the exterior of a cell's 'outer membrane', otherwise known as the 'plasma membrane'. Insulin interacts with muscle and liver cells by means of the insulin receptor to rapidly remove excess blood sugar when the glucose level in the blood is higher than the upper limit of the normal physiologic range. Recognized functions of insulin include stimulating cells to take up glucose from the blood, convert glucose to glycogen (an extensively branched glucose storage polysaccharide molecule), to facilitate the cells in the body to utilize glucose to generate biochemically usable energy, and to stimulate fat cells to take up glucose and synthesize fat.

[0011] Diabetes Mellitus may develop in an individual as the result of one or more factors. Causes of diabetes mellitus may include: (1) mutation of the insulin gene itself causing miscoding, which results in the production of ineffective insulin molecules; (2) mutations to genes that code for the 'transcription factors' needed for transcription of the insulin gene in the DNA to create messenger RNAs which facilitates the manufacture of the insulin molecule; (3) mutations of the gene encoding for the insulin receptor, which produces inactive or an insufficient number of insulin receptors; (4) mutation to the gene encoding for glucokinase, the enzyme that phosphorylates glucose in the first step of glycolysis; (5) mutations to the genes encoding portions of the potassium channels in the plasma membrane of the beta cells, preventing proper closure of the channel, thus blocking insulin release; (6) mutations to mitochondrial genes that as a result, decreases the energy available to be used facilitate the release of insulin, therefore reducing insulin secretion; (7) failure of glucose transporters to properly permit the facilitated diffusion of glucose from plasma into the cells of the body.

[0012] A eukaryote refers to a nucleated cell. Eukaryotes comprise nearly all animal and plant cells. A human eukaryote or nucleated cell is comprised of an exterior lipid bilayer plasma membrane, cytoplasm, a nucleus, and organelles. The exterior plasma membrane defines the perimeter of the cell, regulates the flow of nutrients, water and regulating molecules in and out of the cell, and has embedded into its structure cell-surface receptors that the cell uses to detect properties of the environment surrounding the cell membrane. Cytoplasm refers to the entire contents inside the cell except for the nucleus and acts as a filling medium inside the boundaries of the plasma cell membrane. Cytosol refers to the semifluid portion of the cytoplasm minus the mitochondria and the endoplasmic reticulum. The nucleus, organelles, and ribosomes are suspended in the cytosol. Nutrients such as amino acids, oxygen and glucose are present in the cytosol. The nucleus contains the majority of the cell's genetic information in the form of double stranded deoxyribonucleic acid (DNA). Organelles generally carry out specialized functions for the cell and include such structures as the mitochondria, the endoplasmic reticulum, storage vacuoles, lysosomes and Golgi complex. Floating in the cytoplasm, but also located in the endoplasmic reticulum and mitochondria are ribosomes. Ribosomes are protein structures comprised of several strands of proteins that combine and couple to a messenger ribonucleic acid (mRNA) molecule. More than one ribosome may be attached to a single mRNA at a time. Ribosomes decode genetic information coded in a mRNA molecule and manufacture proteins to the specifications of the instruction code physically present in the mRNA molecule.

[0013] The majority of the deoxyribonucleic acid (DNA) in a cell is present in the form of chromosomes, the double stranded helical structures located in the nucleus of the cell. DNA in a circular form, can also be found in the mitochondria, the powerhouse of the cell, an organelle that assists in converting glucose into usable energy molecules. DNA represents the genetic information a cell needs to manufacture the materials it requires to develop to its mature form, sustain life and to replicate. Genetic information is stored in the DNA by arrangements of four nucleotides referred to as: adenine, thymine, guanine and cytosine. DNA represents instruction coding, that in the process known as transcription, the DNA's genetic information is decoded by transcription protein complexes referred to as polymerases, to produce ribonucleic acid (RNA). RNA is a single strand of genetic information comprised of coded arrangements of four nucleotides: adenine, uracil, guanine and cytosine. The physical difference in the construction of a DNA molecule versus a RNA molecule is that DNA utilizes the nucleotide 'thymine', while RNA molecules utilize the nucleotide 'uracil'. RNAs are generally classified as messenger RNAs (mRNA), transport RNAs (tRNA) and ribosomal RNAs (rRNA).

[0014] Mitochondrion ('mitochondria' pleural) is a cellular organelle that is considered the energy producing organelle of the cell. Mitochondria assist in generating energy for cell metabolism by producing ATP molecules from glucose. Within the cytoplasm and outer wall of the mitochondria sugar molecules undergo the process of glycolysis, and then inside the mitochondria byproducts of glucose are further broken down in the tricarboxylic acid (TCA) cycle and by oxidative phosphorylation to produce useable forms of energy molecules.

[0015] The exterior of a mitochondrion is known as an external membrane. Inside the outer membrane is an inner membrane. Folds in the inner membrane create crista, which expands the surface of the inner membrane and enhances the mitochondrion's ability to create ATP molecules. Inside the inner membrane is the mitochondrion matrix. The mitochondrion matrix contains a highly concentrated mixture of enzymes, ribosomes, tRNA and mitochondrial DNA. Glycolysis occurs in the cytosol of the cell and membrane of the mitochondrion. The tricarboxylic acid cycle functions within the inner chambers and matrix of the mitochondrion. Oxidative phosphorylation occur within the boundaries of the outer and inner membranes of the mitochondrion.

[0016] Many of the intermediates of the processes of glycolysis and the tricarboxylic acid cycle exist as anions at the pH found in cells, and readily associate with H^+ to form acids. The intermediates of glycolysis and the tricarboxylic acid cycle are therefore often written as either an anion or an acid. For the purposes of this description, the intermediates of the processes of glycolysis and the tricarboxylic acid cycle are generally written as anions (as an example pyruvate versus pyruvic acid).

[0017] As a result of the biochemical process of glycolysis during aerobic (oxygen available) respiration conditions glucose is converted to pyruvate. The abbreviated processes of glycolysis include: (1) Glucose is converted to glucose-6-phosphate by the enzyme 'hexokinase'. (2) Glucose-6-phosphate is converted to fructose-6-phosphate by the enzyme 'glucose-6-phosphate isomerase'. (3) Fructose-6-phosphate is converted to fructose 1,6-diphosphate by the enzyme 'phosphofructo kinase'. (4) Fructose 1,6-diphosphate is converted to two different entities including dihydroxyacetone-3-phosphate and glyceraldehydes-3-phosphate by the enzyme 'fructose bisphosphate aldolase'. (5) Dihydroacetone-3-phosphate converts to D-glyceraladehyde-3-phosphate by the enzyme 'triose-phosphate isomerase'. (6) Glyceraldehyde-3-phosphate is converted to 1,3-diphosphoglycerate by the enzyme 'glyceraldehyde-3-phosphate dehydrogenase'. (7) 1,3-diphosphoglycerate is converted to 3-phosphoglycerate by the enzyme 'phosphoglycerate kinase'. (8) 3-phosphoglycerate is converted to 2-phosphoglycerate by the enzyme 'phosphoglycerate mutase'. (9) 2-phosphoglycerate is converted to phosphoenolpyruvate by the enzyme 'enolase'. (10) Phosphoenolpyruvate is converted to pyruvate by the enzyme complex referred to as 'pyruvate kinase'.

[0018] Pyruvate is then oxidized to an acetyl group, which is combined with Coenzyme A and produces acetyl Coenzyme A (acetyl-CoA). Pyruvate dehydrogenase which metabolizes pyruvate to acetyl-CoA is comprised of a multi-enzyme complex. The three protein complexes of pyruvate dehydrogenase are designated E1 (pyruvate dehydrogenase), E2 (dihydrolipoamide S-acetyltransferase), and E3 (dihydrolipoamide dehydrogenase). Acetyl-CoA enters the tricarboxylic acid cycle. Under aerobic respiration conditions from one glucose molecule the process of glycolysis generates 8 ATP molecules, conversion of pyruvate to acetyl CoA generates an additional 6 ATP molecules.

[0019] The tricarboxylic acid cycle otherwise known as the citric acid cycle or the Krebs cycle, was discovered in 1937 by Sir Hans Krebs, and is a biochemical process that provides complete oxidation of acetyl-CoA, which may be derived from sources such as fats, carbohydrates and lipids. For purposes of this discussion, acetyl-CoA is a byproduct of glucose metabolism during glycolysis, and enters the tricarboxylic acid cycle and (1) combines with oxaloacetate (also known as oxaloacetic acid) by the action of the enzyme 'citrate synthetase' which produces citrate (also known as citric acid). (2) Citrate is converted to cis-aconitate per the enzyme 'aconitase'. (3) Cis-aconitate is converted to iso-citrate (also known as isocitur acid) again by the enzyme aconitase. (4) Iso-citrate is converted to alpha-ketoglutarate by the enzyme 'isocitrate dehydrogenase'. (5) Alpha-ketoglutaric acid is converted to succinyl CoA by the enzyme '2-oxoglutarate dehydrogenase'. (6) Succinyl CoA is converted to succinate (also known as succinic acid) by the enzyme 'succinyl-CoA synthetase'. (7) Succinate is converted to fumarate (also known as fumaric acid) by the enzyme 'succinate dehydrogenase'. (8) Fumarate is converted to malate (also known as malic acid) by the enzyme 'fumarate hydratase'. (9) Malate is converted to oxaloacetate by the enzyme 'malate dehydrogenase'. The result of metabolism of glucose by glycolysis and the tricarboxylic acid cycle yields ATP molecules and electron donor molecules such as the reduced form of the coenzyme nicotinamide adenine dinucleotide written NADH +H[+]. The tricarboxylic acid cycle also produces electron donor molecules in the form of the reduced co-enzyme flavin adenine dinucleotide written $FADH_2$.

[0020] Oxidative phosphorylation is a metabolic pathway that uses energy released by oxidation to produce adenosine triphosphate (ATP). During oxidative phosphorylation electrons are transferred from electron donors to electron acceptors such as oxygen in redox reactions. In eukaryotes the redox reactions are carried out by a series of protein complexes located within mitochondria. These protein complexes represent a linked set of enzymes referred to as electron transport chains. The protein complexes utilized in oxidative phosphorylation include nicotinamide adenine dinucleotide (NADH) dehydrogenase enzyme molecule, the succinate dehydrogenase enzyme molecule, the cytochrome-c reductase enzyme molecule, the cytochrome-c oxidase enzyme molecule, and the ATP synthase enzyme molecule. Under aerobic respiration conditions one glucose molecule metabolized by the combination of glycolysis, the tricarboxylic acid cycle and oxidative phosphorylation yields as many as 38 ATP molecules.

[0021] An enzyme is a protein generated by cells that acts as a catalyst to induce chemical changes in other substances, itself remaining apparently unchanged in the process. There are several main groups of enzymes including oxidoreductase, transferase, hydrolase, lyase, isomerase, and ligase, sometimes referred to as synthetase. EC is an abbreviation for Enzyme Commission of the International Union of Biochemistry and this is used in conjunction with a unique number to define a specific enzyme identified in the Enzyme Commission's list of enzymes. Oxidoreductases generally have as their first EC identifying number, the number 1. Transferases generally have as their first EC identifying number, the number 2. Hydrolases generally have as their first EC identifying number, the number 3. Lyases generally have as their first EC identifying number, the number 4. Isomerase generally have as their first EC identifying number, the number 5. Ligases generally have as their first EC identifying number, the number 6. Several scientific names often exist to identify the same enzyme.

[0022] Enzymes utilized in the metabolism of glucose in the processes of glycolysis, tricarboxylic acid cycle, and oxidative phosphorylation include the enzymes in the following paragraphs as described.

[0023] Hexokinase (EC 2.7.1.1), is also referred to as hexokinase type IV glucokinase or in some cases simply glucokinase. Hexokinase converts glucose to glucose-6-phosphate in glycolysis.

[0024] Glucose-6-phosphate isomerase (EC 5.3.1.9), is also known as phosphoglucoisomerase. Glucose-6-phosphate isomerase is an enzyme that converts glucose-6-phosphate to fructose-6-phosphate in glycolysis.

[0025] 6-phosphofructokinase (EC 2.7.1.11), is also known as phosphofructokinase. 6-phosphofructokinase is an enzyme that converts fructose-6-phosphate to fructose 1,6-diphosphate in glycolysis.

[0026] Fructose bisphosphate aldolase (EC 4.1.2.13), is also known as aldolase. Fructose bisphosphate aldolase is an enzyme that converts fructose 1,6-diphosphate to two different entities including dihydroxyacetone 3-phosphate and glyceraldehydes 3-phosphate in glycolysis.

[0027] Triose-phosphate isomerase (EC 5.3.1.1). Triose-phosphate isomerase is an enzyme that converts dihydroacetone-3-phosphate converts to D-glyceraladehyde-3-phosphate.

[0028] Glyceraldehyde-3-phosphate dehydrogenase (EC 1.2.1.12), may be abbreviated GAPDH or G3PDH. Glyceralde-hyde-3-phosphate dehydrogenase is an enzyme that converts glyceraldehydes-3-phosphatate to 1,3-diphosphoglycerate in glycolysis.

[0029] Phosphoglycerate kinase (EC 2.7.2.3). Phosphoglycerate kinase is an enzyme that converts 1,3-diphosphoglycerate to 3-phosphoglycerate in glycolysis.

[0030] Phosphoglycerate mutase (EC 5.4.2.1). Phosphoglyc-erate mutase is an enzyme that converts 3-phosphoglycerate to 2-phosphoglycerate in glycolysis.

[0031] Enolase (EC 4.2.1.11). Enolase is an enzyme that converts 2-phosphoglycerate to phosphoenolpyruvate in glycolysis.

[0032] Pyruvate kinase (EC 2.7.1.40). Pyruvate kinase is an enzyme that converts phosphoenolpyruvate to pyruvate in glycolysis.

[0033] Pyruvate dehydrogenase is comprised of three units. The three units include E1 (EC 1.2.4.1), (EC 1.2.1.51), E2 dihydrolipoamide S-acetyltransferase (EC 2.3.1.12), and E3 dihydrolipoamide dehydrogenase (EC 1.8.1.4). Pyruvate dehydrogenase molecular complex catalyzes the conversion of pyruvate to acetyl-CoA.

[0034] Citrate synthetase (EC 4.1.3.7). Citrate synthetase is an enzyme that converts acetyl-CoA combines with oxaloacetate to produce citrate in the tricarboxylic acid cycle.

[0035] Aconitase (EC 4.2.1.3). Aconitase exists in two isoenzyme forms in eukaryotes: mitochondrial and cytosolic. Aconitase is an enzyme that converts citrate to cis-aconitate in the Tricarboxylic acid cycle and converts cis-aconitate to iso-citrate in the tricarboxylic acid cycle.

[0036] Isocitrate dehydrogenase (EC 1.1.1.41). Isocitrate dehydrogenase is an enzyme that converts isocitrate to alpha-ketoglutaric acid in the tricarboxylic acid cycle.

[0037] 2-oxoglutarate dehydrogenase is a protein complex comprised of three units. The three units include E1 (EC 1.2.4.2), E2 (EC 2.3.1.61), and E3 (EC 1.8.1.4). 2-oxoglutarate dehydrogenase is an enzyme complex that converts alpha-ketoglutaric to succinyl CoA in the tricarboxylic acid cycle.

[0038] Succinyl-CoA synthetase (EC 6.2.1.5). Succinyl-CoA synthetase is an enzyme that converts succinyl CoA to succinate in the tricarboxylic acid cycle.

[0039] Succinate dehydrogenase (EC 1.3.5.1). Succinate dehydrogenase is an enzyme that converts succinate to fumarate in the tricarboxylic acid cycle.

[0040] Fumarate hydratase (EC 4.2.1.2). Fumarate hydratase is an enzyme that converts fumarate to malate in the tricarboxylic acid cycle.

[0041] Malate dehydrogenase (EC 1.1.1.37). Malate dehydrogenase is an enzyme that converts malate to oxaloacetate in the tricarboxylic acid cycle.

[0042] During conditions were sufficient oxygen is available, metabolism of glucose generally occurs through the processes of glycolysis, tricarboxylic acid cycle, and oxidative phosphorylation. When oxygen is not readably available, anaerobic respiration occurs. The enzyme lactate dehydrogenase provides an alternative pathway to produce ATP when sufficient oxygen is not available by converting pyruvate to lactic acid. The anaerobic pathway lactate dehydrogenase catalyzes is much less efficient means of producing energy molecules than the aerobic pathway that takes advantage of oxygen dependent processes of tricarboxylic acid cycle and oxidative phosphorylation.

[0043] Proteins are comprised of a series of amino acids bonded together in a linear strand, sometimes referred to as a chain; a protein may be further modified to be a structure comprised of one or more similar or differing strands of amino acids bonded together. A protein comprised of one or more strands of amino acids (referred to as subunits) may be referred to as a protein complex. Insulin is a protein structure comprised of two strands of amino acids, one strand comprised of 21 amino acids long and the second strand comprised of 30 amino acids; the two strands attached by two disulfide bridges. There are an estimated 30,000 different proteins the cells of the human body may manufacture. The human body is comprised of a wide variety of cells, many with specialized functions requiring unique combinations of proteins and protein structures such as glycoproteins (a protein combined with a carbohydrate) to accomplish the required task or tasks a specialized cell is designed to perform. Forms of glycoproteins are known to be utilized as cell-surface receptors.

[0044]   Messenger RNAs (mRNA) are created by transcription of DNA. Messenger RNA generated by transcription of nuclear DNA, migrate out of the nucleus of the cell, and are utilized as protein manufacturing templates by ribosomes.   Different mRNAs code for different proteins. As previously mentioned, there are as many as 30,000 varieties of proteins, therefore there are at least 30,000 different mRNA molecules. A ribosome is a protein complex that manufactures proteins by deciphering the instruction code located in a mRNA molecule. When a specific protein is needed, pieces of the ribosome complex bind around the strand of mRNA that carries the specific instruction code that will generate the required protein. The ribosome traverses the mRNA strand and deciphers the genetic information coded into the sequence of nucleotides that comprise the mRNA molecule.

[0045]   Transport RNAs (tRNA) are constructed in the nucleus or in the mitochondria, and are coded for one of the 20 amino acids the cells of the human body use to construct proteins. Once a tRNA is created by transcription of the DNA, the tRNA seeks out the type of amino acid it has been coded for and attaches to that specific amino acid. The tRNA then delivers the amino acid it carries to a ribosome that is waiting for that specific amino acid. Proteins are manufactured by the ribosomes binding together sequences of amino acids. The order by which the amino acids are bonded together is dictated by the way the mRNA is constructed and how the ribosome interprets the information encoded in the string of nucleotides present in the mRNA strand.

[0046] A sequence of three nucleotides present in a mRNA molecule represents a unit of information referred to as a codon. Codons code for all of the 20 amino acids used to construct protein molecules and also for START and STOP commands. In the process known as translation, the ribosome decodes the codons present in the mRNA, initiating the protein manufacturing process at a START codon, then interfacing with tRNAs carrying the amino acids that match the sequence of codons in the mRNA as the ribosome traverses the length of the mRNA molecule. The ribosome functions as a protein factory by taking amino acids delivered by tRNAs and binding the amino acids together in the order dictated by the sequence of codon instructions coded into the mRNA template as directed by the manner of the nucleic acid arrangement in the mRNA molecule. Protein synthesis ceases when a ribosome encounters a STOP code. Once complete, the protein molecule is released by the ribosome.

[0047] The insulin molecule is a protein produced by beta cells located in the pancreas. The 'insulin messenger RNA' is created in a cell by transcribing the insulin gene from nuclear DNA in the nucleus of the cell. The native messenger RNA (mRNA) for insulin then travels to the endoplasmic reticulum, where numerous ribosomes engage these mRNA molecules. Many ribosomes may be attached to a single strand of mRNA simultaneously, each generating an identical copy of the protein as dictated by the information encoded in the mRNA. Insulin is produced by ribosomes translating the information in a mRNA molecule coded for the insulin protein, which produce strands of amino acids that are coded for an immature form of the biologically active insulin molecule referred to as 'pro-insulin'. Once the pro-insulin molecule is generated it then undergoes modification by several enzymes including prohormone convertase one (PC1), prohormone convertase two (PC2) and carboxypeptidase E, which results in the production of a biologically active insulin molecule. Once the biologically active insulin protein is generated, it is stored in a vacuole in the beta cell to await being released into the blood stream.

[0048] The insulin receptor, prohormone convertase one (PC1), prohormone convertase two (PC2) and carboxypeptidase E are produced in a similar fashion as to how pro-insulin and insulin are produced in a beta cell. A messenger RNA is transcribed from DNA, specific for either the insulin receptor, prohormone convertase one (PC1), prohormone convertase two (PC2) or carboxypeptidase E. When a messenger RNA coded for an insulin receptor is present and available, ribosomes will attach to the mRNA and generate insulin receptor proteins. When a messenger RNA coded for either prohormone convertase one (PC1), prohormone convertase two (PC2) or carboxypeptidase E is present and available, ribosomes will attach to the mRNA, decode the instructions in the mRNA molecule and generate the protein.

[0049] Insulin receptors, which appear on the surface of cells, offer binding sites for insulin circulating in the blood. When insulin binds to an insulin receptor, the biologic response inside the cell causes glucose to undergo processing in the cytoplasm. Processed glucose molecules then enter the mitochondrion. The mitochondrion further processes the modified glucose molecules to produce usable energy in the form of adenosine triphosphate molecules (ATP). Thirty-eight ATP molecules may be generated from one molecule of glucose during the process of aerobic respiration. ATP molecules are utilized as an energy source by biologic processes throughout the cell.

[0050] The current medical therapeutic approach to the management of diabetes mellitus has produced limited results. Patients with diabetes generally struggle with an inadequate production of insulin, or an ineffective release of biologically active insulin molecules, or a release of an insufficient number of biologically active insulin molecules, or an insufficient production of cell-surface receptors, or a production of ineffective cell-surface receptors, or a production of ineffective insulin molecules that are unable to interact properly with insulin receptors on cells to produce the required biologic effect. Type One diabetes requires administration of exogenous insulin. The traditional approach to Type Two diabetes has generally first been to adjust the diet to limit the caloric intake the individual consumes. Exercise is used as an initial approach to both Type One and Type Two diabetes as a means of up-regulating the utilization of fats and sugar so as to reduce the amount of circulating plasma glucose. When diet and exercise are inadequate in properly managing Type Two diabetes, oral medications are often introduced. The action of sulfonylureas, a commonly prescribed class of oral medication, is to stimulate the beta cells to produce additional insulin receptors and enhance the insulin receptors' response to insulin. Biguanides, another form of oral treatment, inhibit gluconeogenesis, the production of glucose in the liver, thereby attempting to reduce plasma glucose levels. Thiazolidinediones (TZDs) lower blood sugar levels by activating peroxisome proliferator-activated receptor gamma (PPAR-γ), a transcription factor, which when activated regulates the activity of various target genes, particularly ones involved in glucose and lipid metabolism. If diet, exercise and oral medications do not produce a satisfactory control of the level of blood glucose in a diabetic patient, exogenous insulin is injected into the body in an effort to normalize the amount of glucose present in the serum. Insulin, a protein, has not successfully been made available as an oral medication to date due to the fact that proteins in general become degraded when they encounter the acid environment present in the stomach.

[0051] Despite strict monitoring of blood glucose and potentially multiple doses of insulin injected throughout the day sometimes augmented with oral medications, many patients with diabetes mellitus still experience devastating adverse effects from elevated blood glucose levels. Microvascular damage and elevated tissue sugar levels contribute to such complications as renal failure, retinopathy involving the eyes, neuropathy, and accelerated heart disease despite aggressive efforts to maintain the blood sugar within the physiologic normal range using exogenous insulin by itself or a combination of exogenous insulin and one or more oral medications. Diabetes remains the number one cause of renal failure in this country. Especially in diabetic patients that are dependent upon administering exogenous insulin into their body, though dosing of the insulin may be four or more times a day and even though this may produce adequate control of the blood glucose level to prevent the clinical symptoms of hyperglycemia; this does not unerringly supplement the body's natural capacity to monitor the blood sugar level minute to minute, twenty-four hours a day, and deliver an immediate response to a rise in blood glucose by the release of insulin from beta cells as required. The deleterious effects of diabetes may still evolve despite strict and persistent exogenous control of the glucose level in the blood stream.

[0052] The strategy to treat obesity has been founded in encouraging the overweight individual to diet and exercise. When the traditional approach does not suffice and the patient is severely overweight, the strategy may take the form of surgically altering the size of the stomach to physically limit the consumption of food. All three approaches may be successful, but often there exists restrictions, which limit the use or success of these strategies.

[0053] Both obesity and weight related diabetes are to some effect related to a decline in the metabolism in the body, as a person ages. It has been identified that in individuals between the ages of 35 to 50 years old, the energy production generated by the mitochondria in human cells declines by 50%. Between the ages of 65 to 90 years old, energy production by the mitochondria declines by another 39%. Certainly if the energy supplied to human cells is reduced by such drastic percentages, this in part contributes to a decline in the overall metabolic rate of the cell and the body in general.

[0054]   If a patient consumes a diet comprised of relatively the same amount of calories during their youth as they do in their middle age years and the utilization of the consumed sugar declines due to a significant decrease in the function of the mitochondria, the body has no alternative but to store the excess sugar and convert it to fat, thus resulting in the medical state of obesity. When the serum glucose level exceeds the upper limit for the normal range due to both a lack of adequate insulin production and a decline in glucose utilization by the mitochondria, diabetes emerges as a result.

[0055]   The current treatment of diabetes may be augmented by the unique approach to utilizing modified viruses as vehicles to transport biologically active messenger ribonucleic acids (mRNA) coded to facilitate the manufacture of insulin receptors and the enzymes required to conduct the processes of glycolysis, the tricarboxylic acid cycle, oxidative phosphorylation and anaerobic respiration.

[0056]   Viruses are obligate parasites. Viruses simply represent a carrier of genetic material and by themselves viruses are unable to replicate or carry on any form of biologic function outside their host cell. Viruses are generally comprised of one or more shells constructed of one or more layers of protein or lipid material, and inside the outer shell or shells, a virus carries a genetic payload that represents the instruction code necessary to replicate the virus, and protein enzymes to help facilitate the genetic payload in the function of replicating copies of the virus once the genetic payload has been delivered to a host cell. Located on the outer shell or envelope of a virus are probes. The function of a virus's probes is to locate and engage a host cell's receptors. The virus's surface probes are designed to detect, make contact with and functionally engage one or more receptors located on the exterior of a cell type that will offer the virus the proper environment in which to construct copies of itself. A host cell is a cell that provides the virus the proper biochemical machinery for the virus to successfully replicate itself.

[0057]   Protected by the outer coat generally comprised of an envelope or capsid or envelope and capsid, viruses carry a genetic payload in the form of deoxyribonucleic acid (DNA) or ribonucleic acid (RNA).   Once a virus's exterior probes locate and functionally engage the surface receptor or receptors on a host cell, the virus inserts its genetic payload into the interior of the host cell.   In the event a virus is carrying a DNA payload, the virus's DNA travels to the host cell's nucleus and is known to become inserted into the host cell's own native DNA.   In the case where a virus is carrying its genetic payload as RNA, the virus inserts the RNA payload into the host cell and may also insert one or more enzymes to facilitate the RNA being utilized properly to replicate copies of the virus.   Once inside the host cell, some species of virus facilitate their RNA being converted to DNA.   Once the viral RNA has been converted to DNA, the virus's DNA travels to the host cell's nucleus and is known to become inserted into the host cell's native DNA.   Once a virus's genetic material has been inserted into the host cell's native DNA, the virus's genetic material takes command of certain cell functions and redirects the resources of the host cell to generate copies of the virus.   Other forms of RNA viruses bypass the need to use the host cell's nuclear DNA and simply utilize portions of its viral genome to act as messenger RNA (mRNA).   RNA viruses that bypass the host cell's DNA, cause the cell, in general, to generate copies of the necessary parts of the virus directly from the virus's RNA genome.   When a virus's genome directly acts as a template, then similar to the cell's messenger RNA, the virus's RNA is read by the cell's ribosomes and proteins necessary to complete the virus's replication process are generated.

[0058]   The Hepatitis C virus (HCV) is a positive sense RNA virus, meaning a type of RNA that is capable of bypassing the need for involving the host cell's nucleus by having its RNA genome function as messenger RNA. Hepatitis C virus infects liver cells. The Hepatitis C viral genome becomes divided once it gains access to the interior of a liver host cell. Portions of the subdivisions of the Hepatitis C viral genome directly interact with host liver cell's ribosomes to produce proteins necessary to construct copies of the virus.

[0059] HCV belongs to the Flaviviridae family and is the only member of the Hepacivirus genus. There are considered to be at least 100 different strains of Hepatitis C virus based on genome sequencing variability.

[0060] HCV is comprised of an outer lipoprotein envelope and an internal nucleocapsid. The genetic payload is carried within the nucleocapsid. In its natural state, present on the surface of the outer envelope of the Hepatitis C virus are probes that detect receptors present on the surface of liver cells. The glycoprotein E1 probe and the glycoprotein E2 probe have been identified to be affixed to the surface of HCV. The E2 probe binds with high affinity to the large external loop of a CD81 cell-surface receptor. CD81 is found on the surface of many cell types including liver cells. Once the E2 probe has engaged the CD81 cell-surface receptor, cofactors on the surface of HCV's exterior envelope engage either or both the low density lipoprotein receptor (LDLR) or the scavenger receptor class B type I (SR-BI) present on the liver cell in order to activate the mechanism to facilitate HCV breaching the cell membrane and inserting its RNA genome payload through the plasma cell membrane of the liver cell into the liver cell. Upon successful engagement of the HCV surface probes with a liver cell's cell-surface receptors, HCV inserts the single strand of RNA and other payload elements it carries into the liver cell targeted to be a host cell. The HCV RNA genome then interacts with enzymes and ribosomes inside the liver cell in a translational process to produce the proteins required to construct copies of the protein components of HCV. The HCV genome undergoes a method of transcription to replicate copies of the virus's RNA genome. Inside the host, pieces of the HCV virus are assembled together and ultimately loaded with a copy of the HCV genome. Replicas of the original HCV then escape the host cell and migrate the environment in search of additional host liver cells to infect and continue the replication process.

[0061] The HCV's naturally occurring genetic payload consists of a single molecule of linear positive sense, single stranded RNA approximately 9600 nucleotides in length. By means of a translational process a polyprotein of approximately 3000 amino acids is generated. This polyprotein is cleaved post translation by host and viral proteases into individual viral proteins which include: the structural proteins of C, E1, E2, the nonstructural proteins NS1, NS2, NS3, NS4A, NS4B, NS5A, NS5B, p7 and ARFP/F protein. Hepatitis C virus's proteins direct the host liver cell to construct copies of the Hepatitis C virus. A membrane associated replicase complex consisting of the virus's nonstructural proteins NS3 and NS5B facilitate the replication of the viral genome. The membrane of the endoplasmic reticulum appears to be the site of protein maturation and viral assembly. Once copies of the Hepatitis C Virus are generated, they exit the host cell and each copy of HCV migrates in search of another appropriate liver cell that will act as a host to continue the replication process.

[0062] Hepatitis C virus offers a naturally occurring vehicle mechanism to transport and insert medically therapeutic messenger ribonucleic acid (mRNA) molecules into liver cells and other specifically targeted cells of the human body. The naturally occurring Hepatitis C virus already is equipped with the means of seeking out liver cells and delivering to liver cells its genetic payload. Further, the surface probes present on the Hepatitis C virus's outer protein coat can be modified to seek out specific receptors on specific target cells. Once the modified Hepatitis C virus's probes properly engage the cell-surface receptors on a target cell, the modified Hepatitis

C virus would insert into the target cell one or more medically therapeutic mRNAs for the purpose of having the target cell generate proteins to achieve a medical therapeutic response.

[0063] The Hepatitis C virus is one of several viruses that have been identified that possess the natural capacity to locate and infect liver cells with the genome the virus carries, thus including a liver cell as part of its reproductive cycle. Hepatitis A virus (HAV), Hepatitis C virus (HCV), Hepatitis D virus (HDV), Hepatitis E virus (HEV), and Hepatitis G virus (HGV) have been identified to carry their genome as RNA. The Hepatitis G virus is considered to be very similar to the Hepatitis C virus. The Hepatitis F virus and Hepatitis H viruses at this point are not considered to exist. The Hepatitis B virus (HBV) is believed to carry its genome as DNA. These alternative hepatitis viruses may also be utilized to act as alternative vehicles to deliver medically therapeutic messenger RNA molecules to liver cells or specific target cells.

[0064] Current state of gene therapy generally refers to efforts directed toward inserting an exogenous subunit of DNA into a vehicle such as a virus. The vehicle is intended to insert the exogenous subunit of DNA into a target cell. The exogenous DNA subunit then migrates to the target cell's nucleus. The exogenous DNA subunit then inserts into the native DNA of the cell. This represents a permanent alteration of the cell's nuclear DNA. At some point, the nuclear transcription proteins read the exogenous DNA subunit's nucleotide coding to produce the intended cellular response. The approach described within the scope of this text involves RNA versus DNA. DNA is comprised of the nucleotides adenine, thymine, guanine and cytosine. RNA is composed of the nucleotides adenine, uracil, guanine and cytosine. DNA codes for the manufacture of RNAs, which are composed of nucleotides. RNA codes for the manufacture of proteins, which are composed of amino acids. The virus chosen as the example of a transport vehicle,

Hepatitis C virus, is a RNA virus versus a virus that naturally carries a DNA genome.

[0065] It would seem an important element involved in the development of obesity, diabetes, lack of energy or reduced metabolism is linked to the failure of the mitochondria to properly utilize glucose to produce energy in the form of ATP.

[0066] The proteins manufactured by the ribosomes participate in the chemical reactions of glycolysis, the tricarboxylic acid cycle, oxidative phosphorylation and anaerobic respiration by acting as enzymes to catalyze these reactions or as other support proteins.

[0067] If the mitochondria's energy producing mechanisms fail to operate at an optimal level, overall cell function suffers due to a decline in the supply of available energy. Glucose may indeed be available for utilization by the mitochondria, but actual utilization rate of the glucose will be reduced if the cell's mitochondria are not functioning properly, with the result that the necessary supply of ATP molecules may not be adequate to supply the needs of the cell, thus limiting the function and survivability of the cell.

[0068] Developing a method of correcting the cause of the decline in mitochondrial function would lead to increasing the body's utilization of glucose, which would result in a more optimal management of diabetes, obesity, the sense of fatigue some individuals experience and the deleterious effects of the aging process.

[0069] Essential function of the mitochondrion relies on mRNA being decoded by the ribosomes in order to produce proteins that act as enzymes and catalyze the biologic reactions of aerobic respiration. It does not appear that the mitochondrial DNA creates the majority of the required mRNAs to generate the enzymes required for aerobic respiration. The mRNAs are then either produced by the cell nucleus and sent to the mitochondria or the required mRNAs are created at the time a new mitochondrion is constructed. Loss of proper regulation of the chemical pathways inside a mitochondrion may be related to degradation of the necessary mRNAs. Since a significant portion of the population is obese and a significant portion of the population is diagnosed with diabetes, if the mRNAs do indeed degrade and are not adequately replenished, obesity and diabetes may be related to lack of proper function of the mitochondria due to the fact that one or more mRNA molecules are not present in sufficient quantity to interact with ribosomes and thus not available to produce the required enzymes needed for the chemical pathways involved in the optimal metabolism of glucose.

[0070] A treatment of diabetes, obesity, chronic fatigue and aging may be approached by a method utilizing viruses as vehicles to transport biologically active mRNAs to mitochondria to bolster function of the mitochondria of all cells or possibly only certain cells in the body.

[0071] A Hepatitis C virus modified to carry a therapeutic mRNA payload could be introduced into the blood stream, travel the blood stream, engage the receptors on a liver cell with its surface probes, and then insert the genetic payload it carries into the liver cell. A genetic payload such as one or more messenger RNAs could be used to enhance proper protein production by cells deficient in a particular protein. In the case of a deficiency of a protein, production of a deficient protein could be enhanced by inserting one or more messenger RNAs into liver cells to stimulate production of the required protein. In the case of diabetes mellitus, utilizing a modified Hepatitis C virus as a vehicle, messenger RNA molecules could be inserted into liver cells, coded for any protein the liver cells are deficient in producing, with the intention of generating an adequate response to insulin and an optimal utilization of glucose.

[0072] The utilization of positive sense messenger RNA, does not permanently alter the cell's DNA. Messenger RNAs degrade and become unusable after a time. Use of RNA as a therapeutic modality offers a therapeutic opportunity that could have a reversible or an attenuatable effect when required. Messenger RNA also bypasses the action of decoding the DNA and errors or deficiencies that might occur during transcription phase in the nucleus. By employing a medically therapeutic virus to carry messenger RNA to cells, deficiencies of any of the approximately 30,000 proteins that comprise the tissues that exist in the body and on the surface of the body can be successfully treated or averted.

BRIEF SUMMARY OF THE INVENTION

[0073] The method by which a modified virus or virus-like structure is used as a transport medium to carry a payload of one or more messenger ribonucleic acid (RNA) molecules to cells in the body. The modified virus or virus-like structure makes contact with a specific target cell by means of the virus's exterior probes or virus-like structure's exterior probes. Once the exterior probes engage the target cell's receptors, the modified virus or virus-like structure inserts into the target cell one or more messenger ribonucleic acid (mRNA) molecules it is carrying. Messenger RNA molecules inserted into the cell act similar to native messenger RNA molecules and either interact with the cell's ribosomes in the process of protein synthesis or interacts with the cell's native enzymes and undergoes further modification until the delivered messenger RNA molecule is capable of interacting with the cell's ribosomes in the process of protein synthesis. Medical disease states such as diabetes mellitus, obesity, chronic fatigue and aging, that are the result of a deficiency of one or more proteins, can be successfully treated by utilizing viruses or virus-like structures to insert the proper messenger RNA molecules into specific cells to enhance the production of proteins that are identified as being deficient, thus correcting the deficiency. Improved utilization of glucose and optimal production of energy molecules resulting from a robust and efficient metabolism of glucose will enhance the cells' capacity to carryout life sustaining functions and lead to a healthier individual.

DETAILED DESCRIPTION

[0074] Diabetes mellitus, obesity, chronic fatigue syndrome, and aging may all be linked to the common pathway of degradation in an individual's capacity to metabolize glucose through the process of aerobic respiration. Errors in the DNA or errors that occur in the process that generates the messenger RNA or a deficiency in the number of messenger RNA or a deficiency in the number of biologically active messenger RNA results in a deficiency in cellular capacity to construct of the enzymes involved in the biologic respiratory processes of glycolysis, tricarboxylic acid cycle and phosphorylation and result in the medical conditions of diabetes mellitus, obesity, chronic fatigue and aging. Supplying the cells of the body with the means to produce sufficient quantities of biologically active enzymes to insure that the biologic respiratory processes of glycolysis, tricarboxylic acid cycle and oxidative phosphorylation occur at an optimal rate in cells would treat the medical conditions of diabetes mellitus, obesity, chronic fatigue and aging.

[0075] Viruses or virus-like structures can be fashioned to act as transport vehicles to carry and delver messenger ribonucleic acid (mRNA) molecules to cells. The mRNA molecules carried by therapeutic viruses would supply the cells of the body with the genetic templates to construct the proteins the cell would be deficient in producing on its own.

[0076] Naturally occurring viruses can be altered by replacing the genetic material the virus would carry, with mRNA molecules that would have a beneficial medically therapeutic effect on cells. The naturally occurring virus would then carry and deliver to its natural target cell the payload of medically therapeutic mRNA molecules. As an example, Hepatitis viruses could be altered to carry medically therapeutic mRNA molecules to liver cells. The naturally occurring virus then, instead of causing disease associated with delivering its own genome to stimulate its own replication process, would instead act as a method to deliver a quantity of medically therapeutic mRNA molecules which would provide the target cell an enhanced capacity to generate proteins to carryout beneficial biologic processes to accomplish a medically therapeutic outcome.

[0077] Naturally occurring viruses can be further modified to have their naturally occurring glycoprotein surface probes replaced by glycogen surface probes that target specific cells in the body. Viruses modified to carry and deliver medically therapeutic mRNA molecules as the payload, further modified to have their glycoprotein surface probes, that cause the modified virus to engage specific cells in the body, provides a method whereby specific cells in the body can be targeted and this method embodies a means of providing to specific type of cell in the body an enhanced capacity to generate proteins to carryout beneficial biologic processes to accomplish a medically therapeutic outcome.

[0078] Virus-like structures can be constructed with similar physical characteristics to naturally occurring viruses and be fashioned to carry medically therapeutic mRNA molecules as the payload and have located on the surface glycoprotein probes that engage specific cells in the body. Viruses-like structures carrying medically therapeutic mRNA molecules as the payload, constructed to have their glycoprotein surface probes engage specific cells in the body, and deliver to those specific cells the mRNA the virus-like structures carry is a method whereby specific cells in the body can be targeted and this method embodies a means of providing to specific type of cell in the body an enhanced capacity to generate proteins to carryout beneficial biologic processes to accomplish a medically therapeutic outcome. The advantage of a virus-like structure is that the physical dimensions of the virus-like structure can be adjusted to accommodate variations in the physical size of the payload of medically therapeutic mRNA molecules, yet maintain a means of engaging targeted cells in the body and delivering to those targeted cells the mRNA molecules required to accomplish the desired medical therapeutic outcome.

[0079] The Hepatitis C virus virion provides a naturally occurring specimen to illustrate the feasibility of the method described in this text. The Hepatitis C virus (HCV) virion is comprised of an outer lipoprotein envelope and an internal nucleocapsid. The virus's genetic payload is carried within its core, the nucleocapsid. The HCV's naturally occurring genetic payload consists of a single molecule of linear positive sense, single stranded RNA approximately 9600 nucleotides in length, which includes: the structural proteins of C, E1, E2, the nonstructural proteins NS1, NS2, NS3, NS4A, NS4B, NS5A, NS5B, p7 and ARFP/F protein. Present on the surface of the outer envelope of the Hepatitis C virus virion are probes that detect receptors present on the surface of liver cells. The glycoproteins E1 and E2 have been identified to be affixed to the surface of HCV virion. Portions of the Hepatitis C virus genome, when separated into individual pieces, behave like messenger RNA. The naturally occurring HCV virion is constructed with surface probes fashioned to recognize a receptor on the surface of a liver cell. Once the naturally occurring HCV's surface probe E2 engages a liver cell's CD81 receptor, and cofactors on the surface of HCV's exterior envelope engage the low density lipoprotein receptor (LDLR) or the scavenger receptor class B type I (SR-BI) on the liver cell, the HCV virion then has the opportunity to insert its RNA genetic payload into the engaged target liver cell.

[0080] The Hepatitis C virus virion carrying an mRNA payload, infects liver cells with its payload for the purpose of causing the now infected cell to generate a variety of proteins that will be assembled into copies resembling the original HCV virion. The copies of the HCV virion are then released from the infected cell to migrate in search of other host cells. Variations in the Hepatitis C virus are based on variations that occur in the strand of mRNA molecule the HCV virion carries as it genome. HCV virions may therefore carry differing mRNA molecules as its genetic payload and deliver these mRNA molecules to specific liver cells in the body to cause these cells to produce proteins to accomplish the task of replication of similar HCV virions.

[0081]   Replicating viruses and constructing viruses to carry DNA payloads is a form of manufacturing technology that has already been well established and is in use facilitating the concept of gene therapy. Replicating viruses and designing these viruses to carry messenger ribonucleic acid as the genetic payload would incorporate similar techniques as already proven useful in current DNA gene therapy technologies.

[0082]   To carry out the process to manufacture a modified medically therapeutic Hepatitis C virus, messenger RNA that would code for the general physical outer structures of the Hepatitis C virus would be inserted into a host. The host may include devices such as a host cell or a hybrid host cell. The host may utilize DNA or RNA or a combination of genetic instructions in order to accomplish the construction of medically therapeutic virus virions. The DNA or messenger RNA molecules to create the medically therapeutic hepatitis virus would direct the cells to generate copies of the medically therapeutic virus carrying a medically therapeutic mRNA payload. In some cases DNA or messenger RNA would be inserted into the host that would be coded to cause the production of surface probes that would be affixed to the surface of the virus virion that would target the surface receptors on specific cells in the body other than the liver cells the Hepatitis C virus naturally targets. DNA or messenger RNA would direct the host to generate copies of the messenger RNA that would provide a therapeutic action, this medically therapeutic messenger RNA would take the place of the Hepatitis C virus's innate genome as its payload. The medical treatment form of the Hepatitis C virus carrying the medically therapeutic messenger RNA would be produced, assembled and released from a host. Virus-like structures would be generated in similar fashion using a host such as host-cells or hybrid host cells. The copies of the medically therapeutic hepatitis virus or virus-like structures would be collected, stored and utilized as a medical treatment as necessary.

[0083]   To treat the various different forms of diabetes mellitus various combinations of messenger RNA would be inserted into the host, and the host would produce copies of modified Hepatitis C virus that target liver cells and carry a genetic payload consisting of messenger RNA molecules that would consist of one or more copies of a messenger RNA that codes for the insulin receptor, the enzymes utilized in the processes of glucose metabolism including glycolysis, tricarboxylic acid cycle and oxidative phosphorylation.   Depending upon the physical size of the messenger RNAs and the available space inside the modified Hepatitis C virus more than one type of messenger RNA may be packaged into a single modified Hepatitis C virus, which would produce one or more therapeutic actions in a cell. In some cases enzymes that catalyze the chemical reactions in aerobic and anaerobic respiration pathways are comprised of more than one protein molecule and would require the action of several mRNA molecules to create the enzyme in its entirety.

[0084]   The modified Hepatitis C virus and virus-like structures would be incapable of replication on its own due to the fact that the messenger RNA that would code for the replication process to produce copies of the virus or virus-like structure would not be present in the modified form of the Hepatitis C virus or virus-like structure. The modified form of the Hepatitis C virus or virus-like structure would carry messenger RNA that would be coded for generating for a variety of enzymes that would produce a medically therapeutic and beneficial result.   Such enzymes the messenger RNA would code for would include the enzymes as described in the following paragraphs.

[0085] Hexokinase (EC 2.7.1.1) also referred to as hexokinase type IV glucokinase or simply glucokinase. Hexokinase converts glucose to glucose-6-phosphate in the process of glycolysis.

[0086] Glucose-6-phosphate isomerase (EC 5.3.1.9) also known as glucose-6-phosphate isomerase. Glucose-6-phosphate isomerase is an enzyme that converts glucose-6-phosphate to fructose-6-phosphate in the process of glycolysis.

[0087] Phosphofructokinase (EC 2.7.1.11) also known as 6-phosphofructokinase. Phosphofructokinase is an enzyme that converts fructose-6-phosphate to Fructose 1,6-diphosphate in the process of glycolysis.

[0088] Fructose bisphosphate aldolase (EC 4.1.2.13), also known as aldolase. Fructose bisphosphate aldolase is an enzyme that converts fructose 1,6-diphosphate to two different entities including dihydroxyacetone 3-phosphate and glyceraldehydes 3-phosphate in the process of glycolysis.

[0089] Triose-phosphate dehydrogenase (EC 5.3.1.1). Triose-phosphate dehydrogenase is an enzyme that converts glyceraldehydes 3-phosphat to 1,3-diphosphoglycerate in the process of glycolysis.

[0090] Phosphoglycerate kinase (EC 2.7.2.3). Phosphoglycerate kinase is an enzyme that converts 1,3-diphosphoglycerate to 3-phosphoglycerate in the process of glycolysis.

[0091] Phosphoglycerate mutase (EC 5.4.2.1). Phosphoglycerate mutase is an enzyme that converts 3-phosphoglycerate to 2-phosphoglycerate in the process of glycolysis.

[0092] Enolase (EC 4.2.1.11). Enolase is an enzyme that converts 2-phosphoglycerate to phosphoenolpyruvate in the process of glycolysis.

[0093] Pyruvate kinase (EC 2.7.2.3). Pyruvate kinase is an enzyme that converts phosphoenolpyruvate to pyruvate in the process of glycolysis.

[0094] Pyruvate dehydrogenase is comprised of three units. The three units include E1 (EC 1.2.4.1), (EC 1.2.1.51), E2 dihydrolipoamide S-acetyltransferase (EC 2.3.1.12), and E3 dihydrolipoamide dehydrogenase (EC 1.8.1.4). Pyruvate dehydrogenase molecular complex catalyzes the conversion of pyruvate to acetyl-CoA.

[0095] Citrate synthetase (EC 4.1.3.7). Citrate synthetase is an enzyme that converts acetyl-CoA combines with oxaloacetate to produce citrate in the tricarboxylic acid cycle.

[0096] Aconitase (EC 4.2.1.3). Aconitase is an enzyme that converts citrate to cis-aconitate in the tricarboxylic acid cycle. Aconitase is an enzyme that converts cis-aconitate to iso-citrate in the tricarboxylic acid cycle.

[0097] Isocitrate dehydrogenase (EC 1.1.1.41). Isocitrate dehydrogenase is an enzyme that converts isocitrate to alpha-ketoglutaric acid in the tricarboxylic acid cycle.

[0098] 2-oxoglutarate dehydrogenase is protein complex comprised of three units. The three units include E1 (EC 1.2.4.2), E2 (EC 2.3.1.61), and E3 (EC 1.8.1.4). 2-oxoglutarate dehydrogenase is an enzyme complex that converts alpha-ketoglutaric to succinyl-CoA in the tricarboxylic acid cycle.

[0099] Succinyl-CoA synthetase (EC 6.2.1.5). Succinyl-CoA synthetase is an enzyme that converts succinyl CoA to succinate in the tricarboxylic acid cycle.

[0100] Succinate dehydrogenase (EC 1.3.5.1). Succinate dehydrogenase is an enzyme that converts succinate to fumarate in the tricarboxylic acid cycle.

[0101] Fumarate hydratase (EC 4.2.1.2). Fumarate hydratase is an enzyme that converts fumarate to malate in the tricarboxylic acid cycle.

[0102] Malate dehydrogenase (EC 1.1.1.37). Malate dehydrogenase is an enzyme that converts malate to oxaloacetate in the tricarboxylic acid cycle.

[0103] NADH dehydrogenase (EC 1.6.5.3) molecule, also referred to as NADH-coenzyme Q oxidoreductase or complex I, is utilized in oxidative phosphorylation.

[0104] Succinate dehydrogenase (EC 1.3.5.1) molecule, also referred to as succinate oxidoreductase or complex II, is utilized in oxidative phosphorylation.

[0105] Cytochrome-c reductase (EC 1.10.2.2) molecule, also referred to as complex III, is utilized in oxidative phosphorylation.

[0106] Cytochrome-c oxidase (EC 1.9.3.1) molecule, also referred to as complex IV, is utilized in oxidative phosphorylation.

[0107] ATP synthase (EC 3.6.1.34) molecule is utilized in oxidative phosphorylation.

[0108] Lactate dehydrogenase (EC 1.1.1.27) molecule is utilized to convert pyruvate to lactic acid in anaerobic respiration.

[0109] In review, the method described in this text includes taking a naturally occurring virus and altering its payload so that it transports medically therapeutic messenger RNA to cells it was naturally designed to infect, but instead of delivering its own genetic payload, it delivers the medically therapeutic messenger RNA it is carrying so that those cells may benefit from being able to produce protein molecules the messenger RNA are coded for, <u>and</u> the method described in this text includes taking a naturally occurring virus and altering its payload so that it carries medically therapeutic messenger RNA to cells and alter the virus's glycoprotein probes so that it is capable of infecting specifically targeted cells, but instead of delivering its own genetic payload, it delivers the medically therapeutic messenger RNA it is carrying so that those cells may benefit from being able to produce protein molecules the messenger RNA is coded for, <u>and</u> the method described in this text includes taking a virus-like structure, which carries medically therapeutic messenger RNA to cells, affixed to the surface glycoprotein probes so that it is capable of delivering medically therapeutic messenger RNA it is carrying to specific target cells so that those cells may benefit from being able to produce protein molecules the messenger RNA is coded for. Diabetes mellitus, obesity, chronic fatigue, and aging may all be linked to the vital process of glucose metabolism and aerobic respiration. Providing the body with the means of maintaining an optimum level of glucose metabolism and conducting aerobic respiration, in some cases anaerobic respiration, may provide the means to effectively manage the above-mentioned four major health conditions.

[0110] As mentioned above, the method to improve the current glucose management to enhance the treatment diabetes mellitus, a quantity of modified virus virions, such as Hepatitis C virus virions would be introduced into a patient's blood stream or tissues so that the modified virus could deliver the medially therapeutic mRNA payload that it carries to targeted cells in the body, such as liver cells. Once the modified virus virions insert their medically therapeutic payload consisting of messenger RNA into the cell the modified virus virion has been targeted for the cell's biologic function of producing insulin receptors or metabolizing glucose by way of glycolysis, tricarboxylic acid cycle, oxidative phosphorylation or anaerobic respiration are to be enhanced. Improvement in the metabolism of glucose inside cells will reduce circulating levels of glucose in the blood stream and decrease a patient's likelihood of diabetes mellitus.

[0111]   As mentioned above, the method to improve the current glucose management to enhance the treatment obesity, a quantity of modified virus virions, such as Hepatitis C virus virions, would be introduced into a patient's blood stream or tissues so that the modified virus could deliver the medically therapeutic mRNA payload that it carries to targeted cells in the body, such as liver cells. Once the modified virus virions insert their medically therapeutic payload consisting of messenger RNA into the cell the modified virus virion has been targeted for, the cell's biologic function of producing insulin receptors or metabolizing glucose by way of glycolysis, tricarboxylic acid cycle, oxidative phosphorylation or anaerobic respiration are to be enhanced. Improvement in the metabolism of glucose inside cells will reduce circulating levels of glucose in the blood stream and decrease a patient's likelihood of obesity by increasing the cellular consumption of glucose and fats.

[0112]   As mentioned above, the method to improve the current glucose management so as to enhance the treatment chronic fatigue, a quantity of modified virus virions would be introduced into a patient's blood stream or tissues so that the modified virus could deliver the medically therapeutic mRNA payload that it carries to targeted cells in the body, such as muscle cells. Once the modified virus virions insert their medically therapeutic payload consisting of messenger RNA into the targeted cells, the cells' biologic function of producing insulin receptors or metabolizing glucose by way of glycolysis, tricarboxylic acid cycle, oxidative phosphorylation or anaerobic respiration are to be enhanced.   Improvement in the metabolism of glucose inside cells will increase the production of ATP, the result of which will be increasing the available energy resources cells have to conduct biologic processes inside the cell, which will lead to less fatigue in patients.

[0113] As mentioned above, the method to improve the current glucose management so as to enhance the treatment aging, a quantity of modified virus virions would be introduced into a patient's blood stream or tissues so that the modified virus could deliver the medically therapeutic mRNA payload that it carries to targeted cells in the body, such as chondrocytes located in bone. Once the modified virus virions insert their medically therapeutic payload consisting of messenger RNA into the targeted cells, the cells' biologic function of producing insulin receptors or metabolizing glucose by way of glycolysis, tricarboxylic acid cycle, oxidative phosphorylation or anaerobic respiration are to be enhanced. Improvement in the metabolism of glucose inside cells will increase the production of ATP, the result of which will be increasing the available energy resources cells have to conduct biologic processes inside the cell, which will lead to a decline in the failure rate of cells in the body which will forestall and may reverse the process of aging in patients.

[0114] By utilizing the described method to provide the cells of the body with the above-mentioned medically therapeutic messenger RNA molecules and enhancing the capacity of cells to carry out the biologic processes of glycolysis, tricarboxylic acid cycle, oxidative phosphorylation and anaerobic respiration, will result in an efficient means to control the glucose levels in the blood stream and utilize glucose to produce energy molecules such as ATP molecules in the cells of the body, such as liver cells, on a constant and persistent basis by utilizing innate regulatory mechanisms, and will result in effectively managing diabetes mellitus, obesity, chronic fatigue and aging for the betterment of patients.

CLAIMS: Reserved.

B3: A MEDICAL DEVICE FOR TREATING DIABETES MELLITUS, OBESITY, CHRONIC FATIGUE, AGING, AND OTHER MEDICAL CONDITIONS BY UTILIZING MODIFIED VIRUS VIRIONS TO INSERT MESSENGER RIBONUCLEIC ACID MOLECULES INTO CELLS

INDIVIDUALS REQUESTING PATENT: Dr. Lane B. Scheiber, ScD and Dr. Lane B. Scheiber II, MD

NUMBER OF CLAIMS: 3 independent claims, 17 dependent claims

ABSTRACT

The common link between diabetes mellitus, obesity, chronic fatigue and even aging may be related to deficiencies involving a body's metabolism of glucose and the ability to optimally conduct the necessary biologic processes of aerobic respiration. Utilizing a medical device comprised of a modified form of virus to deliver to cells in the body the messenger RNA molecules needed to construct insulin receptors and generate the enzymes that participate in the processes of glycolysis, the tricarboxylic acid cycle, oxidative phosphorylation and anaerobic respiration will lead to greater utilization of blood glucose and a more efficient and sustained production of the energy molecules that fuel the metabolic processes of the cell. Greater utilization of blood glucose will significantly advance the effort to correct the medical problems associated with diabetes, obesity, chronic fatigue, and aging.

BACKGROUND OF THE INVENTION

Field of the Invention

This invention relates to any medical device intended to correct a protein deficiency in the body by increasing the intracellular production of the deficient protein by utilizing a modified virus to insert one or more messenger ribonucleic acid molecules into one or more cells of the body.

Description of Background Art

[0001] Diabetes and obesity represent two very widespread and extremely important health issues across the United States. Both conditions affect a significant portion of the population and result in significant morbidity and mortality. In the United States, about 16 million people suffer from diabetes mellitus. Every year, about 650,000 additional people are diagnosed with the disease. Diabetes mellitus is the seventh leading cause of all deaths. According to the National Institutes of Health, in the United States, 97 million adults are overweight or obese. About 22.5 percent of the population is obese, up from 13 percent in 1960. Obesity and diabetes mellitus are linked disorders in many patients. Studies show that individuals who are 20 percent or more overweight run a greater risk of developing diabetes mellitus, hypertension, coronary heart disease, stroke, arthritis, and some forms of cancer.

[0002] Chronic fatigue syndrome (CFS) is characterized by extreme fatigue that has persisted in excess of six months. CFS occurs most commonly in people in their 40s and 50s. CFS is estimated to affect one million people in the United States, with estimated tens of millions with similar symptoms of fatigue that do not meet the strict criteria to make a formal diagnosis. CFS results in significant loss of productivity by the individuals affected by this condition, thus having a negative impact on the work-force in general.

[0003] Aging affects the entire scope of the population. The characteristics of aging may be related to a lack of sufficient sustained energy production and therefore a progressive decline in an individual's cellular capacity to sufficiently fuel biologic processes requiring energy. The mitochondria are the powerhouses of the cells, converting sugars such as glucose to energy molecules such as adenosine triphosphate (ATP). A liver cell may contain as many as 2500 mitochondria. If the mitochondria lack a sufficient amount of any of the required enzymes to complete the process of metabolizing glucose to energy molecules such as ATP, necessary biologic functions may not be available to engage in cellular functions as needed. It has been estimated that in a person's lifetime, between the ages of 35 to 50 years old, there occurs a fifty percent decline in the mitochondria's capacity to produce energy. As an individual ages, there is a further decline in mitochondrial output capacity.

[0004] Diabetes mellitus, obesity, chronic fatigue, and aging may all be linked to the vital process of glucose metabolism. Providing the body with the means of maintaining an optimum level of glucose metabolism and anaerobic respiration may provide the means to effectively manage the above-mentioned four major health conditions.

[0005] Diabetes mellitus represents a state of hyperglycemia, which is generally defined as a serum blood sugar that is higher than what is considered the normal range for humans. Glucose, a six-carbon molecule, represents a form of sugar. Glucose is absorbed by the cells of the body through passive diffusion and is converted to energy by the biologic processes of glycolysis, the tricarboxylic acid (TCA) cycle and oxidative phosphorylation. Insulin, a protein, facilitates the absorption of glucose into cells. Normal range for blood glucose in humans is generally defined as a fasting blood plasma glucose level of between 70 to 110 mg/dl. An alternative means of measuring the blood glucose level is by measuring the glucose level stored inside red blood cells in the blood, which provides information regarding the average blood glucose spanning several weeks, rather than a real-time blood glucose level represented in a blood plasma glucose level. Measurement of glycated hemoglobin (Hgb A1C) provides an estimate of diabetic control over the preceding three months, with a normal value for nondiabetic patients being approximately 6% and values for a poorly controlled diabetic being 7-12%. For purposes of this description the terms "plasma' and 'serum' refer to the same substance, which is the fluid (noncellular) portion of blood.

[0006] Diabetes mellitus is generally classified as Type One and Type Two. Type One diabetes mellitus is insulin dependent, and refers to the condition where there is an insufficient quantity of insulin molecules circulating in the blood stream compared to the quantity required to maintain the blood glucose level within the recognized normal range. In Type One diabetes mellitus insulin must be provided to the body in order to properly regulate the blood plasma glucose level. When insulin is required to regulate the blood glucose level in the body, this condition is often referred to as insulin dependent diabetes mellitus (IDDM). Type Two diabetes mellitus is not dependent upon insulin and is often referred to as noninsulin dependent diabetes mellitus (NIDDM), meaning the blood glucose level can be managed without treatment with exogenous insulin, and is generally managed by means of diet, exercise or intervention with oral medications. Type Two diabetes mellitus is considered a progressive disease, with the underlying pathogenic mechanisms including pancreatic beta cell (often designated as β-Cell) dysfunction and insulin resistance.

[0007] The pancreas serves as an endocrine gland and an exocrine gland. Functioning as an endocrine gland, the pancreas produces and secretes hormones including the hormones insulin and glucagon. Insulin acts to reduce levels of glucose circulating in the blood. Beta cells secrete insulin into the blood when a higher than normal level of glucose is detected in the serum. Glucagon is an antagonistic hormone to insulin, which acts to stimulate an increase in glucose circulating in the blood. Alpha cells in the pancreas secrete glucagon into the blood when a low level of glucose is detected in the blood.

[0008] Glucose generally enters the body and then the blood stream as a result of the digestion of food. For purposes of this description, 'blood' and 'blood stream' refer to the same substance, which is generally considered to be blood as a whole including plasma and blood cells. The beta cells of the Islets of Langerhans continuously sense the level of glucose in the blood and respond to elevated levels of blood glucose by secreting insulin into the blood. Beta cells produce the protein 'insulin' in the endoplasmic reticulum and store the insulin in vacuoles until the insulin is needed. When beta cells detect an increase in the glucose level in the blood, the beta cells release insulin into the blood plasma from said storage vacuoles.

[0009] Insulin is a protein. An insulin molecule consists of two chains of amino acids, an alpha chain and a beta chain, linked by two disulfide (S-S) bridges. The alpha chain consists of 21 amino acids. The beta chain consists of 30 amino acids.

[0010] Insulin interacts with the cells of the body by means of a cell-surface receptor termed the 'insulin receptor' located on the exterior of a cell's 'outer membrane', often referred to as the 'plasma membrane'. Insulin interacts with muscle and liver cells by means of the insulin receptor to rapidly remove excess blood sugar when the glucose level in the blood is higher than the upper limit of the normal physiologic range. Recognized functions of insulin include stimulating cells to take up glucose from the blood, convert glucose to glycogen (an extensively branched glucose storage polysaccharide molecule), to facilitate the cells in the body to utilize glucose to generate biochemically usable energy, and to stimulate fat cells to take up glucose and synthesize fat.

[0011] Diabetes Mellitus may develop in an individual as the result of one or more factors. Causes of diabetes mellitus may include: (1) mutation of the insulin gene itself causing miscoding, which results in the production of ineffective insulin molecules; (2) mutations to genes that code for the 'transcription factors' needed for transcription of the insulin gene in the DNA to create messenger RNAs which facilitates the manufacture of the insulin molecule; (3) mutations of the gene encoding for the insulin receptor, which produces inactive or an insufficient number of insulin receptors; (4) mutation to the gene encoding for glucokinase, the enzyme that phosphorylates glucose in the first step of glycolysis; (5) mutations to the genes encoding portions of the potassium channels in the plasma membrane of the beta cells, preventing proper closure of the channel, thus blocking insulin release; (6) mutations to mitochondrial genes that as a result, decreases the energy available to be used facilitate the release of insulin, therefore reducing insulin secretion; (7) failure of glucose transporters to properly permit the facilitated diffusion of glucose from plasma into the cells of the body.

[0012] A eukaryote refers to a nucleated cell. Eukaryotes comprise nearly all animal and plant cells. A human eukaryote or nucleated cell is comprised of an exterior lipid bilayer plasma membrane, cytoplasm, a nucleus, and organelles. The exterior plasma membrane defines the perimeter of the cell, regulates the flow of nutrients, water and regulating molecules in and out of the cell, and has embedded into its structure cell-surface receptors that the cell uses to detect properties of the environment surrounding the cell membrane. Cytoplasm refers to the entire contents inside the cell except for the nucleus and acts as a filling medium inside the boundaries of the plasma cell membrane. Cytosol refers to the semifluid portion of the cytoplasm minus the mitochondria and the endoplasmic reticulum. The nucleus, organelles, and ribosomes are suspended in the cytosol. Nutrients such as amino acids, oxygen and glucose are present in the cytosol. The nucleus contains the majority of the cell's genetic information in the form of double stranded deoxyribonucleic acid (DNA). Organelles generally carry out specialized functions for the cell and include such structures as the mitochondria, the endoplasmic reticulum, storage vacuoles, lysosomes and Golgi complex. Floating in the cytoplasm, but also located in the endoplasmic reticulum and mitochondria are ribosomes. Ribosomes are protein structures comprised of several strands of proteins that combine and couple to a messenger ribonucleic acid (mRNA) molecule. More than one ribosome may be attached to a single mRNA at a time. Ribosomes decode genetic information coded in a mRNA molecule and manufacture proteins to the specifications of the instruction code physically present in the mRNA molecule.

[0013]   The majority of the deoxyribonucleic acid (DNA) in a cell is present in the form of chromosomes, the double stranded helical structures located in the nucleus of the cell. DNA in a circular form, can also be found in the mitochondria, the powerhouse of the cell, an organelle that assists in converting glucose into usable energy molecules. DNA represents the genetic information a cell needs to manufacture the materials it requires to develop to its mature form, sustain life and to replicate. Genetic information is stored in the DNA by arrangements of four nucleotides referred to as: adenine, thymine, guanine and cytosine. DNA represents instruction coding, that in the process known as transcription, the DNA's genetic information is decoded by transcription protein complexes referred to as polymerases, to produce ribonucleic acid (RNA). RNA is a single strand of genetic information comprised of coded arrangements of four nucleotides: adenine, uracil, guanine and cytosine. The physical difference in the construction of a DNA molecule versus a RNA molecule is that DNA utilizes the nucleotide 'thymine', while RNA molecules utilize the nucleotide 'uracil'. RNAs are generally classified as messenger RNAs (mRNA), transport RNAs (tRNA) and ribosomal RNAs (rRNA).

[0014] Mitochondrion ('mitochondria' pleural) is a cellular organelle that is considered the energy producing organelle of the cell. Mitochondria assist in generating energy for cell metabolism by producing ATP molecules from glucose. Within the cytoplasm and outer wall of the mitochondria sugar molecules undergo the process of glycolysis, and then inside the mitochondria byproducts of glucose are further broken down in the tricarboxylic acid (TCA) cycle and by oxidative phosphorylation to produce useable forms of energy molecules.

[0015] The exterior of a mitochondrion is known as an external membrane. Inside the outer membrane is an inner membrane. Folds in the inner membrane create crista, which expands the surface of the inner membrane and enhances the mitochondrion's ability to create ATP molecules. Inside the inner membrane is the mitochondrion matrix. The mitochondrion matrix contains a highly concentrated mixture of enzymes, ribosomes, tRNA and mitochondrial DNA. Glycolysis occurs in the cytosol of the cell and membrane of the mitochondrion. The tricarboxylic acid cycle functions within the inner chambers and matrix of the mitochondrion. Oxidative phosphorylation occurs within the boundaries of the outer and inner membranes of the mitochondrion.

[0016] Many of the intermediates of the processes of glycolysis and the tricarboxylic acid cycle exist as anions at the pH found in cells, and readily associate with H^+ to form acids. The intermediates of glycolysis and the tricarboxylic acid cycle are therefore often written as either an anion or an acid. For the purposes of this description, the intermediates of the processes of glycolysis and the tricarboxylic acid cycle are generally written as anions (as an example pyruvate versus pyruvic acid).

[0017] As a result of the biochemical process of glycolysis during aerobic (oxygen available) respiration conditions glucose is converted to pyruvate. The abbreviated processes of glycolysis include: (1) Glucose is converted to glucose-6-phosphate by the enzyme 'hexokinase'. (2) Glucose-6-phosphate is converted to fructose-6-phosphate by the enzyme 'glucose-6-phosphate isomerase'. (3) Fructose-6-phosphate is converted to fructose 1,6-diphosphate by the enzyme 'phosphofructo kinase'. (4) Fructose 1,6-diphosphate is converted to two different entities including dihydroxyacetone-3-phosphate and glyceraldehydes-3-phosphate by the enzyme 'fructose bisphosphate aldolase'. (5) Dihydroacetone-3-phosphate converts to D-glyceraladehyde-3-phosphate by the enzyme 'triose-phosphate isomerase'. (6) Glyceraldehyde-3-phosphate is converted to 1,3-diphosphoglycerate by the enzyme 'glyceraldehyde-3-phosphate dehydrogenase'. (7) 1,3-diphosphoglycerate is converted to 3-phosphoglycerate by the enzyme 'phosphoglycerate kinase'. (8) 3-phosphoglycerate is converted to 2-phosphoglycerate by the enzyme 'phosphoglycerate mutase'. (9) 2-phosphoglycerate is converted to phosphoenolpyruvate by the enzyme 'enolase'. (10) Phosphoenolpyruvate is converted to pyruvate by the enzyme complex referred to as 'pyruvate kinase'.

[0018] Pyruvate is then oxidized to an acetyl group, which is combined with Coenzyme A and produces acetyl Coenzyme A (acetyl-CoA). Pyruvate dehydrogenase, which metabolizes pyruvate to acetyl-CoA is comprised of a multi-enzyme complex. The three protein complexes of pyruvate dehydrogenase are designated E1 (pyruvate dehydrogenase), E2 (dihydrolipoamide S-acetyltransferase), and E3 (dihydrolipoamide dehydrogenase). Acetyl-CoA enters the tricarboxylic acid cycle. Under aerobic respiration conditions from one glucose molecule the process of glycolysis generates 8 ATP molecules, conversion of pyruvate to acetyl CoA generates an additional 6 ATP molecules.

[0019] The tricarboxylic acid cycle otherwise known as the citric acid cycle or the Krebs cycle, was discovered in 1937 by Sir Hans Krebs, and is a biochemical process that provides complete oxidation of acetyl-CoA, which may be derived from sources such as fats, carbohydrates and lipids. For purposes of this discussion, acetyl-CoA is a byproduct of glucose metabolism during glycolysis, and enters the tricarboxylic acid cycle and (1) combines with oxaloacetate (also known as oxaloacetic acid) by the action of the enzyme 'citrate synthetase' which produces citrate (also known as citric acid). (2) Citrate is converted to cis-aconitate per the enzyme 'aconitase'. (3) Cis-aconitate is converted to iso-citrate (also known as isocitur acid) again by the enzyme aconitase. (4) Iso-citrate is converted to alpha-ketoglutarate by the enzyme 'isocitrate dehydrogenase'. (5) Alpha-ketoglutaric acid is converted to succinyl CoA by the enzyme '2-oxoglutarate dehydrogenase'. (6) Succinyl CoA is converted to succinate (also known as succinic acid) by the enzyme 'succinyl-CoA synthetase'. (7) Succinate is converted to fumarate (also known as fumaric acid) by the enzyme 'succinate dehydrogenase'. (8) Fumarate is converted to malate (also known as malic acid) by the enzyme 'fumarate hydratase'. (9) Malate is converted to oxaloacetate by the enzyme 'malate dehydrogenase'. The result of metabolism of glucose by glycolysis and the tricarboxylic acid cycle yields ATP molecules and electron donor molecules such as the reduced form of the coenzyme nicotinamide adenine dinucleotide written NADH +H$^+$. The tricarboxylic acid cycle also produces electron donor molecules in the form of the reduced co-enzyme flavin adenine dinucleotide written FADH$_2$.

[0020] Oxidative phosphorylation is a metabolic pathway that uses energy released by oxidation to produce adenosine triphosphate (ATP). During oxidative phosphorylation electrons are transferred from electron donors to electron acceptors such as oxygen in redox reactions. In eukaryotes the redox reactions are carried out by a series of protein complexes located within mitochondria. These protein complexes represent a linked set of enzymes referred to as electron transport chains. The protein complexes utilized in oxidative phosphorylation include nicotinamide adenine dinucleotide (NADH) dehydrogenase enzyme molecule, the succinate dehydrogenase enzyme molecule, the cytochrome-c reductase enzyme molecule, the cytochrome-c oxidase enzyme molecule, and the ATP synthase enzyme molecule. Under aerobic respiration conditions one glucose molecule metabolized by the combination of glycolysis, the tricarboxylic acid cycle and oxidative phosphorylation yields as many as 38 ATP molecules.

[0021] An enzyme is a protein generated by cells that acts as a catalyst to induce chemical changes in other substances, itself remaining apparently unchanged in the process. There are several main groups of enzymes including oxidoreductase, transferase, hydrolase, lyase, isomerase, and ligase, sometimes referred to as synthetase. EC is an abbreviation for Enzyme Commission of the International Union of Biochemistry and this is used in conjunction with a unique number to define a specific enzyme identified in the Enzyme Commission's list of enzymes. Oxidoreductases generally have as their first EC identifying number, the number 1. Transferases generally have as their first EC identifying number, the number 2. Hydrolases generally have as their first EC identifying number, the number 3. Lyases generally have as their first EC identifying number, the number 4. Isomerase generally have as their first EC identifying number, the number 5. Ligases generally have as their first EC identifying number, the number 6. Several scientific names often exist to identify the same enzyme.

[0022] Enzymes (followed by their Enzyme Commission of the International Union of Biochemistry number) utilized in the metabolism of glucose in the processes of glycolysis, tricarboxylic acid cycle, and oxidative phosphorylation are described in the following paragraphs.

[0023] Hexokinase (EC 2.7.1.1), is also referred to as hexokinase type IV glucokinase or in some cases simply glucokinase. Hexokinase converts glucose to glucose-6-phosphate in glycolysis.

[0024] Glucose-6-phosphate isomerase (EC 5.3.1.9), is also known as phosphoglucoisomerase. Glucose-6-phosphate isomerase is an enzyme that converts glucose-6-phosphate to fructose-6-phosphate in glycolysis.

[0025] 6-phosphofructokinase (EC 2.7.1.11), is also known as phosphofructokinase. 6-phosphofructokinase is an enzyme that converts fructose-6-phosphate to fructose 1,6-diphosphate in glycolysis.

[0026] Fructose bisphosphate aldolase (EC 4.1.2.13), is also known as aldolase. Fructose bisphosphate aldolase is an enzyme that converts fructose 1,6-diphosphate to two different entities including dihydroxyacetone 3-phosphate and glyceraldehydes 3-phosphate in glycolysis.

[0027] Triose-phosphate isomerase (EC 5.3.1.1). Triose-phosphate isomerase is an enzyme that converts dihydroacetone-3-phosphate converts to D-glyceraladehyde-3-phosphate.

[0028] Glyceraldehyde-3-phosphate dehydrogenase (EC 1.2.1.12), may be abbreviated GAPDH or G3PDH. Glyceraldehyde-3-phosphate dehydrogenase is an enzyme that converts glyceraldehydes-3-phosphatate to 1,3-diphosphoglycerate in glycolysis.

[0029] Phosphoglycerate kinase (EC 2.7.2.3). Phosphoglycerate kinase is an enzyme that converts 1,3-diphosphoglycerate to 3-phosphoglycerate in glycolysis.

[0030] Phosphoglycerate mutase (EC 5.4.2.1). Phosphoglycerate mutase is an enzyme that converts 3-phosphoglycerate to 2-phosphoglycerate in glycolysis.

[0031] Enolase (EC 4.2.1.11). Enolase is an enzyme that converts 2-phosphoglycerate to phosphoenolpyruvate in glycolysis.

[0032] Pyruvate kinase (EC 2.7.1.40). Pyruvate kinase is an enzyme that converts phosphoenolpyruvate to pyruvate in glycolysis.

[0033] Pyruvate dehydrogenase is comprised of three units. The three units include E1 (EC 1.2.4.1), (EC 1.2.1.51), E2 dihydrolipoamide S-acetyltransferase (EC 2.3.1.12), and E3 dihydrolipoamide dehydrogenase (EC 1.8.1.4). Pyruvate dehydrogenase molecular complex catalyzes the conversion of pyruvate to acetyl-CoA.

[0034] Citrate synthetase (EC 4.1.3.7). Citrate synthetase is an enzyme that converts acetyl-CoA combines with oxaloacetate to produce citrate in the tricarboxylic acid cycle.

[0035] Aconitase (EC 4.2.1.3). Aconitase exists in two isoenzyme forms in eukaryotes: mitochondrial and cytosolic. Aconitase is an enzyme that converts citrate to cis-aconitate in the Tricarboxylic acid cycle and converts cis-aconitate to iso-citrate in the tricarboxylic acid cycle.

[0036] Isocitrate dehydrogenase (EC 1.1.1.41). Isocitrate dehydrogenase is an enzyme that converts isocitrate to alpha-ketoglutaric acid in the tricarboxylic acid cycle.

[0037] 2-oxoglutarate dehydrogenase is a protein complex comprised of three units. The three units include E1 (EC 1.2.4.2), E2 (EC 2.3.1.61), and E3 (EC 1.8.1.4). 2-oxoglutarate dehydrogenase is an enzyme complex that converts alpha-ketoglutaric to succinyl CoA in the tricarboxylic acid cycle.

[0038] Succinyl-CoA synthetase (EC 6.2.1.5). Succinyl-CoA synthetase is an enzyme that converts succinyl CoA to succinate in the tricarboxylic acid cycle.

[0039] Succinate dehydrogenase (EC 1.3.5.1). Succinate dehydrogenase is an enzyme that converts succinate to fumarate in the tricarboxylic acid cycle.

[0040] Fumarate hydratase (EC 4.2.1.2). Fumarate hydratase is an enzyme that converts fumarate to malate in the tricarboxylic acid cycle.

[0041] Malate dehydrogenase (EC 1.1.1.37). Malate dehydrogenase is an enzyme that converts malate to oxaloacetate in the tricarboxylic acid cycle.

[0042] During conditions were sufficient oxygen is available, metabolism of glucose generally occurs through the processes of glycolysis, tricarboxylic acid cycle, and oxidative phosphorylation. When oxygen is not readably available, anaerobic respiration occurs. The enzyme lactate dehydrogenase provides an alternative pathway to produce ATP when sufficient oxygen is not available by converting pyruvate to lactic acid. The anaerobic pathway lactate dehydrogenase catalyzes is much less efficient means of producing energy molecules than the aerobic pathway that takes advantage of oxygen dependent processes of tricarboxylic acid cycle and oxidative phosphorylation.

[0043] Proteins are comprised of a series of amino acids bonded together in a linear strand, sometimes referred to as a chain; a protein may be further modified to be a structure comprised of one or more similar or differing strands of amino acids bonded together. A protein comprised of more than one strand of amino acids (referred to as subunits) may be referred to as a protein complex. Insulin is a protein structure comprised of two strands of amino acids, one strand comprised of 21 amino acids long and the second strand comprised of 30 amino acids; the two strands attached by two disulfide bridges. There are an estimated 30,000 different proteins the cells of the human body may manufacture. The human body is comprised of a wide variety of cells, many with specialized functions requiring unique combinations of proteins and protein structures such as glycoproteins (a protein combined with a carbohydrate) to accomplish the required task or tasks a specialized cell is designed to perform. Forms of glycoproteins are known to be utilized as cell-surface receptors.

[0044] Messenger RNAs (mRNA) are created by transcription of DNA. Messenger RNA generated by transcription of nuclear DNA, migrate out of the nucleus of the cell, and are utilized as protein manufacturing templates by ribosomes. Different mRNAs code for different proteins. As previously mentioned, there are as many as 30,000 varieties of proteins, therefore there are at least 30,000 different mRNA molecules. A ribosome is a protein complex that manufactures proteins by deciphering the instruction code located in a mRNA molecule. When a specific protein is needed, pieces of the ribosome complex bind around the strand of mRNA that carries the specific instruction code that will generate the required protein. The ribosome traverses the mRNA strand and deciphers the genetic information coded into the sequence of nucleotides that comprise the mRNA molecule.

[0045] Transport RNAs (tRNA) are constructed in the nucleus or in the mitochondria, and are coded for one of the 20 amino acids the cells of the human body use to construct proteins. Once a tRNA is created by transcription of the DNA, the tRNA seeks out the type of amino acid it has been coded for and attaches to that specific amino acid. The tRNA then delivers the amino acid it carries to a ribosome that is waiting for that specific amino acid. Proteins are manufactured by the ribosomes binding together sequences of amino acids. The order by which the amino acids are bonded together is dictated by the way the mRNA is constructed and how the ribosome interprets the information encoded in the string of nucleotides present in the mRNA strand.

[0046]   A sequence of three nucleotides present in a mRNA molecule represents a unit of information referred to as a codon. Codons code for all of the 20 amino acids used to construct protein molecules and also for START and STOP commands. In the process known as translation, the ribosome decodes the codons present in the mRNA, initiating the protein manufacturing process at a START codon, then interfacing with tRNAs carrying the amino acids that match the sequence of codons in the mRNA as the ribosome traverses the length of the mRNA molecule. The ribosome functions as a protein factory by taking amino acids delivered by tRNAs and binding the amino acids together in the order dictated by the sequence of codon instructions coded into the mRNA template as directed by the manner of the nucleic acid arrangement in the mRNA molecule. Protein synthesis ceases when a ribosome encounters a STOP code. Once complete, the protein molecule is released by the ribosome.

[0047]   The insulin molecule is a protein produced by beta cells located in the pancreas. The 'insulin messenger RNA' is created in a cell by transcribing the insulin gene from nuclear DNA in the nucleus of the cell. The native messenger RNA (mRNA) for insulin then travels to the endoplasmic reticulum, where numerous ribosomes engage these mRNA molecules. Many ribosomes may be attached to a single strand of mRNA simultaneously, each generating an identical copy of the protein as dictated by the information encoded in the mRNA. Insulin is produced by ribosomes translating the information in a mRNA molecule coded for the insulin protein, which produce strands of amino acids that are coded for an immature form of the biologically active insulin molecule referred to as 'pro-insulin'. Once the pro-insulin molecule is generated it then undergoes modification by several enzymes including prohormone convertase one (PC1), prohormone convertase two (PC2) and carboxypeptidase E, which results in the production of a biologically active insulin molecule. Once the biologically active insulin protein is generated, it is stored in a vacuole in the beta cell to await being released into the blood stream.

[0048] The insulin receptor, prohormone convertase one (PC1), prohormone convertase two (PC2) and carboxypeptidase E are produced in a similar fashion as to how pro-insulin and insulin are produced in a beta cell. A messenger RNA is transcribed from DNA, specific for either the insulin receptor, prohormone convertase one (PC1), prohormone convertase two (PC2) or carboxypeptidase E. When a messenger RNA coded for an insulin receptor is present and available, ribosomes will attach to the mRNA and generate insulin receptor proteins. When a messenger RNA coded for either prohormone convertase one (PC1), prohormone convertase two (PC2) or carboxypeptidase E is present and available, ribosomes will attach to the mRNA, decode the instructions in the mRNA molecule and generate the protein.

[0049] Insulin receptors, which appear on the surface of cells, offer binding sites for insulin circulating in the blood. When insulin binds to an insulin receptor, the biologic response inside the cell causes glucose to undergo processing in the cytoplasm. Processed glucose molecules then enter the mitochondrion. The mitochondrion further processes the modified glucose molecules to produce usable energy in the form of adenosine triphosphate molecules (ATP). Thirty-eight ATP molecules may be generated from one molecule of glucose during the process of aerobic respiration. ATP molecules are utilized as an energy source by biologic processes throughout the cell.

[0050] The current medical therapeutic approach to the management of diabetes mellitus has produced limited results. Patients with diabetes generally struggle with an inadequate production of insulin, or an ineffective release of biologically active insulin molecules, or a release of an insufficient number of biologically active insulin molecules, or an insufficient production of cell-surface receptors, or a production of

373

ineffective cell-surface receptors, or a production of ineffective insulin molecules that are unable to interact properly with insulin receptors on cells to produce the required biologic effect. Type One diabetes requires administration of exogenous insulin. The traditional approach to Type Two diabetes has generally first been to adjust the diet to limit the caloric intake the individual consumes. Exercise is used as an initial approach to both Type One and Type Two diabetes as a means of up-regulating the utilization of fats and sugar so as to reduce the amount of circulating plasma glucose. When diet and exercise are inadequate in properly managing Type Two diabetes, oral medications are often introduced. The action of sulfonylureas, a commonly prescribed class of oral medication, is to stimulate the beta cells to produce additional insulin receptors and enhance the insulin receptors' response to insulin. Biguanides, another form of oral treatment, inhibit gluconeogenesis, the production of glucose in the liver, thereby attempting to reduce plasma glucose levels. Thiazolidinediones (TZDs) lower blood sugar levels by activating peroxisome proliferator-activated receptor gamma (PPAR-γ), a transcription factor, which when activated regulates the activity of various target genes, particularly ones involved in glucose and lipid metabolism. If diet, exercise and oral medications do not produce a satisfactory control of the level of blood glucose in a diabetic patient, exogenous insulin is injected into the body in an effort to normalize the amount of glucose present in the serum. Insulin, a protein, has not successfully been made available as an oral medication to date due to the fact that proteins in general become degraded when they encounter the acid environment present in the stomach.

[0051] Despite strict monitoring of blood glucose and potentially multiple doses of insulin injected throughout the day sometimes augmented with oral medications, many patients with diabetes mellitus still experience devastating adverse effects from elevated blood glucose levels. Microvascular damage and elevated tissue sugar levels contribute to such complications as renal failure, retinopathy involving the eyes, neuropathy, and accelerated heart disease despite aggressive efforts to maintain the blood sugar within the physiologic normal range using exogenous insulin by itself or a combination of exogenous insulin and one or more oral medications. Diabetes remains the number one cause of renal failure in this country. Especially in diabetic patients that are dependent upon administering exogenous insulin into their body, though dosing of the insulin may be four or more times a day and even though this may produce adequate control of the blood glucose level to prevent the clinical symptoms of hyperglycemia; this does not unerringly supplement the body's natural capacity to monitor the blood sugar level minute to minute, twenty-four hours a day, and deliver an immediate response to a rise in blood glucose by the release of insulin from beta cells as required. The deleterious effects of diabetes may still evolve despite strict and persistent exogenous control of the glucose level in the blood stream.

[0052] The strategy to treat obesity has been founded in encouraging the overweight individual to diet and exercise. When the traditional approach does not suffice and the patient is severely overweight, the strategy may take the form of surgically altering the size of the stomach to physically limit the consumption of food. All three approaches may be successful, but often there exists restrictions, which limit the use or success of these strategies.

[0053] Both obesity and weight related diabetes are to some effect related to a decline in the metabolism in the body, as a person ages. As mentioned previously, it has been identified that in individuals between the ages of 35 to 50 years old, the energy production generated by the mitochondria in human cells declines by 50%. Between the ages of 65 to 90 years old, energy production by the mitochondria declines by another 39%. Certainly if the energy supplied to human cells is reduced by such drastic percentages, this in part contributes to a decline in the overall metabolic rate of the cell and the body in general.

[0054] If a patient consumes a diet comprised of relatively the same amount of calories during their youth as they do in their middle age years and the utilization of the consumed sugar declines due to a significant decrease in the function of the mitochondria, the body has no alternative but to store the excess sugar and convert it to fat, thus resulting in the medical state of obesity. When the serum glucose level exceeds the upper limit for the normal range due to both a lack of adequate insulin production and a decline in glucose utilization by the mitochondria, diabetes emerges as a result.

[0055] The current treatment of diabetes may be augmented by the unique approach to utilizing modified viruses as vehicles to transport biologically active messenger ribonucleic acids (mRNA) coded to facilitate the manufacture of insulin receptors and the enzymes required to conduct the processes of glycolysis, the tricarboxylic acid cycle, oxidative phosphorylation and anaerobic respiration.

[0056] Viruses are obligate parasites. Viruses simply represent a carrier of genetic material and by themselves viruses are unable to replicate or carry on any form of biologic function outside their host cell. Viruses are generally comprised of one or more shells constructed of one or more layers of protein or lipid material, and inside the outer shell or shells, a virus carries a genetic payload that represents the instruction code necessary to replicate the virus, and protein enzymes to help facilitate the genetic payload in the function of replicating copies of the virus once the genetic payload has been delivered to a host cell. Located on the outer shell or envelope of a virus are probes. The function of a virus's probes is to locate and engage a host cell's receptors. The virus's surface probes are designed to detect, make contact with and functionally engage one or more receptors located on the exterior of a cell type that will offer the virus the proper environment in which to construct copies of itself. A host cell is a cell that provides the virus the proper biochemical machinery for the virus to successfully replicate itself.

[0057] Protected by the outer coat generally comprised of an envelope or capsid or envelope and capsid, viruses carry a genetic payload in the form of deoxyribonucleic acid (DNA) or ribonucleic acid (RNA). Once a virus's exterior probes locate and functionally engage the surface receptor or receptors on a host cell, the virus inserts its genetic payload into the interior of the host cell. In the event a virus is carrying a DNA payload, the virus's DNA travels to the host cell's nucleus and is known to become inserted into the host cell's own native DNA. In the case where a virus is carrying its genetic payload as RNA, the virus inserts the RNA payload into the host cell and may also insert one or more enzymes to facilitate the RNA being utilized properly to replicate copies of the virus. Once inside the host cell, some species of virus facilitate their RNA being converted to DNA. Once the viral RNA has been converted to DNA, the virus's DNA travels to the host cell's nucleus and is known to become inserted into the host cell's native DNA. Once a virus's genetic material has been inserted into the host cell's native DNA, the virus's genetic material takes command of certain cell functions and redirects the resources of the host cell to generate copies of the virus. Other forms of RNA viruses bypass the need to use the host cell's nuclear DNA and simply utilize portions of its innate viral genome to act as messenger RNA (mRNA). RNA viruses that bypass the host cell's DNA, cause the cell, in general, to generate copies of the necessary parts of the virus directly from the virus's RNA genome. When a virus's genome directly acts as a template, then similar to the cell's messenger RNA, the virus's RNA is read by the cell's ribosomes and proteins necessary to complete the virus's replication process are generated.

[0058]   The Hepatitis C virus (HCV) is a positive sense RNA virus, meaning a type of RNA that is capable of bypassing the need for involving the host cell's nucleus by having its RNA genome function as messenger RNA. Hepatitis C virus infects liver cells. The Hepatitis C viral genome becomes divided once it gains access to the interior of a liver host cell. Portions of the subdivisions of the Hepatitis C viral genome directly interact with host liver cell's ribosomes to produce the proteins necessary to construct copies of the virus.

[0059] HCV belongs to the Flaviviridae family and is the only member of the Hepacivirus genus. There are considered to be at least 100 different strains of Hepatitis C virus based on genome sequencing variability.

[0060] HCV is comprised of an outer lipoprotein envelope and an internal nucleocapsid. The genetic payload is carried within the nucleocapsid. In its natural state, present on the surface of the outer envelope of the Hepatitis C virus are probes that detect receptors present on the surface of liver cells. The glycoprotein E1 probe and the glycoprotein E2 probe have been identified to be affixed to the surface of HCV. The E2 probe binds with high affinity to the large external loop of a CD81 cell-surface receptor. CD81 is found on the surface of many cell types including liver cells. Once the E2 probe has engaged the CD81 cell-surface receptor, cofactors on the surface of HCV's exterior envelope engage either or both the low density lipoprotein receptor (LDLR) or the scavenger receptor class B type I (SR-BI) present on the liver cell in order to activate the mechanism to facilitate HCV breaching the cell membrane and inserting its RNA genome payload through the plasma cell membrane of the liver cell into the liver cell. Upon successful engagement of the HCV surface probes with a liver cell's cell-surface receptors, HCV inserts the single strand of RNA and other payload elements it carries into the liver cell targeted to be a host cell. The HCV RNA genome then interacts with enzymes and ribosomes inside the liver cell in a translational process to produce the proteins required to construct copies of the protein components of HCV. The HCV genome undergoes a method of transcription to replicate copies of the virus's RNA genome. Inside the host, pieces of the HCV virus are assembled together and ultimately loaded with a copy of the HCV genome. Replicas of the original HCV then escape the host cell and migrate the environment in search of additional host liver cells to infect and continue the replication process.

[0061] The HCV's naturally occurring genetic payload consists of a single molecule of linear positive sense, single stranded RNA approximately 9600 nucleotides in length. By means of a translational process a polyprotein of approximately 3000 amino acids is generated. This polyprotein is cleaved post translation by host and viral proteases into individual viral proteins which include: the structural proteins of C, E1, E2, the nonstructural proteins NS1, NS2, NS3, NS4A, NS4B, NS5A, NS5B, p7 and ARFP/F protein. Hepatitis C virus's proteins direct the host liver cell to construct copies of the Hepatitis C virus. A membrane associated replicase complex consisting of the virus's nonstructural proteins NS3 and NS5B facilitate the replication of the viral genome. The membrane of the endoplasmic reticulum appears to be the site of protein maturation and viral assembly. Once copies of the Hepatitis C Virus are generated, they exit the host cell and each copy of HCV migrates in search of another appropriate liver cell that will act as a host to continue the replication process.

[0062] Hepatitis C virus offers a naturally occurring vehicle mechanism to transport and insert medically therapeutic messenger ribonucleic acid (mRNA) molecules into liver cells and other specifically targeted cells of the human body. The naturally occurring Hepatitis C virus already is equipped with the means of seeking out liver cells and delivering to liver cells its genetic payload. Further, the surface probes present on the Hepatitis C virus's outer protein coat can be modified to seek out specific receptors on specific target cells. Once the modified Hepatitis C virus's probes properly engage the cell-surface receptors on a target cell, the modified Hepatitis

C virus would insert into the target cell one or more medically therapeutic mRNAs for the purpose of having the target cell generate proteins to achieve a medical therapeutic response.

[0063] The Hepatitis C virus is one of several viruses that have been identified that possess the natural capacity to locate and infect liver cells with the genome the virus carries, thus including a liver cell as part of its reproductive cycle. Hepatitis A virus (HAV), Hepatitis C virus (HCV), Hepatitis D virus (HDV), Hepatitis E virus (HEV), and Hepatitis G virus (HGV) have been identified to carry their genome as RNA. The Hepatitis G virus is considered to be very similar to the Hepatitis C virus. The Hepatitis F virus and Hepatitis H viruses at this point are not considered to exist, though this is controversial. The Hepatitis B virus (HBV) is believed to carry its genome as DNA. These alternative hepatitis viruses may also be utilized to act as alternative vehicles to deliver medically therapeutic messenger RNA molecules to liver cells or specific target cells.

[0064] Current state of gene therapy generally refers to efforts directed toward inserting an exogenous subunit of DNA into a vehicle such as a virus. The vehicle is intended to insert the exogenous subunit of DNA into a target cell. The exogenous DNA subunit then migrates to the target cell's nucleus. The exogenous DNA subunit then inserts into the native DNA of the cell. This represents a permanent alteration of the cell's nuclear DNA. At some point, the nuclear transcription proteins read the exogenous DNA subunit's nucleotide coding to produce the intended cellular response. The medical device described within the scope of this text involves RNA versus DNA as a modified virus virion's payload. DNA is comprised of the nucleotides adenine, thymine, guanine and cytosine. RNA is composed of the nucleotides adenine, uracil, guanine and cytosine. DNA codes for the manufacture of RNAs, which are composed of nucleotides. RNA codes for the manufacture of proteins, which are composed of amino acids. The virus chosen as the example of a the transport vehicle, Hepatitis

C virus, is a RNA virus versus a virus that naturally carries a DNA genome.

[0065] It would seem an important element involved in the development of obesity, diabetes, lack of energy or reduced metabolism is linked to the failure of the mitochondria to properly utilize glucose to produce energy in the form of ATP.

[0066] The proteins manufactured by the ribosomes participate in the chemical reactions of glycolysis, the tricarboxylic acid cycle, oxidative phosphorylation and anaerobic respiration by acting as enzymes to catalyze these reactions or as other support proteins.

[0067] If the mitochondria's energy producing mechanisms fail to operate at an optimal level, overall cell function suffers due to a decline in the supply of available energy. Glucose may indeed be available for utilization by the mitochondria, but actual utilization rate of the glucose will be reduced if the cell's mitochondria are not functioning properly, with the result that the necessary supply of ATP molecules may not be adequate to supply the needs of the cell, thus limiting the function and survivability of the cell.

[0068] Creating a device to act as a means of correcting the cause of the decline in mitochondrial function would lead to increasing the body's utilization of glucose, which would result in a more optimal management of diabetes, obesity, the sense of fatigue some individuals experience, and the deleterious effects of the aging process.

[0069] Essential function of the mitochondrion relies on a variety of mRNAs being decoded by the ribosomes in order to the many produce proteins that act as enzymes and catalyze the biologic reactions of aerobic respiration. It does not appear that the mitochondrial DNA creates the majority of the required mRNAs to generate the enzymes required for aerobic respiration. The mRNAs are then either produced by the cell nucleus and sent to the mitochondria or the required mRNAs are created at the time a new mitochondrion is constructed. Loss of proper regulation of the chemical pathways inside the mitochondrion may be related to degradation of the necessary mRNAs. Since a significant portion of the population is obese and a significant portion of the population is diagnosed with diabetes, if the mRNAs do indeed degrade and are not adequately replenished, obesity and diabetes may be related to lack of proper function of mitochondria due to the fact that one or more mRNA molecules are not present in sufficient quantity to interact with ribosomes and thus not available to produce a sufficient quantity of the required enzymes needed to maintain the chemical pathways involved in the optimal metabolism of glucose.

[0070] A treatment of diabetes, obesity, chronic fatigue and aging may be approached by a medical device utilizing viruses as vehicles to transport biologically active mRNAs to mitochondria to bolster function of the mitochondria of all cells or possibly only certain cells in the body.

[0071] A Hepatitis C virus modified to carry a therapeutic mRNA payload could be introduced into the blood stream, travel the blood stream, engage the receptors on a liver cell with its surface probes, and then insert the genetic payload it carries into the liver cell. A genetic payload such as a quantity of messenger RNAs could be used to enhance proper protein production by cells deficient in a particular protein. In the case of a deficiency of a protein, production of a deficient protein could be enhanced by inserting a quantity of messenger RNAs into liver cells to stimulate production of the required protein. In the case of diabetes mellitus, utilizing a modified Hepatitis C virus as a vehicle, messenger RNA molecules could be inserted into liver cells, coded for any protein the liver cells are deficient in producing, with the intention of generating an adequate response to insulin and an optimal utilization of glucose.

[0072]   The utilization of positive sense messenger RNA, does not permanently alter the cell's DNA. Messenger RNAs degrade and become unusable after a time. Use of RNA as a therapeutic modality offers a therapeutic opportunity that could have a reversible or an attenuatable effect when required. Exogenous messenger RNAs could begin producing the required proteins they are coded for as soon as they are inserted into a cell; where exogenous DNA would first need to be inserted into a nuclear chromosome, then read by a polymerase molecule in order to generate an endogenous messenger RNA that would be capable of stimulating the production of a desired protein. Messenger RNA also bypasses the action of decoding the DNA and errors or deficiencies that might occur during transcription phase in the nucleus. By employing a medically therapeutic virus to carry messenger RNA to cells, deficiencies of any of the approximately 30,000 proteins that comprise the tissues that exist in the body and on the surface of the body can be successfully treated or averted.

BRIEF SUMMARY OF THE INVENTION

[0073]   The medical device by which a modified virus or virus-like structure is used as a transport medium to carry a payload of one or more messenger ribonucleic acid (RNA) molecules to cells in the body. The modified virus or virus-like structure makes contact with a specific target cell by means of the virus's exterior probes or virus-like structure's exterior probes. Once the exterior probes engage the target cell's receptors, the modified virus or virus-like structure inserts into the target cell one or more messenger ribonucleic acid (mRNA) molecules it is carrying. Messenger RNA molecules inserted into the cell act similar to native messenger RNA molecules and either interact with the cell's ribosomes in the process of protein synthesis or interacts with the cell's native enzymes and undergoes further modification until the delivered messenger RNA molecule is capable of interacting with the cell's ribosomes in the process of protein synthesis. Medical disease states such as diabetes mellitus, obesity, chronic fatigue and aging, that are the result of a deficiency of one or more proteins, can be successfully treated by utilizing viruses or virus-like structures to insert the proper messenger RNA molecules into specific cells to enhance the production of proteins that are identified as being deficient, thus correcting the deficiency. Improved utilization of glucose and optimal production of energy molecules resulting from a robust and efficient metabolism of glucose will enhance the cells' capacity to carryout life sustaining functions and lead to a healthier individual.

DETAILED DESCRIPTION

[0074] Diabetes mellitus, obesity, chronic fatigue syndrome, and aging may all be linked to the common pathway of degradation in an individual's capacity to metabolize glucose through the process of aerobic respiration. Errors in the DNA or errors that occur in the process that generates the messenger RNA or a deficiency in the number of messenger RNA or a deficiency in the number of biologically active messenger RNA results in a deficiency in cellular capacity to construct the enzymes involved in the biologic respiratory processes of glycolysis, tricarboxylic acid cycle and phosphorylation, which results in the medical conditions of diabetes mellitus, obesity, chronic fatigue and aging. Supplying the cells of the body with the means to produce sufficient quantities of biologically active enzymes to insure that the biologic respiratory processes of glycolysis, tricarboxylic acid cycle and oxidative phosphorylation occur at an optimal rate in cells would treat the medical conditions of diabetes mellitus, obesity, chronic fatigue and aging.

[0075] Viruses or virus-like structures can be fashioned to act as transport vehicles to carry and deliver messenger ribonucleic acid (mRNA) molecules to cells. The mRNA molecules carried by therapeutic viruses would supply the cells of the body with the genetic templates to construct the proteins the cell would be deficient in producing on its own.

[0076] Naturally occurring viruses can be altered by replacing the genetic material the virus would carry, with mRNA molecules that would have a beneficial medically therapeutic effect on cells. The naturally occurring virus would then carry and deliver to its natural target cell the payload of medically therapeutic mRNA molecules. As an example, Hepatitis viruses could be altered to carry medically therapeutic mRNA molecules to liver cells. The naturally occurring virus then, instead of causing disease associated with delivering its own genome to stimulate its own replication process, would instead act as a medical device to deliver a quantity of medically therapeutic mRNA molecules which would provide the target cell an enhanced capacity to generate proteins to carryout beneficial biologic processes to accomplish a medically therapeutic outcome.

[0077] Naturally occurring viruses can be further modified to have their naturally occurring glycoprotein surface probes replaced by glycogen surface probes that target specific cells in the body. Viruses modified to carry and deliver medically therapeutic mRNA molecules as the payload, further modified to have their glycoprotein surface probes, that cause the modified virus to engage specific cells in the body, provides a method whereby specific cells in the body can be targeted and this method embodies a means of providing to specific type of cell in the body an enhanced capacity to generate proteins to carryout beneficial biologic processes to accomplish a medically therapeutic outcome.

[0078] Virus-like structures can be constructed with similar physical characteristics to naturally occurring viruses and be fashioned to carry medically therapeutic mRNA molecules as the payload and have located on the surface glycoprotein probes that engage specific cells in the body. Viruses-like structures carrying medically therapeutic mRNA molecules as the payload, constructed to have their glycoprotein surface probes engage specific cells in the body, and deliver to those specific cells the mRNA the virus-like structures carry is a medical device whereby specific cells in the body can be targeted and this medical device embodies a means of providing to specific type of cell in the body an enhanced capacity to generate proteins to carryout beneficial biologic processes to accomplish a medically therapeutic outcome. The advantage of a virus-like structure is that the physical dimensions of the virus-like structure can be adjusted to accommodate variations in the physical size of the payload of medically therapeutic mRNA molecules, yet maintain a means of engaging targeted cells in the body and delivering to those targeted cells the mRNA molecules required to accomplish the desired medical therapeutic outcome. A second advantage of utilizing virus-like structures is to be able to change the surface characteristics of the transport vehicle to prevent the body's immune system from reacting to the presence of the therapeutic modified virus and destroying the modified virus before it is able to deliver the payload it carries to the cells it has been designed to target. HIV utilizes an exterior envelope comprised of the surface membrane of its host, the T-Helper cell, which acts as a disguise to fool the body's immune system detection resources. Virus-like structures could be fashioned, similar to HIV, to have as an exterior envelope a surface that resembles a cell's outer membrane in order to avoid detection by the body's immune system to improve survivability of the virus-like structure.

[0079] The Hepatitis C virus virion provides a naturally occurring specimen to illustrate the feasibility of the medical device described in this text. The Hepatitis C virus (HCV) virion is comprised of an outer lipoprotein envelope and an internal nucleocapsid. The virus's genetic payload is carried within its core, the nucleocapsid. The HCV's naturally occurring genetic payload consists of a single molecule of linear positive sense, single stranded RNA approximately 9600 nucleotides in length, which includes: the structural proteins of C, E1, E2, the nonstructural proteins NS1, NS2, NS3, NS4A, NS4B, NS5A, NS5B, p7 and ARFP/F protein. Present on the surface of the outer envelope of the Hepatitis C virus virion are probes that detect receptors present on the surface of liver cells. The glycoproteins E1 and E2 have been identified to be affixed to the surface of HCV virion. Portions of the Hepatitis C virus genome, when separated into individual pieces, behave like messenger RNA. The naturally occurring HCV virion is constructed with surface probes fashioned to recognize receptors on the surface of a liver cell. Once the naturally occurring HCV's surface probe E2 engages a liver cell's CD81 receptor, and cofactors on the surface of HCV's exterior envelope engage the low density lipoprotein receptor (LDLR) or the scavenger receptor class B type I (SR-BI) on the liver cell, the HCV virion then has the opportunity to insert its RNA genetic payload into the engaged target liver cell.

[0080]   The Hepatitis C virus virion carrying a mRNA payload, infects liver cells with its payload for the purpose of causing the now infected cell to generate a variety of proteins that will be assembled into copies resembling the original HCV virion. The copies of the HCV virion are then released from the infected cell to migrate in search of other host cells. Variations in the Hepatitis C virus are based on variations that occur in the strand of mRNA molecule the HCV virion carries as it genome. HCV virions may therefore carry differing mRNA molecules as its genetic payload and deliver these mRNA molecules to specific liver cells in the body to cause these cells to produce proteins to accomplish the task of replication of similar HCV virions.

[0081]   Replicating viruses and constructing viruses to carry DNA payloads is a form of manufacturing technology that has already been well established and is in use facilitating the concept of gene therapy. Replicating viruses and designing these viruses to carry messenger ribonucleic acid as the genetic payload would incorporate similar techniques as already proven useful in current DNA gene therapy technologies.

[0082] To carry out the process to manufacture a modified medically therapeutic Hepatitis C virus, messenger RNA that would code for the general physical outer structures of the Hepatitis C virus would be inserted into a host. The host may include devices such as a host cell or a hybrid host cell. The host may utilize DNA or RNA or a combination of genetic instructions in order to accomplish the construction of medically therapeutic modified virus virions. The DNA or messenger RNA molecules to create the medically therapeutic hepatitis virus would direct the cells to generate copies of the medically therapeutic virus carrying a medically therapeutic mRNA payload. In some cases DNA or messenger RNA would be inserted into the host that would be coded to cause the production of surface probes that would be affixed to the surface of the virus virion that would target the surface receptors on specific cells in the body other than the liver cells the Hepatitis C virus naturally targets. DNA or messenger RNA would direct the host to generate copies of the messenger RNA that would provide a therapeutic action, this medically therapeutic messenger RNA would take the place of the Hepatitis C virus's innate genome as its payload. The medical treatment form of the Hepatitis C virus carrying the medically therapeutic messenger RNA would be produced, assembled and released from a host. Virus-like structures would be generated in similar fashion using a host such as host-cells or hybrid host cells. The copies of the medically therapeutic hepatitis virus or virus-like structures, upon exiting the host, would be collected, stored and utilized as a medical treatment as necessary.

[0083] To treat the various different forms of diabetes mellitus various combinations of messenger RNA would be inserted into the host, and the host would produce copies of modified Hepatitis C virus that target liver cells and carry a genetic payload consisting of messenger RNA molecules that would consist of one or more copies of a messenger RNA that codes for the insulin receptor, the enzymes utilized in the processes of glucose metabolism including glycolysis, tricarboxylic acid cycle and oxidative phosphorylation. Depending upon the physical size of the messenger RNAs and the available space inside the modified Hepatitis C virus more than one type of messenger RNA may be packaged into a single modified Hepatitis C virus, which would produce one or more therapeutic actions in a cell. In some cases enzymes that catalyze the chemical reactions in aerobic and anaerobic respiration pathways are comprised of more than one protein molecule and would require the action of several mRNA molecules to create the physical entity of the enzyme in its entirety.

[0084] The modified Hepatitis C virus and virus-like structures would be incapable of replication on its own due to the fact that the messenger RNA that would code for the replication process to produce copies of the modified virus or virus-like structure would not be present in the modified form of the Hepatitis C virus or virus-like structure. The modified form of the Hepatitis C virus or virus-like structure would carry messenger RNA that would be coded for generating a variety of enzymes that would produce a medically therapeutic and beneficial result. Enzymes such messenger RNA would code for would include the enzymes listed in the following paragraphs.

[0085] Hexokinase (EC 2.7.1.1) also referred to as hexokinase type IV glucokinase or simply glucokinase. Hexokinase converts glucose to glucose-6-phosphate in the process of glycolysis.

[0086] Glucose-6-phosphate isomerase (EC 5.3.1.9) also known as glucose-6-phosphate isomerase. Glucose-6-phosphate isomerase is an enzyme that converts glucose-6-phosphate to fructose-6-phosphate in the process of glycolysis.

[0087] Phosphofructokinase (EC 2.7.1.11) also known as 6-phosphofructokinase. Phosphofructokinase is an enzyme that converts fructose-6-phosphate to Fructose 1,6-diphosphate in the process of glycolysis.

[0088] Fructose bisphosphate aldolase (EC 4.1.2.13), also known as aldolase. Fructose bisphosphate aldolase is an enzyme that converts fructose 1,6-diphosphate to two different entities including dihydroxyacetone 3-phosphate and glyceraldehydes 3-phosphate in the process of glycolysis.

[0089] Triose-phosphate dehydrogenase (EC 5.3.1.1). Triose-phosphate dehydrogenase is an enzyme that converts glyceraldehydes 3-phosphat to 1,3-diphosphoglycerate in the process of glycolysis.

[0090] Phosphoglycerate kinase (EC 2.7.2.3). Phosphoglycerate kinase is an enzyme that converts 1,3-diphosphoglycerate to 3-phosphoglycerate in the process of glycolysis.

[0091] Phosphoglycerate mutase (EC 5.4.2.1). Phosphoglycerate mutase is an enzyme that converts 3-phosphoglycerate to 2-phosphoglycerate in the process of glycolysis.

[0092] Enolase (EC 4.2.1.11). Enolase is an enzyme that converts 2-phosphoglycerate to phosphoenolpyruvate in the process of glycolysis.

[0093] Pyruvate kinase (EC 2.7.2.3). Pyruvate kinase is an enzyme that converts phosphoenolpyruvate to pyruvate in the process of glycolysis.

[0094] Pyruvate dehydrogenase is comprised of three units. The three units include E1 (EC 1.2.4.1), (EC 1.2.1.51), E2 dihydrolipoamide S-acetyltransferase (EC 2.3.1.12), and E3 dihydrolipoamide dehydrogenase (EC 1.8.1.4). Pyruvate dehydrogenase molecular complex catalyzes the conversion of pyruvate to acetyl-CoA.

[0095] Citrate synthetase (EC 4.1.3.7). Citrate synthetase is an enzyme that converts acetyl-CoA combines with oxaloacetate to produce citrate in the tricarboxylic acid cycle.

[0096] Aconitase (EC 4.2.1.3). Aconitase is an enzyme that converts citrate to cis-aconitate in the tricarboxylic acid cycle. Aconitase is an enzyme that converts cis-aconitate to iso-citrate in the tricarboxylic acid cycle.

[0097] Isocitrate dehydrogenase (EC 1.1.1.41). Isocitrate dehydrogenase is an enzyme that converts isocitrate to alpha-ketoglutaric acid in the tricarboxylic acid cycle.

[0098] 2-oxoglutarate dehydrogenase is protein complex comprised of three units. The three units include E1 (EC 1.2.4.2), E2 (EC 2.3.1.61), and E3 (EC 1.8.1.4). 2-oxoglutarate dehydrogenase is an enzyme complex that converts alpha-ketoglutaric to succinyl-CoA in the tricarboxylic acid cycle.

[0099] Succinyl-CoA synthetase (EC 6.2.1.5). Succinyl-CoA synthetase is an enzyme that converts succinyl CoA to succinate in the tricarboxylic acid cycle.

[0100] Succinate dehydrogenase (EC 1.3.5.1). Succinate dehydrogenase is an enzyme that converts succinate to fumarate in the tricarboxylic acid cycle.

[0101] Fumarate hydratase (EC 4.2.1.2). Fumarate hydratase is an enzyme that converts fumarate to malate in the tricarboxylic acid cycle.

[0102] Malate dehydrogenase (EC 1.1.1.37). Malate dehydrogenase is an enzyme that converts malate to oxaloacetate in the tricarboxylic acid cycle.

[0103] NADH dehydrogenase (EC 1.6.5.3) molecule, also referred to as NADH-coenzyme Q oxidoreductase or complex I, is utilized in oxidative phosphorylation.

[0104] Succinate dehydrogenase (EC 1.3.5.1) molecule, also referred to as succinate oxidoreductase or complex II, is utilized in oxidative phosphorylation.

[0105] Cytochrome-c reductase (EC 1.10.2.2) molecule, also referred to as complex III, is utilized in oxidative phosphorylation.

[0106] Cytochrome-c oxidase (EC 1.9.3.1) molecule, also referred to as complex IV, is utilized in oxidative phosphorylation.

[0107] ATP synthase (EC 3.6.1.34) molecule is utilized in oxidative phosphorylation.

[0108] Lactate dehydrogenase (EC 1.1.1.27) molecule is utilized to convert pyruvate to lactic acid in anaerobic respiration.

[0109] In review, the medical device described in this text includes taking a naturally occurring virus and altering its payload so that it transports medically therapeutic messenger RNA to cells it was naturally designed to infect, but instead of delivering its own genetic payload, it delivers the medically therapeutic messenger RNA it is carrying so that those cells may benefit from being able to produce protein molecules the messenger RNA are coded for, and the medical device described in this text includes taking a naturally occurring virus and altering its payload so that it carries medically therapeutic messenger RNA to cells and alter the virus's glycoprotein probes so that it is capable of infecting specifically targeted cells, but instead of delivering its own genetic payload, it delivers to specific cells the medically therapeutic messenger RNA it is carrying so that those cells may benefit from being able to produce protein molecules the messenger RNA is coded for, <u>and</u> the medical device described in this text includes taking a virus-like structure, which carries medically therapeutic messenger RNA to cells, affixed to the surface glycoprotein probes so that it is capable of delivering medically therapeutic messenger RNA it is carrying to specific target cells so that those cells may benefit from being able to produce protein molecules the messenger RNA is coded for once the messenger RNA is delivered to the specific cells. Diabetes mellitus, obesity, chronic fatigue, and aging may all be linked to the vital process of glucose metabolism and aerobic respiration. Providing the body with the means of maintaining an optimum level of glucose metabolism and conducting aerobic respiration, in some cases anaerobic respiration, may provide the means to effectively manage the above-mentioned four major health conditions.

[0110] As mentioned above, the medical device to improve the current glucose management to enhance the treatment diabetes mellitus, a quantity of modified virus virions, such as modified Hepatitis C virus virions or virus-like structures would be introduced into a patient's blood stream or tissues so that the modified virus could deliver the medically therapeutic mRNA payload that it carries to targeted cells in the body, such as liver cells. Once the modified virus virions insert their medically therapeutic payload consisting of messenger RNA into the cell the modified virus virion has been targeted for the cell's biologic function of producing insulin receptors or metabolizing glucose by way of glycolysis, tricarboxylic acid cycle, oxidative phosphorylation or anaerobic respiration are to be enhanced. Improvement in the metabolism of glucose inside cells will reduce circulating levels of glucose in the blood stream and decrease a patient's likelihood of diabetes mellitus.

[0111] As mentioned above, the medical device to improve the current glucose management to enhance the treatment obesity, a quantity of modified virus virions, such as modified Hepatitis

C virus virions or virus-like structures, would be introduced into a patient's blood stream or tissues so that the modified virus could deliver the medically therapeutic mRNA payload that it carries to targeted cells in the body, such as liver cells. Once the modified virus virions insert their medically therapeutic payload consisting of messenger RNA into the cell the modified virus virion has been targeted for, the cell's biologic function of producing insulin receptors or metabolizing glucose by way of glycolysis, tricarboxylic acid cycle, oxidative phosphorylation or anaerobic respiration are to be enhanced. Improvement in the metabolism of glucose inside cells will reduce circulating levels of glucose in the blood stream and decrease a patient's likelihood of obesity by increasing the cellular consumption of glucose and fats.

[0112]   As mentioned above, the medical device to improve the current glucose management so as to enhance the treatment chronic fatigue, a quantity of modified virus virions, such as modified Hepatitis C virus virions or virus-like structures, would be introduced into a patient's blood stream or tissues so that the modified virus could deliver the medically therapeutic mRNA payload that it carries to targeted cells in the body, such as muscle cells. Once the modified virus virions insert their medically therapeutic payload consisting of messenger RNA into the targeted cells, the cells' biologic function of producing insulin receptors or metabolizing glucose by way of glycolysis, tricarboxylic acid cycle, oxidative phosphorylation or anaerobic respiration are to be enhanced. Improvement in the metabolism of glucose inside cells will increase the production of ATP, the result of which will be increasing the available energy resources cells have to conduct biologic processes inside the cell, which will lead to less fatigue in patients.

[0113]   As mentioned above, the medical device to improve the current glucose management so as to enhance the treatment aging, a quantity of modified virus virions, such as modified Hepatitis C virus virions or virus-like structures, would be introduced into a patient's blood stream or tissues so that the modified virus could deliver the medically therapeutic mRNA payload that it carries to targeted cells in the body, such as chondrocytes, cells responsible for the production of cartilage on the joint surfaces of bone. Once the modified virus virions insert their medically therapeutic payload consisting of messenger RNA into the targeted cells, the cells' biologic function of producing insulin receptors or metabolizing glucose by way of glycolysis, tricarboxylic acid cycle, oxidative phosphorylation or anaerobic respiration are to be enhanced. Improvement in the metabolism of glucose inside cells will increase the production of ATP, the result of which will be increasing the available energy resources cells have to conduct biologic processes inside the cell, which will lead to a decline in the failure rate of cells in the body which will forestall and may reverse the process of aging in patients.

[0114] By utilizing the described medical device to provide the cells of the body with the above-mentioned medically therapeutic messenger RNA molecules and enhancing the capacity of cells to carry out the biologic processes of glycolysis, tricarboxylic acid cycle, oxidative phosphorylation and anaerobic respiration, will result in an efficient means to control the glucose levels in the blood stream and utilize glucose to produce energy molecules such as ATP molecules in the cells of the body, such as liver cells, on a constant and persistent basis by utilizing innate regulatory mechanisms, will result in effectively managing diabetes mellitus, obesity, chronic fatigue and aging for the betterment of the medical care of patients.

CLAIMS: Reserved.

APPENDIX C:
Patent Applications for Innovative Means for Intervention in Heart Attacks, Stroke, Diabetic Crisis, and Cancer

C1: METHOD FOR TREATING HEART ATTACKS, STROKES AND DIABETIC CRISIS BY UTILIZING MODIFIED VIRUS VIRIONS TO INSERT NECESSARY PROTEIN MOLECULES AND VITAL NUTRIENTS INTO TARGETED CELLS

INDIVIDUALS REQUESTING PATENT: Dr. Lane B. Scheiber, ScD and Dr. Lane B. Scheiber II, MD

NUMBER OF CLAIMS: 3 independent claims, 15 dependent claims

ABSTRACT

The common link between incurring a heart attack, suffering a stroke or diabetic crisis is related to deficiencies involving a body's metabolism of glucose and the ability to optimally conduct the necessary biologic processes of aerobic respiration to produce energy molecules. Utilizing a medical treatment method comprised of a modified form of virus to deliver to cells in the body the protein molecules and nutrients needed to enhance the processes of glycolysis, the tricarboxylic acid cycle, oxidative phosphorylation and anaerobic respiration will save lives. Providing an alternative means for brain cells and heart muscle cells to have access to proteins, nutrients such as glucose and oxygen, and energy molecules by providing these tissues with viruses that carry these vital elements to these tissues will greatly improve the survivability of individuals experiencing a heart attack, a stroke or a diabetic crisis.

BACKGROUND OF THE INVENTION

Field of the Invention

Any medical treatment method intended to correct a protein or nutrient deficiency in the body by utilizing a modified virus to insert a quantity of protein molecules or a quantity of nutrient molecules into one or more cells of the body.

Description of Background Art

[0001] The medical conditions where a heart attack or a stroke occurs generally is associated with or the result of a lack of sufficient supply of oxygenated blood to the heart in the case of a heart attack or to the brain in case of a stroke. One of the vital functions of blood is to act as the vehicle, by way of hemoglobin residing in the red blood cells that circulate in blood, to carry oxygen to the tissues where individual cells can utilize the oxygen for the purpose of aerobic respiration. Other important functions of blood include supplying the body's cells with nutrients such as glucose and the removal of waste products such as carbon dioxide from cells. Oxygen becomes critical as demonstrated in the brain, where at a normal body temperature, brain cells cannot be without a sufficient supply of oxygen for more than five minutes before irreversible damage to brain cells begins to occur. Other tissues in the body, including heart cells, demonstrate a chronic need for an adequate supply of oxygen, and when not enough oxygen is supplied to the tissues of the body, damage occurs to those cells. If an ample amount of oxygen is unable to reach and nourish cells in the body in a timely fashion, cells die for lack of being able to generate a sufficient amount of energy to sustain life.

[0002] Oxygen and glucose are two vital consumable nutrients that provide all cells in the body the raw materials to generate energy in the form of adenosine triphosphate (ATP). ATP is the common energy medium used throughout the cell, and in all cells of the body, to power the biologic processes that sustain life in the cell. Both oxygen and glucose are transported by the blood to the cells of the body. Inside the cell, glucose is transformed by the biologic process of glycolysis into pyruvate. For generation of maximum number of ATP molecules from the parent molecule glucose, pyruvate then is metabolized by the tricarboxylic acid cycle and oxidative phosphorylation. Oxygen is vital participant in oxidative phosphorylation. When sufficient oxygen is available to the cell, by means of aerobic respiration one glucose molecule can yield 36 ATP molecules in nerve and muscle cells, as many as 38 ATP molecules in liver and heart cells. In circumstances where an insufficient amount of oxygen is available to the cell, pyruvate is diverted to an anaerobic respiration process and is converted to lactic acid by the enzyme lactate dehydrogenase. The conversion of pyruvate to lactic acid yields 2 ATP molecules.

[0003] Diabetic crisis occurs due to cells not being able to sufficiently utilize circulating glucose. The level of glucose rises in the blood due to the cells not being capable of adequately transporting glucose efficiently from the blood into cells, resulting in the cells of the body not being able to efficiently process the glucose through aerobic respiration including glycolysis, tricarboxylic acid cycle and oxidative phosphorylation to produce energy molecules.

[0004]   A method of treatment to reduce damage to cells at times when there exits a state where a lack of sufficient aerobic respiration threatens the health of cells due to an adequate supply of oxygenated blood, such as a heart attack, stroke or diabetic crisis, is to optimize the overall respiration process or increase the anaerobic respiration process or provide an alternate means to supply the vital nutrients such as oxygen and glucose or energy molecules to the cells being threatened. The respiration process is comprised of a chain of biologic reactions that occur due to the presence of enzymes that catalyze the reactions.   Increasing the number of available enzymes that would participate in the respiration process would help to maximize the utilization of glucose in cells that are stressed.

[0005]   For aerobic respiration, which is dependent upon the presence of both oxygen and glucose, increasing only the number of enzymes would force a utilization of all available oxygen and glucose inside the cell, but aerobic respiration would cease once the consumable nutrients were utilized. Two options to optimize survival of cells threatened by a lack of sufficient oxygen supplied by blood are to increase the efficiency of a means of producing energy that is not dependent upon oxygen, therefore increase the output of the anaerobic respiratory process inside the threatened cells, or provide an alternative means of supplying the cells with oxygen and glucose or energy molecules. Supplying cells cut off from a supply of oxygenated blood, with an alternative supply of energy molecules, could sustain such threatened cells until the deficiency in the supply of oxygenated blood is corrected.

[0006]   A method of optimizing the respiratory process inside cells would be to utilize modified virus virions as a vehicle to transport necessary enzymes, nutrients such as oxygen and glucose molecules and even energy molecules to cells threatened by a lack of oxygen during periods of crisis such in the event of a heart attack, stroke or diabetic crisis.

[0007]   A virus is an obligate parasite. A virus is comprised of generally one or two shells, glycoprotein probes affixed to the outermost shell, one or more genetic material and in some cases enzymes to assist in the replication process are carried in the core of the virus.   An intact, individual form of a virus, as it exists outside the boundaries of a host cell, is generally referred to as a 'virion'.

[0008]   Glucose, a six-carbon molecule, represents a form of sugar. Glucose is absorbed by the cells of the body through passive diffusion and is converted to energy by the biologic processes of glycolysis, the tricarboxylic acid (TCA) cycle and oxidative phosphorylation. Insulin, a protein, facilitates the absorption of glucose into cells. Normal range for blood glucose in humans is generally defined as a fasting blood plasma glucose level of between 70 to 110 mg/dl.

[0009]   Glucose generally enters the body and then the blood stream as a result of the digestion of food. For purposes of this description, 'blood' and 'blood stream' refer to the same substance, which is generally considered to be blood as a whole including plasma and blood cells. The beta cells of the Islets of Langerhans continuously sense the level of glucose in the blood and respond to elevated levels of blood glucose by secreting insulin into the blood. Beta cells produce the protein 'insulin' in the endoplasmic reticulum and store the insulin in vacuoles until the insulin is needed. When beta cells detect an increase in the glucose level in the blood, the beta cells release insulin into the blood plasma from said storage vacuoles.

[0010]   Insulin is a protein; proteins are comprised of amino acids. An insulin molecule consists of two chains of amino acids, an alpha chain and a beta chain, linked by two disulfide (S-S) bridges. The alpha chain consists of 21 amino acids. The beta chain consists of 30 amino acids.

[0011] A eukaryote refers to a nucleated cell. Eukaryotes comprise nearly all animal and plant cells. A human eukaryote or nucleated cell is comprised of an exterior lipid bilayer plasma membrane, cytoplasm, a nucleus, and organelles. The exterior plasma membrane defines the perimeter of the cell, regulates the flow of nutrients, water and regulating molecules in and out of the cell, and has embedded into its structure cell-surface receptors that the cell uses to detect properties of the environment surrounding the cell membrane. Cytoplasm refers to the entire contents inside the cell except for the nucleus and acts as a filling medium inside the boundaries of the plasma cell membrane. Cytosol refers to the semifluid portion of the cytoplasm minus the mitochondria and the endoplasmic reticulum. The nucleus, organelles, and ribosomes are suspended in the cytosol. Nutrients such as amino acids, oxygen and glucose are present in the cytosol. The nucleus contains the majority of the cell's genetic information in the form of double stranded deoxyribonucleic acid (DNA). Organelles generally carry out specialized functions for the cell and include such structures as the mitochondria, the endoplasmic reticulum, storage vacuoles, lysosomes and Golgi complex. Floating in the cytoplasm, but also located in the endoplasmic reticulum and mitochondria are ribosomes. Ribosomes are protein structures comprised of several strands of proteins that combine and couple to a messenger ribonucleic acid (mRNA) molecule. More than one ribosome may be attached to a single mRNA at a time. Ribosomes decode genetic information coded in a mRNA molecule and manufacture proteins to the specifications of the instruction code physically present in the mRNA molecule.

[0012] The majority of the deoxyribonucleic acid (DNA) in a cell is present in the form of chromosomes, the double stranded helical structures located in the nucleus of the cell. DNA in a circular form, can also be found in the mitochondria, the powerhouse of the cell, an organelle that assists in converting glucose into usable energy molecules. DNA represents the genetic information a cell needs to manufacture the materials it requires to develop to its mature form, sustain life and to replicate. Genetic information is stored in the DNA by arrangements of four nucleotides referred to as: adenine, thymine, guanine and cytosine. DNA represents instruction coding, that in the process known as transcription, the DNA's genetic information is decoded by transcription protein complexes referred to as polymerases, to produce ribonucleic acid (RNA). RNA is a single strand of genetic information comprised of coded arrangements of four nucleotides: adenine, uracil, guanine and cytosine. The physical difference in the construction of a DNA molecule versus an RNA molecule is that DNA utilizes the nucleotide 'thymine', while RNA molecules utilize the nucleotide 'uracil'. RNAs are generally classified as messenger RNAs (mRNA), transport RNAs (tRNA) and ribosomal RNAs (rRNA).

[0013] Mitochondrion ('mitochondria' pleural form) is a cellular organelle that is considered the energy producing organelle of the cell. Mitochondria assist in generating energy for cell metabolism by producing ATP molecules from glucose. Within the cytoplasm and outer wall of the mitochondria sugar molecules undergo the process of glycolysis, and then inside the mitochondria byproducts of glucose are further broken down in the tricarboxylic acid (TCA) cycle and by oxidative phosphorylation to useable energy molecules.

[0014] The exterior of a mitochondrion is known as an external membrane. Inside the outer membrane is an inner membrane. Folds in the inner membrane create crista, which expands the surface of the inner membrane and enhances the mitochondrion's ability to create the energy molecules referred to as adenosine triphosphate molecules or ATP molecules. Inside the inner membrane is the mitochondrion matrix. The mitochondrion matrix contains a highly concentrated mixture of enzymes, ribosomes, tRNA and mitochondrial DNA. Glycolysis occurs in the cytosol of the cell and membrane of the mitochondrion. The tricarboxylic acid cycle functions within the inner chambers and matrix of the mitochondrion. Oxidative phosphorylation occurs within the outer and inner membranes of the mitochondrion.

[0015] Many of the intermediates of the processes of glycolysis and the tricarboxylic acid cycle exist as anions at the pH found in cells, and readily associate with H^+ to form acids. The intermediates of glycolysis and the tricarboxylic acid cycle are therefore often written as either an anion or an acid. For the purposes of this description, the intermediates of the processes of glycolysis and the tricarboxylic acid cycle are generally written as anions (as an example pyruvate versus pyruvic acid).

[0016] As a result of the biochemical process of glycolysis during aerobic (oxygen sufficiently available) respiration conditions glucose is converted to pyruvate. The abbreviated processes of glycolysis include: (1) Glucose is converted to glucose-6-phosphate by the enzyme 'hexokinase'. (2) Glucose-6-phosphate is converted to fructose-6-phosphate by the enzyme 'glucose-6-phosphate isomerase'. (3) Fructose-6-phosphate is converted to fructose 1,6-diphosphate by the enzyme 'phosphofructo kinase'. (4) Fructose 1,6-diphosphate is converted to two different entities including dihydroxyacetone-3-phosphate and glyceraldehydes-3-phosphate by the enzyme 'fructose bisphosphate aldolase'. (5) Dihydroacetone-3-phosphate converts to D-glyceraladehyde-3-phosphate by the enzyme 'triose-phosphate isomerase'. (6) Glyceraldehyde-3-phosphate is converted to 1,3-diphosphoglycerate by the enzyme 'glyceraldehyde-3-phosphate dehydrogenase'. (7) 1,3-diphosphoglycerate is converted to 3-phosphoglycerate by the enzyme 'phosphoglycerate kinase'. (8) 3-phosphoglycerate is converted to 2-phosphoglycerate by the enzyme 'phosphoglycerate mutase'. (9) 2-phosphoglycerate is converted to phosphoenolpyruvate by the enzyme 'enolase'. (10) Phosphoenolpyruvate is converted to pyruvate by the enzyme complex referred to as 'pyruvate kinase'.

[0017] Pyruvate is then oxidized to an acetyl group, which is combined with Coenzyme A and produces acetyl Coenzyme A (acetyl-CoA). Pyruvate dehydrogenase, which metabolizes pyruvate to acetyl-CoA is comprised of a multi-enzyme complex. The three protein complexes of pyruvate dehydrogenase are designated E1 (pyruvate dehydrogenase), E2 (dihydrolipoamide S-acetyltransferase), and E3 (dihydrolipoamide dehydrogenase). Acetyl-CoA enters the tricarboxylic acid cycle. Under aerobic respiration conditions from one glucose molecule the process of glycolysis generates 8 ATP molecules, conversion of pyruvate to acetyl CoA generates an additional 6 ATP molecules.

[0018] The tricarboxylic acid cycle otherwise known as the citric acid cycle or the Krebs cycle, was discovered in 1937 by Sir Hans Krebs, and is a biochemical process that provides complete oxidation of acetyl-CoA, which may be derived from sources such as fats, carbohydrates and lipids. For purposes of this discussion, acetyl-CoA is a byproduct of glucose metabolism during glycolysis, and enters the tricarboxylic acid cycle and (1) combines with oxaloacetate (also referred to as oxaloacetic acid) by the action of the enzyme 'citrate synthetase' which produces citrate (also referred to as citric acid).   (2) Citrate is converted to cis-aconitate (also referred to as cis-aconitic acid) per the enzyme 'aconitase'. (3) Cis-aconitate is converted to iso-citrate (also referred to as isocitric acid) again by the enzyme aconitase. (4) Iso-citrate is converted to alpha-ketoglutarate (also referred to as alpha-ketoglutaric acid) by the enzyme 'isocitrate dehydrogenase'. (5) Alpha-ketoglutarate is converted to succinyl CoA by the enzyme '2-oxoglutarate dehydrogenase'. (6) Succinyl CoA is converted to succinate (also referred to as succinic acid) by the enzyme 'succinyl-CoA synthetase'. (7) Succinate is converted to fumarate (also referred to as fumaric acid) by the enzyme 'succinate dehydrogenase'. (8) Fumarate is converted to malate (also referred to as malic acid) by the enzyme 'fumarate hydratase'. (9) Malate is converted to oxaloacetate by the enzyme 'malate dehydrogenase'.   The result of metabolism of glucose by glycolysis and the tricarboxylic acid cycle yields ATP molecules and electron donor molecules such as the reduced form of the coenzyme nicotinamide adenine dinucleotide written NADH +H$^+$. The tricarboxylic acid cycle also produces electron donor molecules in the form of the reduced co-enzyme flavin adenine dinucleotide written FADH$_2$.

[0019]   Oxidative phosphorylation is a metabolic pathway that uses energy released by oxidation to produce adenosine triphosphate (ATP) molecules.   During oxidative phosphorylation electrons are transferred from electron donors to electron acceptors such as oxygen in redox reactions. In eukaryotes the redox reactions are carried out by a series of protein complexes located within mitochondria. These protein complexes represent a linked set of enzymes referred to as electron transport chains.   The protein complexes utilized in oxidative phosphorylation include nicotinamide adenine dinucleotide (NADH) dehydrogenase enzyme molecule, the succinate dehydrogenase enzyme molecule, the cytochrome-c reductase enzyme molecule, the cytochrome-c oxidase enzyme molecule, and the ATP synthase enzyme molecule. Under aerobic respiration conditions one glucose molecule metabolized by the combination of glycolysis, the tricarboxylic acid cycle and oxidative phosphorylation yields as many as 38 ATP molecules in liver and heart cells; 36 ATP molecules in some tissues such as nerve and muscle cells.

[0020]   An enzyme is a protein generated by cells that acts as a catalyst to induce chemical changes in other substances, itself remaining apparently unchanged in the process. There are several main groups of enzymes including oxidoreductase, transferase, hydrolase, lyase, isomerase, and ligase, sometimes referred to as synthetase. EC is an abbreviation for Enzyme Commission of the International Union of Biochemistry and this is used in conjunction with a unique number to define a specific enzyme identified in the Enzyme Commission's list of enzymes. Oxidoreductases generally have as their first EC identifying number, the number 1. Transferases generally have as their first EC identifying number, the number 2. Hydrolases generally have as their first EC identifying number, the number 3. Lyases generally have as their first EC identifying number, the number 4. Isomerase generally have as their first EC identifying number, the number 5. Ligases generally have as their first EC identifying number, the number 6. Several scientific names often exist to identify the same enzyme.

[0021] Enzymes (followed by their Enzyme Commission of the International Union of Biochemistry number) utilized in the metabolism of glucose in the processes of glycolysis, tricarboxylic acid cycle, and oxidative phosphorylation are described in the following paragraphs.

[0022] Hexokinase (EC 2.7.1.1), is also referred to as hexokinase type IV glucokinase or in some cases simply glucokinase. Hexokinase converts glucose to glucose-6-phosphate in glycolysis.

[0023] Glucose-6-phosphate isomerase (EC 5.3.1.9), is also known as phosphoglucoisomerase. Glucose-6-phosphate isomerase is an enzyme that converts glucose-6-phosphate to fructose-6-phosphate in glycolysis.

[0024] 6-phosphofructokinase (EC 2.7.1.11), is also known as phosphofructokinase. 6-phosphofructokinase is an enzyme that converts fructose-6-phosphate to fructose 1,6-diphosphate in glycolysis.

[0025] Fructose bisphosphate aldolase (EC 4.1.2.13), is also known as aldolase. Fructose bisphosphate aldolase is an enzyme that converts fructose 1,6-diphosphate to two different entities including dihydroxyacetone 3-phosphate and glyceraldehydes 3-phosphate in glycolysis.

[0026] Triose-phosphate isomerase (EC 5.3.1.1). Triose-phosphate isomerase is an enzyme that converts dihydroacetone-3-phosphate converts to D-glyceraladehyde-3-phosphate.

[0027] Glyceraldehyde-3-phosphate dehydrogenase (EC 1.2.1.12), may be abbreviated GAPDH or G3PDH. Glyceraldehyde-3-phosphate dehydrogenase is an enzyme that converts glyceraldehydes-3-phosphatate to 1,3-diphosphoglycerate in glycolysis.

[0028] Phosphoglycerate kinase (EC 2.7.2.3). Phosphoglycerate kinase is an enzyme that converts 1,3-diphosphoglycerate to 3-phosphoglycerate in glycolysis.

[0029] Phosphoglycerate mutase (EC 5.4.2.1). Phosphoglycerate mutase is an enzyme that converts 3-phosphoglycerate to 2-phosphoglycerate in glycolysis.

[0030] Enolase (EC 4.2.1.11). Enolase is an enzyme that converts 2-phosphoglycerate to phosphoenolpyruvate in glycolysis.

[0031] Pyruvate kinase (EC 2.7.1.40). Pyruvate kinase is an enzyme that converts phosphoenolpyruvate to pyruvate in glycolysis.

[0032] Pyruvate dehydrogenase. Pyruvate dehydrogenase is comprised of three units. The three units include E1 (EC 1.2.4.1), (EC 1.2.1.51), E2 dihydrolipoamide S-acetyltransferase (EC 2.3.1.12), and E3 dihydrolipoamide dehydrogenase (EC 1.8.1.4). Pyruvate dehydrogenase molecular complex catalyzes the conversion of pyruvate to acetyl-CoA.

[0033] Citrate synthetase (EC 4.1.3.7). Citrate synthetase is an enzyme that converts acetyl-CoA combines with oxaloacetate to produce citrate in the tricarboxylic acid cycle.

[0034] Aconitase (EC 4.2.1.3). Aconitase exists in two isoenzyme forms in eukaryotes: mitochondrial and cytosolic. Aconitase is an enzyme that converts citrate to cis-aconitate in the tricarboxylic acid cycle and converts cis-aconitate to iso-citrate in the tricarboxylic acid cycle.

[0035] Isocitrate dehydrogenase (EC 1.1.1.41). Isocitrate dehydrogenase is an enzyme that converts isocitrate to alpha-ketoglutaric acid in the tricarboxylic acid cycle.

[0036] 2-oxoglutarate dehydrogenase. 2-oxoglutarate dehydrogenase is a protein complex comprised of three units. The three units include E1 (EC 1.2.4.2), E2 (EC 2.3.1.61), and E3 (EC 1.8.1.4). 2-oxoglutarate dehydrogenase is an enzyme complex that converts alpha-ketoglutaric to succinyl CoA in the tricarboxylic acid cycle.

[0037] Succinyl-CoA synthetase (EC 6.2.1.5). Succinyl-CoA synthetase is an enzyme that converts succinyl CoA to succinate in the tricarboxylic acid cycle.

[0038] Succinate dehydrogenase (EC 1.3.5.1). Succinate dehydrogenase is an enzyme that converts succinate to fumarate in the tricarboxylic acid cycle.

[0039] Fumarate hydratase (EC 4.2.1.2). Fumarate hydratase is an enzyme that converts fumarate to malate in the tricarboxylic acid cycle.

[0040] Malate dehydrogenase (EC 1.1.1.37). Malate dehydrogenase is an enzyme that converts malate to oxaloacetate in the tricarboxylic acid cycle.

[0041] During conditions were sufficient oxygen is available, metabolism of glucose generally occurs through the processes of glycolysis, tricarboxylic acid cycle, and oxidative phosphorylation. When oxygen is not readably available, anaerobic respiration occurs. The enzyme lactate dehydrogenase provides an alternative pathway to produce ATP when sufficient oxygen is not available by converting pyruvate to lactic acid. The anaerobic pathway lactate dehydrogenase catalyzes is much less efficient means of producing energy molecules than the aerobic pathway that takes advantage of oxygen dependent processes of tricarboxylic acid cycle and oxidative phosphorylation.

[0042]   Proteins are comprised of a series of amino acids bonded together in a linear strand, sometimes referred to as a chain; a protein may be further modified to be a structure comprised of one or more similar or differing strands of amino acids bonded together. A protein comprised of more than one strand of amino acids (referred to as subunits) may be referred to as a protein complex. Insulin is a protein structure comprised of two strands of amino acids, one strand comprised of 21 amino acids long and the second strand comprised of 30 amino acids; the two strands attached by two disulfide bridges. There are an estimated 30,000 different proteins the cells of the human body may manufacture. The human body is comprised of a wide variety of cells, many with specialized functions requiring unique combinations of proteins and protein structures such as glycoproteins (a protein combined with a carbohydrate) to accomplish the required task or tasks a specialized cell is designed to perform. Forms of glycoproteins are known to be utilized as cell-surface receptors.

[0043]   Messenger RNAs (mRNA) are created by transcription of DNA. Messenger RNA generated by transcription of nuclear DNA, migrate out of the nucleus of the cell, and are utilized as protein manufacturing templates by ribosomes.   Different mRNAs code for different proteins. As previously mentioned, there are as many as 30,000 varieties of proteins, therefore there are at least 30,000 different mRNA molecules. A ribosome is a protein complex that manufactures proteins by deciphering the instruction code located in a mRNA molecule. When a specific protein is needed, pieces of the ribosome complex bind around the strand of mRNA that carries the specific instruction code that will generate the required protein. The ribosome traverses the mRNA strand and deciphers the genetic information coded into the sequence of nucleotides that comprise the mRNA molecule and generates the protein by binding together amino acids into a chain.

[0044] Viruses are obligate parasites. Viruses simply represent a carrier of genetic material and by themselves viruses are unable to replicate or carry on any form of biologic function outside their host cell. Viruses are generally comprised of one or more shells constructed of one or more layers of protein or lipid material, and inside the outer shell or shells, carries a genetic payload that represents the instruction code necessary to replicate the virus, and protein enzymes to help facilitate the genetic payload in the function of replicating copies of the virus once the genetic payload has been delivered to a host cell. Located on the outer shell or envelope of a virus are probes. The function of a virus's probes is to locate and engage a host cell's receptors. The virus's surface probes are designed to detect, make contact with and functionally engage one or more receptors located on the exterior of a cell type that will offer the virus the proper environment in which to construct copies of itself. A host cell is a cell that provides the virus the proper biochemical machinery for the virus to successfully replicate itself.

[0045] Protected by the outer coat generally comprised of an envelope or capsid or envelope and capsid, viruses carry a genetic payload in the form of deoxyribonucleic acid (DNA) or ribonucleic acid (RNA). Once a virus's exterior probes locate and functionally engage the surface receptor or receptors on a host cell, the virus inserts its genetic payload into the interior of the host cell. In the event a virus is carrying a DNA payload, the virus's DNA travels to the host cell's nucleus and is known to become inserted into the host cell's own native DNA. In the case where a virus is carrying its genetic payload as RNA, the virus inserts the RNA payload into the host cell and may also insert one or more enzymes to facilitate the RNA being utilized properly to replicate copies of the virus. Once inside the host cell, some species of virus facilitate their RNA being converted to DNA. Once the viral RNA has been converted to DNA, the virus's DNA travels to the host cell's nucleus and is known to become inserted into the host cell's native DNA. Once a virus's genetic material has been inserted into the host cell's native DNA, the virus's genetic material takes command of certain cell functions and redirects the resources of the host cell to generate copies of the virus. Other forms of RNA viruses bypass the need to use the host cell's nuclear DNA and simply utilize portions of its viral genome to act as messenger RNA (mRNA). RNA viruses that bypass the host cell's DNA, cause the cell, in general, to generate copies of the necessary parts of the virus directly from the virus's RNA genome.

[0046] The Hepatitis C virus (HCV) is a positive sense RNA virus, meaning a type of RNA that is capable of bypassing the need for involving the host cell's nucleus by having its RNA genome function as messenger RNA. Hepatitis C virus infects liver cells. The Hepatitis C viral genome becomes divided once it gains access to the interior of a liver host cell. Portions of the subdivisions of the Hepatitis C viral genome directly interact with host liver cell's ribosomes to produce proteins necessary to construct copies of the virus.

[0047] HCV belongs to the Flaviviridae family and is the only member of the Hepacivirus genus. There are considered to be at least 100 different strains of Hepatitis C virus based on genome sequencing variability.

[0048] HCV is comprised of an outer lipoprotein envelope and an internal nucleocapsid. The genetic payload is carried within the nucleocapsid. In its natural state, present on the surface of the outer envelope of the Hepatitis C virus are probes that detect receptors present on the surface of liver cells. The glycoprotein E1 probe and the glycoprotein E2 probe have been identified to be affixed to the surface of HCV. The E2 probe binds with high affinity to the large external loop of a CD81 cell-surface receptor. CD81 is found on the surface of many cell types including liver cells. Once the E2 probe has engaged the CD81 cell-surface receptor, cofactors on the surface of HCV's exterior envelope engage either or both the low density lipoprotein receptor (LDLR) or the scavenger receptor class B type I (SR-BI) present on the liver cell in order to activate the mechanism to facilitate HCV breaching the cell membrane and inserting its RNA genome payload through the plasma cell membrane of the liver cell into the liver cell. Upon successful engagement of the HCV surface probes with a liver cell's cell-surface receptors, HCV inserts the single strand of RNA and other payload elements it carries into the liver cell targeted to be a host cell. The HCV RNA genome then interacts with enzymes and ribosomes inside the liver cell in a translational process to produce the proteins required to construct copies of the protein components of HCV. The HCV genome undergoes a method of transcription to replicate copies of the virus's RNA genome. Inside the host, pieces of the HCV virus are assembled together and ultimately loaded with a copy of the HCV genome. Replicas of the original HCV then escape the host cell and migrate the environment in search of additional host liver cells to infect and continue the replication process.

[0049] As an alternative example of how virus's function to locate their host, the Human Immunodeficiency Virus seeks out and engages its host, the T-Helper cell, by utilizing its glycoprotein 120 probe and glycoprotein 41 probe to intercept the CD4 cell-surface receptor and either the CCR5 or CXCR4 cell-surface receptor on the T-Helper cell.

[0050] The HCV's naturally occurring genetic payload consists of a single molecule of linear positive sense, single stranded RNA approximately 9600 nucleotides in length. By means of a translational process a polyprotein of approximately 3000 amino acids is generated. This polyprotein is cleaved post translation by host and viral proteases into individual viral proteins which include: the structural proteins of C, E1, E2, the nonstructural proteins NS1, NS2, NS3, NS4A, NS4B, NS5A, NS5B, p7 and ARFP/F protein. Hepatitis C virus's proteins direct the host liver cell to construction copies of the Hepatitis C virus. A membrane associated replicase complex consisting of the virus's nonstructural proteins NS3 and NS5B facilitate the replication of the viral genome. The membrane of the endoplasmic reticulum appears to be the site of protein maturation and viral assembly. Once copies of the Hepatitis C Virus are generated, they exit the host cell and each copy of HCV migrates in search of another appropriate liver cell that will act as a host to continue the replication process.

[0051] Hepatitis C virus offers a naturally occurring vehicle mechanism to transport and insert medically therapeutic protein molecules, nutrient molecules or energy molecules into liver cells and other specifically targeted cells of the human body. The naturally occurring Hepatitis C virus already is equipped with the means of seeking out liver cells and delivering to liver cells its genetic payload. Further, the surface probes present on the Hepatitis C virus's outer protein coat can be modified to seek out specific receptors on specific target cells other than liver cells. Once the modified Hepatitis C virus's probes properly engage the cell-surface receptors on a target cell, the modified Hepatitis C virus would insert into the target cell its payload of medically therapeutic protein molecules, nutrient molecules or energy molecules for the purpose of achieving a medically therapeutic response.

[0052] The Hepatitis C virus is one of several viruses that have been identified that possess the natural capacity to locate and infect liver cells with the genome the virus carries, thus including a liver cell as part of its reproductive cycle. Hepatitis

A virus (HAV), Hepatitis C virus (HCV), Hepatitis D virus (HDV), Hepatitis E virus (HEV), and Hepatitis G virus (HGV) have been identified to carry their genome as RNA. The Hepatitis G virus is considered to be very similar to the Hepatitis C virus. The Hepatitis F virus and Hepatitis H viruses at this point are not considered to exist, though this is controversial. The Hepatitis B virus (HBV) is believed to carry its genome as DNA. These alternative hepatitis viruses may also be utilized to act as alternative vehicles to deliver medically therapeutic protein molecules, nutrients or energy molecules to liver cells or specific target cells.

[0053] Current state of gene therapy generally refers to efforts directed toward inserting an exogenous subunit of DNA into a vehicle such as a virus. The vehicle is intended to insert the exogenous subunit of DNA into a target cell. The exogenous DNA subunit then migrates to the target cell's nucleus. The exogenous DNA subunit then inserts into the native DNA of the cell. This represents a permanent alteration of the cell's nuclear DNA. The nuclear transcription proteins then read the exogenous DNA subunit's nucleotide coding to generate RNA molecules to produce the intended cellular response. The approach described within the scope of this text involves protein molecules, nutrients or energy molecules versus DNA as a modified virus virion's payload. DNA is comprised of the nucleotides adenine, thymine, guanine and cytosine. RNA is composed of the nucleotides adenine, uracil, guanine and cytosine. DNA codes for the manufacture of RNAs, which are composed of nucleotides. Messenger RNAs code for the manufacture of proteins, which are composed of amino acids. Transport RNAs transport single amino acids to ribosomes. Ribosome RNAs assist with the construction of ribosomes. Proteins are comprised of amino acids. Oxygen is an element. Glucose is a sugar molecule. Energy molecules such as adenosine triphosphate are nucleotide that acts as an energy source. Protein molecules, oxygen, glucose and adenosine triphosphate are physically and functionally different than DNA.

[0054] If the mitochondria's energy producing mechanisms fail to operate at an optimal level, overall cell function suffers due to a decline in the supply of available energy. Glucose may indeed be available for utilization by the mitochondria, but actual utilization rate of the glucose will be reduced if the cell's mitochondria are not functioning properly, with the result being the necessary supply of ATP molecules may not be available for the cell to function properly as required.

[0055] A Hepatitis C virus modified to carry therapeutic protein molecules could be introduced into the blood stream, travel the blood stream, engage the receptors on a liver cell with its surface probes, and then insert the protein molecules it carries as a payload into the liver cells. A payload consisting of a quantity of protein molecules could be used to enhance cellular biochemical reactions in liver cells deficient in a particular protein. Hepatitis C viruses could be further modified to not only carry protein molecules instead of its own RNA genome, but also modified such that the surface probes of the Hepatitis C virions are altered to seek out and engage the surface-receptors on specific cells in the body. Modified Hepatitis C virus virions could be fashioned to deliver medically therapeutic protein molecules, nutrient molecules and energy molecules to specific cells in the body.

[0056] Minutes may be vital to the survival of an individual suffering from a heart attack or a stroke or a diabetic crisis. When cells experience a lack of oxygenated blood such cells run the risk of incurring irreversible damage. Up until now there has been no alternative means to oxygenate cells that are becoming compromised due to a lack of supply of sufficient oxygenated blood to provide needed oxygen and glucose to cells at risk of sustaining irreversible damage to facilitate aerobic respiration in such cells. Utilizing modified virus virions to transport protein molecules, nutrients such as oxygen and glucose, or energy molecules such as ATP, offers an alternate means to relying on oxygenated blood to supply endangered cells with the resources they need to prevent irreversible damage. In cases of a stroke, a needle could be introduced into the spinal canal and viruses transporting vital proteins, nutrients, or ATP molecules could be injected through the needle. The virus virions could traverse the spinal fluid as an alternate means of reaching brain cells rather than by blood vessels and deliver to specific brain cells their payload of vital proteins, nutrients, or ATP molecules. Such an action could provide minutes to hours of life saving support to brain tissues that are in danger of irreversible damage. In the case of a serious life-threatening heart attack, a needle could be passed through the chest wall to the heart and viruses transporting vital proteins, nutrients, or ATP molecules could be injected through needle directly into heart muscle tissue. The virus virions could traverse heart tissues as an alternate means of delivering to heart cells their payload of vital proteins, nutrients, or ATP molecules. Such an action could provide minutes to hours of life saving support to heart tissues that are in danger of irreversible damage. In the case of diabetic crisis, many tissues throughout the body suffer from a dysfunction of glucose metabolism. Virus virions could be introduced into the blood stream fashioned with probes to seek out and engage the tissues of vital organs such as the brain, heart and kidneys to deliver vital proteins, nutrients, or ATP molecules to these tissues until the diabetic crisis has been resolved. In cases of severe oxygen deprivation, the method of utilizing modified viruses to transport the enzyme lactate dehydrogenase to cells in crisis could result in an increase in anaerobic respiration in such cells thus providing cells with some energy production despite a lack of oxygen, to increase their survivability.

BRIEF SUMMARY OF THE INVENTION

[0057]   A medical treatment method which involves modified virus virions to be used as a transport medium to carry a payload of medically therapeutic protein molecules, nutrient molecules or energy molecules to specific cells in the body. The modified virus virions makes contact with target cells by means of the modified virus virions' exterior probes. Once the modified virus virions' exterior probes engage the cell-surface receptors of target cells the modified virus virions inserts into the target cells their payload of medically therapeutic protein molecules, nutrient molecules or energy molecules. Medical conditions such as heart attack, stroke and diabetic crisis are a result of inadequate aerobic respiration due to a lack of oxygen or proper glucose metabolism. The method by utilizing modified virus virions to transport medically therapeutic protein molecules, nutrient molecules or energy molecules to specific cells in the body may support cells in the time of crisis and improve the survivability and functionality of such cells.

DETAILED DESCRIPTION

[0058]   The medical condition where a heart attack or a stroke occurs generally is associated with or the result of a lack of sufficient supply of oxygenated blood to the heart in the case of a heart attack or to the brain in case of a stroke. Diabetic crisis occurs due to cells not being able to sufficiently utilize circulating glucose.   All of these conditions may lead to irreversible damage to cells in the body.

[0059]   The Hepatitis C virus (HCV) is comprised of an outer lipoprotein envelope and an internal nucleocapsid. The virus's genetic payload is carried within the nucleocapsid. The HCV's naturally occurring genetic payload consists of a single molecule of linear positive sense, single stranded RNA approximately 9600 nucleotides in length, which includes: the structural proteins of C, E1, E2, the nonstructural proteins NS1, NS2,

NS3, NS4A, NS4B, NS5A, NS5B, p7 and ARFP/F protein. Present on the surface of the outer envelope of the Hepatitis C virus are probes that detect receptors present on the surface of liver cells. The glycoproteins E1 and E2 have been identified to be affixed to the surface of HCV. Portions of the Hepatitis C virus genome, when separated into individual pieces, behave like messenger RNA. Naturally occurring HCV is constructed with surface probes fashioned to recognize a receptor on the surface of a liver cell. Once the naturally occurring HCV's surface probe E2 engages a liver cell's CD81 receptor, and cofactors on the surface of HCV's exterior envelope engage the low density lipoprotein receptor (LDLR) or the scavenger receptor class B type I (SR-BI) on the liver cell, HCV then has the opportunity to insert its RNA genetic payload into the engaged target liver cell. The Human Immunodeficiency Virus seeks out and engages its host, the T-Helper cell, by utilizing its glycoprotein 120 probe and glycoprotein 41 probe to intercept the CD4 cell-surface receptor and either the CCR5 or CXCR4 cell-surface receptor on the T-Helper cell. Modifying Hepatitis C virus virions to carry therapeutic protein molecules, nutrient molecules, or energy molecules as its payload rather than its own innate genome and modifying the Hepatitis C virus's external probes to target specific cells in the body provides a medically therapeutic method to treat individuals that may potentially suffer from a heart attack, stroke or diabetic crisis. Creating virus-like structures to carry therapeutic protein molecules, nutrient molecules, or energy molecules and constructing the virus-like structures to have affixed to their surface external probes to target specific cells in the body also provides a medically therapeutic method to treat individuals that may potentially suffer from a heart attack, stroke or diabetic crisis.

[0060] Replicating viruses and constructing viruses to carry DNA payloads is a form of manufacturing technology that has already been well established and is in use facilitating gene therapy. Replicating viruses and constructing these viruses to carry messenger ribonucleic acid as the genetic payload would incorporate similar techniques as already proven useful in current gene therapy technologies.

[0061] To carry out the process to manufacture a modified medically therapeutic Hepatitis C virus, messenger RNA that would code for the general physical outer structures of the Hepatitis C virus would be inserted into a host. The host may include devices such as a host cell or a hybrid host cell. The host may utilize DNA or RNA or a combination of genetic instructions in order to accomplish the construction of medically therapeutic modified virus virions. The DNA or messenger RNA molecules to create the medically therapeutic hepatitis virus would direct the cells to generate copies of the medically therapeutic virus carrying a medically therapeutic mRNA payload. In some cases DNA or messenger RNA would be inserted into the host that would be coded to cause the production of surface probes that would be affixed to the surface of the virus virion that would target the surface receptors on specific cells in the body other than the liver cells the Hepatitis C virus naturally targets. DNA or messenger RNA would direct the host to generate copies of the proteins that would provide a therapeutic action, these medically therapeutic proteins would take the place of the Hepatitis C virus's innate genome as its payload. DNA or messenger RNA would direct the host to generate a quantity of the nutrient molecules or energy molecules that would provide a therapeutic action, these medically therapeutic nutrient molecules or energy molecules would take the place of the Hepatitis C virus's innate genome as its payload. Alternatively, artificially, a quantity of protein molecules, nutrient molecules or energy molecules could be inserted into the host so that these medically therapeutic protein molecules, nutrient molecules or energy molecules would take the place of the Hepatitis C virus's innate genome as its payload. The medical treatment form of the Hepatitis C virus carrying the medically therapeutic messenger RNA would be produced, assembled and released from a host. Virus-like structures would be generated in similar fashion using a host such as host-cells or hybrid host cells. The copies of the medically therapeutic hepatitis virus or virus-like structures, upon exiting the host, would be collected, stored and utilized as a medical treatment as necessary.

[0062] To treat tissues suffering from a lack of oxygen in times of a heart attack or a stroke, or times where glucose metabolism is dysfunctional such as in a diabetic crisis modified Hepatitis C virus or virus-like structures could be used to transport medically therapeutic protein molecules, nutrient molecules or energy molecules to specific cells in the body to improve glucose metabolism including glycolysis, tricarboxylic acid cycle and oxidative phosphorylation or cause the cell to engage in anaerobic respiration.

[0063] The modified Hepatitis C virus or virus-like structures would be incapable of replication on its own due to the fact that the messenger RNA that a naturally occurring Hepatitis C virus would normally carry would not be present in the modified form of the Hepatitis C virus or virus-like structure.

[0064] The modified Hepatitis C virus virions or virus-like structures could be fashioned to carry nutrient molecules such as oxygen molecules, glucose molecules, fatty acid molecules, vitamin molecules or mineral molecules. The modified Hepatitis C virus virions or virus-like structures could be fashioned to carry energy molecules such as adenosine triphosphate molecules, adenosine diphosphate molecules, nicotinamide adenine dinucleotide molecules, reduced form of nicotinamide adenine dinucleotide molecules, flavin adenine dinucleotide molecules, or reduced form of flavin adenine dinucleotide molecules. The modified Hepatitis C virus virions or virus-like structures could be fashioned to carry enzymes such as those described in the following paragraphs.

[0065] Hexokinase (EC 2.7.1.1) also referred to as hexokinase type IV glucokinase or simply glucokinase. Hexokinase converts glucose to glucose-6-phosphate in the process of glycolysis.

[0066] Glucose-6-phosphate isomerase (EC 5.3.1.9) also known as glucose-6-phosphate isomerase. Glucose-6-phosphate isomerase is an enzyme that converts glucose-6-phosphate to fructose-6-phosphate in the process of glycolysis.

[0067] Phosphofructokinase (EC 2.7.1.11) also known as 6-phosphofructokinase. Phosphofructokinase is an enzyme that converts fructose-6-phosphate to Fructose 1,6-diphosphate in the process of glycolysis.

[0068] Fructose bisphosphate aldolase (EC 4.1.2.13), also known as aldolase. Fructose bisphosphate aldolase is an enzyme that converts fructose 1,6-diphosphate to two different entities including dihydroxyacetone 3-phosphate and glyceraldehydes 3-phosphate in the process of glycolysis.

[0069] Triose-phosphate dehydrogenase (EC 5.3.1.1). Triose-phosphate dehydrogenase is an enzyme that converts glyceraldehydes 3-phosphat to 1,3-diphosphoglycerate in the process of glycolysis.

[0070] Phosphoglycerate kinase (EC 2.7.2.3). Phosphoglycerate kinase is an enzyme that converts 1,3-diphosphoglycerate to 3-phosphoglycerate in the process of glycolysis.

[0071] Phosphoglycerate mutase (EC 5.4.2.1). Phosphoglycerate mutase is an enzyme that converts 3-phosphoglycerate to 2-phosphoglycerate in the process of glycolysis.

[0072] Enolase (EC 4.2.1.11). Enolase is an enzyme that converts 2-phosphoglycerate to phosphoenolpyruvate in the process of glycolysis.

[0073] Pyruvate kinase (EC 2.7.2.3). Pyruvate kinase is an enzyme that converts phosphoenolpyruvate to pyruvate in the process of glycolysis.

[0074] Pyruvate dehydrogenase. Pyruvate dehydrogenase is comprised of three units. The three units include E1 (EC 1.2.4.1), (EC 1.2.1.51), E2 dihydrolipoamide S-acetyltransferase (EC 2.3.1.12), and E3 dihydrolipoamide dehydrogenase (EC 1.8.1.4). Pyruvate dehydrogenase molecular complex catalyzes the conversion of pyruvate to acetyl-CoA.

[0075] Citrate synthetase (EC 4.1.3.7). Citrate synthetase is an enzyme that converts acetyl-CoA combines with oxaloacetate to produce citrate in the tricarboxylic acid cycle.

[0076] Aconitase (EC 4.2.1.3). Aconitase is an enzyme that converts citrate to cis-aconitate in the tricarboxylic acid cycle. Aconitase is an enzyme that converts cis-aconitate to iso-citrate in the tricarboxylic acid cycle.

[0077] Isocitrate dehydrogenase (EC 1.1.1.41). Isocitrate dehydrogenase is an enzyme that converts isocitrate to alpha-ketoglutaric acid in the tricarboxylic acid cycle.

[0078] 2-oxoglutarate dehydrogenase. 2-oxoglutarate dehydrogenase is protein complex comprised of three units. The three units include E1 (EC 1.2.4.2), E2 (EC 2.3.1.61), and E3 (EC 1.8.1.4). 2-oxoglutarate dehydrogenase is an enzyme complex that converts alpha-ketoglutaric to succinyl-CoA in the tricarboxylic acid cycle.

[0079] Succinyl-CoA synthetase (EC 6.2.1.5). Succinyl-CoA synthetase is an enzyme that converts succinyl CoA to succinate in the tricarboxylic acid cycle.

[0080] Succinate dehydrogenase (EC 1.3.5.1). Succinate dehydrogenase is an enzyme that converts succinate to fumarate in the tricarboxylic acid cycle.

[0081] Fumarate hydratase (EC 4.2.1.2). Fumarate hydratase is an enzyme that converts fumarate to malate in the tricarboxylic acid cycle.

[0082] Malate dehydrogenase (EC 1.1.1.37). Malate dehydrogenase is an enzyme that converts malate to oxaloacetate in the tricarboxylic acid cycle.

[0083] NADH dehydrogenase (EC 1.6.5.3) molecule, also referred to as NADH-coenzyme Q oxidoreductase or complex I, is utilized in oxidative phosphorylation.

[0084] Succinate dehydrogenase (EC 1.3.5.1) molecule, also referred to as succinate oxidoreductase or complex II, is utilized in oxidative phosphorylation.

[0085] Cytochrome-c reductase (EC 1.10.2.2) molecule, also referred to as complex III, is utilized in oxidative phosphorylation.

[0086] Cytochrome-c oxidase (EC 1.9.3.1) molecule, also referred to as complex IV, is utilized in oxidative phosphorylation.

[0087] ATP synthase (EC 3.6.1.34) molecule is utilized in oxidative phosphorylation.

[0088] Lactate dehydrogenase (EC 1.1.1.27) molecule is utilized to convert pyruvate to lactic acid in anaerobic respiration.

[0089] In review, the medical treatment method described in this text includes taking a naturally occurring virus and altering its payload so that it transports medically therapeutic protein molecules, nutrient molecules, or energy molecules to cells it was naturally designed to infect, but instead of delivering its own genetic payload, it delivers the medically therapeutic protein molecules, nutrient molecules, or energy molecules it is carrying, <u>and</u> the medical treatment method described in this text includes taking a naturally occurring virus and altering its payload so that it carries medically therapeutic protein molecules, nutrient molecules, or energy molecules and alter the virus's glycoprotein probes so that it is capable of infecting specifically targeted cells, but instead of delivering its own genetic payload, it delivers to specific cells the medically therapeutic protein molecules, nutrient molecules, or energy molecules it is carrying, <u>and</u> the medical treatment method described in this text includes taking a virus-like structure, which carries medically therapeutic protein molecules, nutrient molecules, or energy molecules, affixed to the surface glycoprotein probes so that it is capable of delivering medically therapeutic protein molecules, nutrient molecules, or energy molecules it is carrying to specific target cells to produce a beneficial medically therapeutic outcome.

[0090] As mentioned above, the medical treatment method to improve glucose metabolism during the threat of a heart attack, stroke, or diabetic crisis, involves a quantity of modified virus virions, such as modified Hepatitis C virus virions or virus-like structures that would be introduced into a patient's blood stream, or into spinal fluid, or directly into the endangered tissues so that the modified virus could deliver the medically therapeutic mRNA payload that it carries to targeted cells in the body. Once the modified virus virions or virus-like structures insert their medically therapeutic payload consisting of medically therapeutic protein molecules, nutrient molecules, energy molecules into the cells the modified virus virions or virus-like structures have been targeted for, the cells' biologic function of metabolizing glucose by way of glycolysis, tricarboxylic acid cycle, oxidative phosphorylation or anaerobic respiration will be enhanced. Improvement in the metabolism of glucose inside cells and the resultant increase in production of energy molecules will reduce the risk of irreversible damage to cells during conditions when oxygen deprivation threatens cells of the body.

CLAIMS: Reserved.

C2: METHOD FOR TREATING CANCER, RHEUMATOID ARTHRITIS AND OTHER MEDICAL DISEASES BY UTILIZING MODIFIED VIRUS VIRIONS TO INSERT MEDICATIONS INTO TARGETED CELLS

INDIVIDUALS REQUESTING PATENT: Dr. Lane B. Scheiber, ScD and Dr. Lane B. Scheiber II, MD

NUMBER OF CLAIMS: 2 independent claims, 8 dependent claims

ABSTRACT

A safer, more effective treatment of many medical diseases may be approached by a method utilizing modified viruses as vehicles to transport medically therapeutic drug molecules to specific cells in the body with the intent to have the drug exert an effect only on those cells to which the modified virus delivers the drug. The modified virus or virus-like structures make contact with specific target cells by means of the modified virus's exterior probes or virus-like structures' exterior probes. Once the exterior probes engage a target cell's receptors, the modified virus or virus-like structure inserts into the target cell the quantity of medically therapeutic drug molecules it is carrying. By delivering the medically therapeutic drug only to specific cells in the body it is assured the drug reaches the site in the body it will be most beneficial and the occurrence of unwanted side effects due the drug are significantly minimized.

BACKGROUND OF THE INVENTION

Field of the Invention

This invention relates to any medical treatment method intended to treat a medical condition in the body by utilizing a modified virus to insert a drug into specific cells of the body.

Description of Background Art

[0001] Treatment of cancer, rheumatoid arthritis and other medical conditions may be approached by a method utilizing modified virus virions as vehicles to transport medically therapeutic drugs to cells to increase the potency of the drug and significantly reduce the deleterious side effects of the drug. An intact, individual form of a virus, as it exists outside the boundaries of a host cell, is generally referred to as a 'virion'.

[0002] The current approach medical drug treatment to manage cancer generally involves administering chemotherapy to an individual afflicted with cancer. The intention of administering the chemotherapy is in theory to poison and kill the cancer cells before causing significant side effects to the individual receiving the chemotherapy. Cancer cells generally grow and multiply at a rate that is faster than normal cells. The side effects patients experience from chemotherapy is often related to the harmful effects of the chemotherapy poisoning the healthy cells of the body as well as the cancer cells.

[0003] One of the most successful approaches to the treatment of rheumatoid arthritis in the last two decades has been the use of a chemotherapy known as methotrexate. Methotrexate is administered to patients either orally or by injection. Methotrexate interferes with the folate metabolism in cells, which results in decreased cellular metabolism and inhibits cellular replication. Methotrexate tends to exert its effect on cells that are growing and multiplying faster than

427

normal. Cancer cells and in rheumatoid arthritis, synovial cells, grow and multiply at a rate that is faster than normal cellular metabolism. In rheumatoid arthritis, low dose methotrexate tends to inhibit the growth of the synovial cells that surround the joints and tendons in the body. The inhibition of synovial cell proliferation results in the disease being put into a state of remission and the crippling effects of the disease being averted.

[0004] Many drugs used to treat medical diseases have limited success and incomplete compliance by patients due to the fact that drugs often cause unwanted side effects when healthy cells suffer delirious effects of the drug. A drug introduced into the body by means of an oral route, inhaled route, rectal suppository or an injectable manner may affect every cell it comes in contact with rather than limiting its effects on the specific tissues or specific cells that the drug is intended to exert an effect on to generate a medically therapeutic outcome. Adverse side effects generated by systemic effects of drugs may be minimized by limiting the delivery of a drug to specific target cells or specific tissues in the body.

[0005] A eukaryote refers to a nucleated cell. Eukaryotes comprise nearly all animal and plant cells. A human eukaryote or nucleated cell is comprised of an exterior lipid bilayer plasma membrane, cytoplasm, a nucleus, and organelles. The exterior plasma membrane defines the perimeter of the cell, regulates the flow of nutrients, water and regulating molecules in and out of the cell, and has embedded into its structure cell-surface receptors that the cell uses to detect properties of the environment surrounding the cell membrane. Cytoplasm refers to the entire contents inside the cell except for the nucleus and acts as a filling medium inside the boundaries of the plasma cell membrane. Cytosol refers to the semifluid portion of the cytoplasm minus the mitochondria and the endoplasmic reticulum. The nucleus, organelles, and ribosomes are suspended in the cytosol. Nutrients such as amino acids, oxygen and glucose are present in the cytosol. The nucleus contains the majority of the cell's genetic information in the form of double stranded deoxyribonucleic acid (DNA). Organelles generally carry out specialized functions for the cell and include such structures as the mitochondria, the endoplasmic reticulum, storage vacuoles, lysosomes and Golgi complex. Floating in the cytoplasm, but also located in the endoplasmic reticulum and mitochondria are ribosomes. Ribosomes are protein structures comprised of several strands of proteins that combine and couple to a messenger ribonucleic acid (mRNA) molecule. More than one ribosome may be attached to a single mRNA at a time. Ribosomes decode genetic information coded in a mRNA molecule and manufacture proteins to the specifications of the instruction code physically present in the mRNA molecule.

[0006] The majority of the deoxyribonucleic acid (DNA) in a cell is present in the form of chromosomes, the double stranded helical structures located in the nucleus of the cell. DNA in a circular form, can also be found in the mitochondria, the powerhouse of the cell, an organelle that assists in converting glucose into usable energy molecules. DNA represents the genetic information a cell needs to manufacture the materials it requires to develop to its mature form, sustain life and to replicate. Genetic information is stored in the DNA by arrangements of four nucleotides referred to as: adenine, thymine, guanine and cytosine. DNA represents instruction coding, that in the process known as transcription, the DNA's genetic information is decoded by transcription protein complexes referred to as polymerases, to produce ribonucleic acid (RNA). RNA is a single strand of genetic information comprised of coded arrangements of four nucleotides: adenine, uracil, guanine and cytosine. The physical difference in the construction of a DNA molecule versus a RNA molecule is that DNA utilizes the nucleotide 'thymine', while RNA molecules utilize the nucleotide 'uracil'. RNAs are generally classified as messenger RNAs (mRNA), transport RNAs (tRNA) and ribosomal RNAs (rRNA).

[0007] Proteins are comprised of a series of amino acids bonded together in a linear strand, sometimes referred to as a chain; a protein may be further modified to be a structure comprised of one or more similar or differing strands of amino acids bonded together. A protein comprised of one or more strands of amino acids (referred to as subunits) may be referred to as a protein complex. Insulin is a protein structure comprised of two strands of amino acids, one strand comprised of 21 amino acids long and the second strand comprised of 30 amino acids; the two strands attached by two disulfide bridges. There are an estimated 30,000 different proteins the cells of the human body may manufacture. The human body is comprised of a wide variety of cells, many with specialized functions requiring unique combinations of proteins and protein structures such as glycoproteins (a protein combined with a carbohydrate) to accomplish the required task or tasks a specialized cell is designed to perform. Forms of glycoproteins are known to be utilized as cell-surface receptors.

[0008] Viruses are obligate parasites. Viruses simply represent a carrier of genetic material and by themselves viruses are unable to replicate or carry on any form of biologic function outside their host cell. Viruses are generally comprised of one or more shells constructed of one or more layers of protein or lipid material, and inside the outer shell or shells, a virus carries a genetic payload that represents the instruction code necessary to replicate the virus, and protein enzymes to help facilitate the genetic payload in the function of replicating copies of the virus once the genetic payload has been delivered to a host cell. Located on the outer shell or envelope of a virus are probes. The function of a virus's probes is to locate and engage a host cell's receptors. The virus's surface probes are designed to detect, make contact with and functionally engage one or more receptors located on the exterior of a cell type that will offer the virus the proper environment in which to construct copies of itself. A host cell is a cell that provides the virus the proper biochemical machinery for the virus to successfully replicate itself.

[0009] Protected by the outer coat generally comprised of an envelope or capsid or envelope and capsid, viruses carry a genetic payload in the form of deoxyribonucleic acid (DNA) or ribonucleic acid (RNA). Once a virus's exterior probes locate and functionally engage the surface receptor or receptors on a host cell, the virus inserts its genetic payload into the interior of the host cell. In the event a virus is carrying a DNA payload, the virus's DNA travels to the host cell's nucleus and is known to become inserted into the host cell's own native DNA. In the case where a virus is carrying its genetic payload as RNA, the virus inserts the RNA payload into the host cell and may also insert one or more enzymes to facilitate the RNA being utilized properly to replicate copies of the virus. Once inside the host cell, some species of virus facilitate their RNA being converted to DNA. Once the viral RNA has been converted to DNA, the virus's DNA travels to the host cell's nucleus and is known to become inserted into the host cell's native DNA. Once a virus's genetic material has been inserted into the host cell's native DNA, the virus's genetic material takes command of certain cell functions and redirects the resources of the host cell to generate copies of the virus. Other forms of RNA viruses bypass the need to use the host cell's nuclear DNA and simply utilize portions of its innate viral genome to act as messenger RNA (mRNA). RNA viruses that bypass the host cell's DNA, cause the cell, in general, to generate copies of the necessary parts of the virus directly from the virus's RNA genome. When a virus's genome directly acts as a template, then similar to the cell's messenger RNA, the virus's RNA is read by the cell's ribosomes and proteins necessary to complete the virus's replication process are generated.

[0010]   The Hepatitis C virus (HCV) is a positive sense RNA virus, meaning a type of RNA that is capable of bypassing the need for involving the host cell's nucleus by having its RNA genome function as messenger RNA. Hepatitis C virus infects liver cells.   The Hepatitis C viral genome becomes divided once it gains access to the interior of a liver host cell. Portions of the subdivisions of the Hepatitis C viral genome directly interact with host liver cell's ribosomes to produce proteins necessary to construct copies of the virus.

[0011]   HCV belongs to the Flaviviridae family and is the only member of the Hepacivirus genus. There are considered to be at least 100 different strains of Hepatitis C virus based on genome sequencing variability.

[0012]   HCV is comprised of an outer lipoprotein envelope and an internal nucleocapsid. The genetic payload is carried within the nucleocapsid. In its natural state, present on the surface of the outer envelope of the Hepatitis C virus are probes that detect receptors present on the surface of liver cells. The glycoprotein E1 probe and the glycoprotein E2 probe have been identified to be affixed to the surface of HCV. The E2 probe binds with high affinity to the large external loop of a CD81 cell-surface receptor. CD81 is found on the surface of many cell types including liver cells. Once the E2 probe has engaged the CD81 cell-surface receptor, cofactors on the surface of HCV's exterior envelope engage either or both the low density lipoprotein receptor (LDLR) or the scavenger receptor class B type I (SR-BI) present on the liver cell in order to activate the mechanism to facilitate HCV breaching the cell membrane and inserting its RNA genome payload through the plasma cell membrane of the liver cell into the liver cell. Upon successful engagement of the HCV surface probes with a liver cell's cell-surface receptors, HCV inserts the single strand of RNA and other payload elements it carries into the liver cell targeted to be a host cell. The HCV RNA genome then interacts with enzymes and ribosomes inside the liver cell in a translational process to produce the proteins required to construct copies of the protein components of HCV. The HCV genome undergoes a method of transcription to replicate copies of the virus's RNA genome. Inside the host, pieces of the HCV virus are assembled together and ultimately loaded with a copy of the HCV genome. Replicas of the original HCV then escape the host cell and migrate the environment in search of additional host liver cells to infect and continue the replication process.

[0013] The HCV's naturally occurring genetic payload consists of a single molecule of linear positive sense, single stranded RNA approximately 9600 nucleotides in length. By means of a translational process a polyprotein of approximately 3000 amino acids is generated. This polyprotein is cleaved post translation by host and viral proteases into individual viral proteins which include: the structural proteins of C, E1, E2, the nonstructural proteins NS1, NS2, NS3, NS4A, NS4B, NS5A, NS5B, p7 and ARFP/F protein. Hepatitis C virus's proteins direct the host liver cell to construct copies of the Hepatitis C virus. A membrane associated replicase complex consisting of the virus's nonstructural proteins NS3 and NS5B facilitate the replication of the viral genome. The membrane of the endoplasmic reticulum appears to be the site of protein maturation and viral assembly. Once copies of the Hepatitis C Virus are generated, they exit the host cell and each copy of HCV migrates in search of another appropriate liver cell that will act as a host to continue the replication process.

[0014] Hepatitis C virus offers a naturally occurring vehicle mechanism to transport and insert medically therapeutic drug molecules into liver cells and other specifically targeted cells of the human body. The naturally occurring Hepatitis C virus already is equipped with the means of seeking out liver cells and delivering to liver cells its genetic payload. Further, the surface probes present on the Hepatitis C virus's outer protein coat can be modified to seek out specific receptors on specific target cells. HCV's innate genetic payload could be replaced by a payload consisting of medically therapeutic drug molecules. Once the modified Hepatitis C virus's probes properly engage the cell-surface receptors on a target cell, the modified Hepatitis C virus would insert into the target cell a medically therapeutic drug for the purpose of achieving a medical therapeutic response.

[0015] The Hepatitis C virus is one of several viruses that have been identified that possess the natural capacity to locate and infect liver cells with the genome the virus carries, thus including a liver cell as part of its reproductive cycle. Hepatitis A virus (HAV), Hepatitis C virus (HCV), Hepatitis D virus (HDV), Hepatitis E virus (HEV), and Hepatitis G virus (HGV) have been identified to carry their genome as RNA. The Hepatitis G virus is considered to be very similar to the Hepatitis C virus. The Hepatitis F virus and Hepatitis H viruses at this point are not considered to exist, though this is controversial. The Hepatitis B virus (HBV) is believed to carry its genome as DNA. These alternative hepatitis viruses may also be utilized to act as alternative vehicles to deliver medically therapeutic drug molecules to liver cells or specific target cells.

[0016] Current state of gene therapy generally refers to efforts directed toward inserting an exogenous subunit of DNA into a vehicle such as a naturally occurring virus. The vehicle is intended to insert the exogenous subunit of DNA into a target cell. The exogenous DNA subunit then migrates to the target cell's nucleus. The exogenous DNA subunit then inserts into the native DNA of the cell. This represents a permanent alteration of the cell's nuclear DNA. At some point, the nuclear transcription proteins read the exogenous DNA subunit's nucleotide coding to produce the intended cellular response. The approach described within the scope of this text involves a medically therapeutic drug as a payload versus DNA or RNA as a payload. DNA is comprised of the nucleotides adenine, thymine, guanine and cytosine. RNA is composed of the nucleotides adenine, uracil, guanine and cytosine. DNA codes acts as a template to code for the manufacture of RNA molecules. RNA acts as a template coding for the manufacture of proteins, which are composed of amino acids. A drug acts to function as a participant in a chemical reaction, as either a catalyst of the reaction or with another substance to produce one or more additional substances, these additional substances often having different properties. The virus chosen as the example of a transport vehicle, Hepatitis C virus, could be outfitted to carry a medically therapeutic drug molecules rather than RNA or DNA molecules.

[0017]   Treatment of cancer may be approached by a method utilizing modified viruses as vehicles to transport medically therapeutic drugs directly to cancer cells with the intent to directly poison cancer cells by having the drug the modified virus virions carry interfere with the metabolism of the cancer cells. Forms of liver cancer, including primary cancers of the liver or secondary cancers due to metastasis, can be treated utilizing modified hepatitis viruses to carry chemotherapy directly to liver cells to terminate cancer cells residing in the liver.

[0018]   Treatment of rheumatoid arthritis may be approached by a method utilizing modified virus virions as vehicles to transport a medically therapeutic drug such as methotrexate directly to the synovial cells associated with joints and tendons with the intent to have the drug interfere with the metabolism of the synovial cells in order to place the disease in remission. Liver and bone marrow toxicity is often an unwanted side effect of methotrexate therapy. To be able to deliver the methotrexate directly to the synovial cells without exposing the cells of the body as a whole to the effects of methotrexate, would significantly decrease the side effects of the drug and provide an effective therapy to many more patients than are currently able to tolerate the drug. In addition delivering glucosamine molecules and chondroitin molecules to chondrocytes, the cells responsible for producing cartilage, will increase cartilage production on the surface of bones. Delivering nonsteroidal anti-inflammatory drug molecules directly to synovial cells and muscle cells will reduce the inflammation associated with arthritis.

[0019] A safer, more effective treatment of many disease may be approached by a method utilizing modified virus virions as vehicles to transport medically therapeutic drug molecules to specific cells in the body with the intent to have the drug exert an effect only on those cells to which the modified virus virions deliver the drug.

BRIEF SUMMARY OF THE INVENTION

[0020] The method by which a quantity of modified virus virions or virus-like structures are used as a transport medium to carry a payload consisting of a quantity of medically therapeutic drug molecules to specific cells in the body. The modified virus virions or virus-like structures make contact with specific target cells by means of the modified virus virions' exterior probes or virus-like structures' exterior probes. Once the exterior probes engage the target cells' receptors, the modified virus virions or virus-like structures insert into the target cells the quantity of medically therapeutic drug molecules they are carrying.

DETAILED DESCRIPTION

[0021] Viruses or virus-like structures can be fashioned to act as transport vehicles to carry and deliver medically therapeutic drug molecules directly to specific cells. The medically therapeutic drug carried by therapeutic modified viruses or virus-like structures would supply the cells of the body with the drug without interfering or harming other cells in the body.

[0022] Naturally occurring viruses can be altered by replacing the genetic material the virus would carry, with medically therapeutic drug molecules that would have a beneficial medically therapeutic effect on cells. The naturally occurring virus would then carry and deliver to its natural target cell the payload of medically therapeutic drug molecules. As an example, hepatitis viruses could be altered to carry medically therapeutic drug molecules to liver cells. The naturally occurring virus then, instead of causing disease associated with delivering its own genome to conduct its replication process, would instead act as a method to deliver a quantity of medically therapeutic drug molecules, which would provide the target cell with a medically therapeutic outcome.

[0023] Naturally occurring viruses can be further modified to have their naturally occurring glycoprotein surface probes replaced by glycoprotein surface probes that target specific cells in the body. Viruses modified to carry and deliver medically therapeutic drug molecules as the payload, further modified to have their glycoprotein surface probes, that cause the modified virus to engage specific cells in the body, provides a method whereby specific cells in the body can be targeted and this method embodies a means of providing to a specific type of cell in the body a drug to participate in chemical reactions with the intent to accomplish a medically therapeutic outcome.

[0024] Virus-like structures can be constructed with similar physical characteristics to naturally occurring viruses and be fashioned to carry medically therapeutic drug molecules as the payload and have located on the surface glycoprotein probes that engage specific cells in the body. Viruses-like structures carrying medically therapeutic drug molecules as the payload, constructed to have their glycoprotein surface probes engage specific cells in the body, and deliver to those specific cells the drug the virus-like structures carry provides a method whereby specific cells in the body can be targeted and this method embodies a means of providing to a specific type of cell in the body a drug to participate in chemical reactions with the intent to accomplish a medically therapeutic outcome. The advantage of a virus-like structure is that the physical dimensions of the virus-like structure can be adjusted to accommodate variations in the physical size of the payload of medically therapeutic drug molecules, yet maintain a means of engaging targeted cells in the body and delivering to those targeted cells the drug molecules required to accomplish the desired medical therapeutic outcome. A second advantage of utilizing virus-like structures is to be able to change the surface characteristics of the transport vehicle to prevent the body's immune system from reacting to the presence of the therapeutic modified virus and destroying the modified virus before it is able to deliver the payload it carries to the cells it has been designed to target. HIV utilizes an exterior envelope comprised of the surface membrane of its host, the T-Helper cell, which acts as a disguise to fool the body's immune system detection resources. Virus-like structures could be fashioned, similar to HIV, to have as an exterior envelope a surface that resembles a cell's outer membrane. Constructing virus-like structures with an exterior envelope that resembles a cell's outer membrane would assist in the virus-like structure being able to avoid detection by the body's immune system to improve survivability of the virus-like structure thus improving the virus-like structures' chances of reaching the cells it is targeted for and delivering to those cells the drug that it carries as a payload.

[0025] The Hepatitis C virus virion provides a naturally occurring specimen to illustrate the feasibility of the method described in this text. The Hepatitis C virus (HCV) virion is comprised of an outer lipoprotein envelope and an internal nucleocapsid. The virus's genetic payload is carried within its core, the nucleocapsid. The HCV's naturally occurring genetic payload consists of a single molecule of linear positive sense, single stranded RNA approximately 9600 nucleotides in length, which includes: the structural proteins of C, E1, E2, the nonstructural proteins NS1, NS2, NS3, NS4A, NS4B, NS5A, NS5B, p7 and ARFP/F protein. Present on the surface of the outer envelope of the Hepatitis C virus virion are probes that detect receptors present on the surface of liver cells. The glycoproteins E1 and E2 have been identified to be affixed to the surface of HCV virion. Portions of the Hepatitis C virus genome, when separated into individual pieces, behave like messenger RNA. The naturally occurring HCV virion is constructed with surface probes fashioned to recognize receptors on the surface of a liver cell. Once the naturally occurring HCV's surface probe E2 engages a liver cell's CD81 receptor, and cofactors on the surface of HCV's exterior envelope engage the low density lipoprotein receptor (LDLR) or the scavenger receptor class B type I (SR-BI) on the liver cell, the HCV virion then has the opportunity to insert its RNA genetic payload into the engaged target liver cell.

[0026] The Hepatitis C virus virion carrying an mRNA payload, infects liver cells with its payload for the purpose of causing the now infected cell to generate a variety of proteins that will be assembled into copies resembling the original HCV virion. The copies of the HCV virion are then released from the infected cell to migrate in search of other host cells. Variations in the Hepatitis C virus are based on variations that occur in the strand of mRNA molecule the HCV virion carries as it genome. HCV virions may therefore carry differing mRNA molecules as its genetic payload and deliver these mRNA molecules specifically to liver cells in the body to cause these cells to produce proteins to accomplish the task of replication of similar HCV virions.

[0027] Replicating viruses and constructing viruses to carry DNA payloads is a form of manufacturing technology that has already been well established and is in use facilitating the concept of gene therapy. Replicating viruses and designing these viruses to carry drug as the genetic payload would incorporate similar techniques as already proven useful in current DNA gene therapy technologies.

[0028] To carry out the process to manufacture a modified medically therapeutic Hepatitis C virus, messenger RNA that would code for the general physical outer structures of the

Hepatitis C virus would be inserted into a host. The host may include devices such as a host cell or a hybrid host cell. The host may utilize DNA or RNA or a combination of genetic instructions in order to accomplish the construction of medically therapeutic modified virus virions. The DNA or messenger RNA molecules to create the medically therapeutic hepatitis virus would direct the cells to generate copies of the medically therapeutic virus carrying a medically therapeutic drug payload. In some cases DNA or messenger RNA would be inserted into the host that would be coded to cause the production of surface probes that would be affixed to the surface of the virus virion that would target the surface receptors on specific cells in the body other than the liver cells the Hepatitis C virus naturally targets. DNA or messenger RNA would direct the host to generate copies of the medically therapeutic drug molecules that would provide a therapeutic action, or alternatively the medically therapeutic drug molecules would be artificially introduced into the host; these medically therapeutic drug molecules would take the place of the Hepatitis C virus's innate genome as its payload. The medical treatment form of the Hepatitis C virus carrying the medically therapeutic drug molecules would be produced, assembled and released from a host. Virus-like structures would be generated in similar fashion using a host such as host-cells or hybrid host cells. The copies of the medically therapeutic hepatitis virus or virus-like structures, upon exiting the host, would be collected, stored and utilized as a medical treatment as necessary.

[0029] The modified Hepatitis C virus and virus-like structures would be incapable of replication on its own due to the fact that the messenger RNA that would code for the replication process to produce copies of the virus or virus-like structure would not be present in the modified form of the Hepatitis C virus or virus-like structure.

[0030] In review, the method described in this text includes taking a naturally occurring virus and altering its payload so that it transports medically therapeutic drug molecules to cells it was naturally designed to infect, but instead of delivering its own genetic payload, it delivers the medically therapeutic drug molecules it is carrying, <u>and</u> the method described in this text includes taking a naturally occurring virus and altering its payload so that it carries medically therapeutic drug molecules to cells and alter the virus's glycoprotein probes so that it is capable of infecting specifically targeted cells, but instead of delivering its own genetic payload, it delivers the medically therapeutic drug molecules it is carrying to specific target cells, <u>and</u> the method described in this text includes taking a virus-like structure, which carries medically therapeutic drug molecules to cells, affixed to the surface glycoprotein probes so that it is capable of delivering medically therapeutic drug molecules it is carrying to specific target cells.

[0031] As mentioned above, a quantity of modified virus virions, such as Hepatitis C virus virions would be introduced into a patient's blood stream or tissues so that the modified virus could deliver the medially therapeutic drug payload that it carries to targeted cells in the body, such as liver cells.

[0032] The medical treatment method will treat medical diseases associated with a variety of cell types including cells comprising a cancer, cells comprising a malignancy, cells comprising a tumor, cells comprising synovial tissues surrounding a joint, cells comprising synovial tissues surrounding a tendon, cells comprising synovial tissues surrounding a rheumatoid nodule, cells comprising the muscles, cells comprising the brain, cells comprising the heart, cells comprising the pancreas, cells comprising the endocrine glands, cells comprising the dermis, cells comprising the mucosa, cells comprising the gastroenteric tract, cells comprising the renal system, cells comprising the skeletal structure, cells comprising the pulmonary system, cells comprising the nervous system, cells comprising the immune system, cells comprising the sex organs, cells comprising the connective tissues, cells comprising the spleen, cells comprising the eyes, cells comprising the reticuloendothelial system, and cells comprising the liver.

[0033] By utilizing the described method to provide the cells of the body with the above-mentioned medically therapeutic drug molecules and enhancing the capacity of cells to treat a variety of medical conditions from cancer to rheumatoid arthritis, which will result the betterment of medical management for patients.

CLAIMS: Reserved.